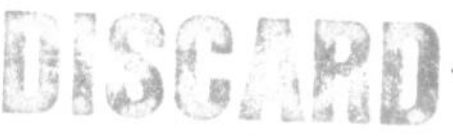
DISCARD

WHEN TUMOR IS THE RUMOR AND CANCER IS THE ANSWER

A comprehensive text for newly diagnosed cancer patients and their families

Kevin P Ryan MD FACP

Foreword by Maurie Markman, MD FACP Senior Vice President of Clinical Affairs & National Director of Medical Oncology, Cancer Treatment Centers Of America

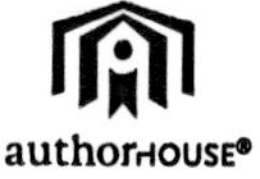

AuthorHouse™
1663 Liberty Drive
Bloomington, IN 47403
www.authorhouse.com
Phone: 1-800-839-8640

Published by AuthorHouse 3/6/2013

ISBN: 978-1-4817-0878-4 (sc)
ISBN: 978-1-4817-0879-1 (hc)
ISBN: 978-1-4817-0880-7 (e)

Library of Congress Control Number: 2013904127

First in line for dedication is my mom. I affectionately refer to her as the Sicilian Tsunami Mommy. She is a ninety-plus-years-young former first-grade teacher who incessantly encouraged me to get this work done. Since the loss of Dad to small-cell lung cancer, she has wisely invested herself as a hospital volunteer. Among the many lessons I have learned from her are a love of knowledge and the belief that failure is unavoidable but one must never, ever quit.

I dedicate this to my patients. I remain humbled by their pluck under fire and unfathomable courage while going toe-to-toe with a fearsome and formidable foe—cancer.

I dedicate this to my wife, whose sensitivity and wisdom are a blessing. We were at Barnes and Noble, perusing books in print with aims similar to the goal I had in mind for mine. We were spying our way through all the volumes written on every aspect of cancer by legions of patients, family, friends, and health-care providers. Feeling increasingly overwhelmed, I mumbled something like, "I really don't believe I am going to do this." My beloved's answer was simple and swift. With a smile that could support all fears and eyes brimming with knowing tears, she quietly said, "You always have been".

Finally, I thank the architect of everything, God. The journey of this book has reinforced fundamental lessons imbedded in our nature and authored by Him that, when remembered, smooth the stones in the journey and level the mountains of anxiety. There is calmness available to the clinical practice of oncology when we see humans as fundamentally not wired differently from each other. None of our emotions at their core are so novel as to escape understanding. They are as universal and sustaining as the breathing of air and the pulsing of your blood. Thus, no matter how intricate the case and no matter how seemingly unique the patient, patients can be understood and reached. There is enormous comfort in knowing this. Although the heart is perhaps an often lonely hunter on a journey whose very beginning and end are quite alone, all stories are filled with folks made of the same stuff.

Thus, I happily thank God. For my nickel, God got the recipe of man's nature just right. Our being heavenly hardwired informs the entire health-care team in their journey of caring for those afraid in their fight against cancer.

Life is not about fairness, and the outcome is predictable. If you seek to control events, you cannot. Bad things will happen to good people. Cancer befalls saint and sinner equally. Once again, the core sameness of humanity by design encourages us that no one rows the treacherous seas of life alone.

Finally, then, this work is dedicated to those friends, family, well-doers, and volunteers who grab an oar in the communal sea of life, pull hard, and, when called upon, lovingly help the less fortunate ashore.

TABLE OF CONTENTS

Foreword .... **xiii**
Maurie Markman, MD, FACP

Introduction .... **xvii**

Read the Directions First **1**
La Dolce Vita (A Recipe) for the Sweet Life 1

Read This Second, but Learn It First **7**
Autonomy 7

Anxiety and Fear **11**

The Enemy **15**

Broad Overview of the Nuts and Bolts of Oncology **19**
Overview of Specialty 20
Specific and Related Fields 21
The Scope Of The Problem 22
Scope of Chemotherapy 24
Scope of Lay Knowledge of Malignancy 37
Scope of Adult Oncology Practice 39
Treatment Setting 40
Prevention 41
Screening 44

Cause 47
Pathophysiology of Cancer 52
Life Cycle of Cancer 53
Tumor Growth Characteristics 55
Rational Naming of Cancers 57
Pathological Diagnosis 58
Signs and Symptoms of Cancer 60
Stage of the Cancer and Prognosis 61
Broad Concepts of Goals and Timing of Treatment 62
Vocabulary of Survival 63

The Oncologist 65
Why Oncology? 65
MD: What Is In a Name? 67
What About Oncologists? 67

Suspect the Diagnosis 77

Diagnosis 85
The Opening Pitch 85
How You Say It 86
Lies, Damn Lies, and Statistics 87
Listening for Those Whispering in the Patient's Ear 89
Preconceived Ideas 92
Assess Patient Goals 93
Psychological Issues 93
Sex and Significant Others 97
Spirituality 97
The Role of the Family 98
Teach Your Children Well 101
Cultural Differences 101
Focus on Symptomatic Relief 102
Introducing Clinical Trials 102
Introduction to Complementary and Alternative Medicine 103
Media Matters 106

Antidotes for Anecdotes 107
Prognosis and the Future 107
Take the Time and Avoid Timelines 108
Remember, Statistics Can Be Your Friends 109
Second Opinions 110
The Contract 110
Remember Autonomy: It Begins and Ends There 111
A Final Few Words 111

Treatments 113
Example of Finding Just One Cancer Cell 113
Beyond Single-Cell Detection 119
Staging 124
Chemotherapy 129
Radiation Therapy 136
Principles of Surgical Oncology 140
Therapeutic Monoclonal Antibodies 143
Other Biological Therapies 149
Angiogenesis Inhibitors 151
Bone Marrow and Stem Cell Transplantation 152
Targeted Cancer Therapies 157
Gene Therapy for Cancer 159
Hyperthermia 161
Laser 164
Photodynamic Therapy 165

Clinical Trials in Oncology 167
Statistics 175

Symptom Control and Side Effects 181
Alopecia 183
Anorexia 184
Bleeding and Thrombocytopenia 185
Constipation 186
Dental Problems 188

Depression 189
Diarrhea 190
Dysphagia 191
Edema 192
Fatigue 193
Flulike Symptoms 195
Heart and Cardiovascular Changes 196
Infertility and Sterility 196
Insomnia 197
Lymphedema 198
Menopausal Symptoms 199
Mucositis 200
Nausea and Vomiting 201
Neutropenia 203
Neurological Symptoms 204
Palmar-Plantar Erythrodesia 205
Photosensitivity Reactions 206
Sexual Dysfunction 207
Xerostomia 209

The Problem of Pain 211

Alternative and Unproven Forms of Cancer Treatment 221
Introduction 221
Types of CAM 226
What Is Really Going On 233
Why 233
Sacred Cow Killing 234
Complementary Exercises for People with Cancer 237
Physician–Patient Communication 238

The Future 241
Understanding Cutting-Edge Therapies 241
New Diagnostic Tools 255

Spiritual Care **257**

Self-Talk **267**
Why Me? 267
Laughter and Beauty 268
Baby Steps 269
Daily Affirmations 269
Toxic Stress 270
Live the Moment 271
Honor Your Thoughts 271
Conspire against Your Emotions 272
Set Goals 273
Support Groups 273
Forgiveness, Gratitude, and Unconditional Love 274

But What Do I Say? **277**

Front Office **287**

Nurses **291**

Inpatient Care **293**

Psychosocial/Hospice/End-of-Life Issues **309**
Psychosocial Issues 309
Hospice Care 314
End-of-Life Care 317

Ethics **323**
Principles 323
Managed Care 324
Truth-Telling 324
Living Wills 325
Discontinuing Care 326

Sedation and Symptom Control 327
Legal Aspects of Oncology 329

The Internet 337

Prognosis 343

What Is a Tumor Registry? 345

Some Final Thoughts 347

The Heroes 349
The Telling 349
Hitting Home 350
Snow Job 352
The Lioness 356
The Flood 360
The Gift 362
A Leprechaun's Laser Light of Life 366
The Connection 370
The Quality of Mercy 377
The Power of We 379

Epilogue 381

Index/ Partial Glossary 383

FOREWORD

On Becoming a Cancer Survivor

Cancer is an intensely personal experience. Yet it routinely involves a variety of social interactions with family, friends, coworkers, and employers. The diagnosis of cancer brings up serious concerns of death, pain, suffering, and loss of control and dignity.

It is an interesting observation that while overall survival following a diagnosis of malignancy is at least equal, if not superior, to that of a diagnosis of heart failure, few people told they have heart disease will declare, "Oh no, I am going to die." However, such a response is not uncommon when the diagnosis is cancer.

No group of diseases generates more fear and anxiety: *Why me? How did I get it? What did I do wrong? Will I transmit the cancer to my children through my genes? Will I experience the same miserable death my mother told me my grandfather experienced when he was diagnosed with some "unknown type of cancer" forty years ago? Can I survive? Will I be able to work during treatment? Does radiation therapy "burn"? How bad will the vomiting be after chemotherapy?*

There are so many questions, with answers desperately sought—some very complex and not answerable, others very direct and simple (such as "Will I lose my hair?"). All of this is rushing into one consciousness over a remarkably short period. It can be truly overwhelming.

Thus we see the important need for a commonsense, straight-talking book that describes the cancer experience to patients and their families, including standard diagnostic and therapeutic techniques, management options, and toxicities of treatment. The book should help the patient and his/her family through this experience, answer commonly asked questions, and point to where one can receive appropriate responses to other concerns (e.g., "Where do I find information I can use to help me understand my cancer?").

Of great importance is that the book have as a major aim the goal of reducing anxiety and helping those confronted with this disease to marshal their internal resources to conquer their natural fears and ultimately learn to become cancer survivors.

Does such a book exist?

You are about to read it.

Maurie Markman, MD, FACP

Senior Vice President of Clinical Affairs and National Director of Medical Oncology, Cancer Treatment Centers Of America

Former Professor and Vice President of Clinical Research and Chairman of the Department of Gynecologic Medical Oncology, MD Anderson Cancer Center

Former Chairman of the Department of Hematology/Oncology and Director of the Taussig Cancer Center at the Cleveland Clinic Foundation

Former Vice-Chair, Department of Medicine, Memorial Sloan Kettering Cancer Center, New York City, New York

Acknowledgments
(in random order)

Frederick J. Meyers, MD, MACP; Lt. General P. K. Carlton, USAF (ret); Robert O Dillman, MD, FACP; Maurie Markman, MD, FACP; James Unger, PhD; Norman DeTullio; Norm Siegel; Andy Amalfitano; Jim Higgins; John Mendelsohn, MD, FACP; Paul Hill, MD (dec); Charles Goldman, MD, FACS; Tom Bradley, MD, PhD; James Long, MD; Col. Ken Ansell, USAF (ret); Dick Witten; Bonnie Karr, RN, ONS; Col. Stephen Jennings, USAF, MC, FACS; Roland Flint, PhD (dec); Madame P; Wild Bill Gresham; Joel Fine, MD; J. Boriskin, PhD; and a few thousand heroes.

INTRODUCTION

So why this book, and who is it for? The odds are over 40% that cancer will touch one's life. Our nation spends over $150 billion dollars directly on cancer care per year. It is one of the largest single expenditures of the national health-care budget. There are over five hundred thousand deaths per year and over one million new cases. Including families, cancer touches almost four million people per year. There are few common medical realities that are surrounded by as much malefaction, mystique, and misunderstanding as cancer is. *When Tumor Is the Rumor and Cancer Is the Answer* helps one see past the understandably macabre mythology.

This work attempts to address the needs for knowledge when receiving the overwhelming news that you may or do have cancer. It attempts to cover not just the fear of the diagnosis or certain aspects of the journey of care but also the entire trek from when tumor is the rumor and cancer is the answer onward. It tries to envelop with knowledge the soul-sucking sense of loss of control, anxiety's favorite fodder and fuel.

Let us just walk around the table of contents. We open by addressing the hit-in-the-gut issues that come up immediately. First are some thoughts about the right recipe for the right mindset in handling the journey. Believe it or not, we are well wired to handle this stress. Thus, in "Read the Directions First," we look at how we might have a recipe for mental and emotional success as we gird up to weather the storm.

Then we specifically address the crucial issue of autonomy—the notion that you are an individual with explicit defined rights and that you can and will be in control.

We then address the problem of anxiety and its distinction from fear, the nature of cancer, and oncologists and the team they will lead in your journey, as well as how their world will become yours. This book teaches that anxiety and fear are not the same and that knowledge in all spheres—not just sterile clinical facts—is power and a therapeutic balm. Informed fear is a call to action, and the more informed you are, the better your clarity of resolve and the less your anxiety.

The section "The Enemy" explains how cancer is almost the perfect medical predator. It introduces the villain for what it is and prepares the stage for our fight against it. That fight starts and ends with defeating ignorance, using knowledge as our greatest weapon. The book addresses suspecting the diagnosis, the diagnosis, standard and alternative treatment, and symptom relief. This is followed by an in depth discussion on the problem of pain, clinical trials, future therapies, spirituality, and self-talk (how to talk with yourself when confronting cancer).

We then move into useful chapters on the ethics of cancer care, challenges of managed care, psychosocial issues with ethical and legal components, and the way end-of-life concerns play a common role in the care of oncology patients. Difficult concepts such as physician-assisted suicide, durable power of attorney, living wills, failure to diagnose, lost opportunities in life, euthanasia, and death by secondary intent (death occurring during a course of treating the patient and alleviating suffering) have led to cancer cases being second in frequency of lawsuits after cases of infant injury or disability.

One team member is largely shrouded in mystery despite his or her core responsibility often being shouldered rather alone. This is the oncologist, and just as orthopedists or pediatricians do, they tend to share similar traits. Understanding those traits can, in general, be both fascinating and fruitful. After all, to some degree these physicians are somewhat boxing with God and against a most mysterious of infirmities that affects all organ systems; all the while, they are engaging deep psychological and spiritual issues. The field is more on the cutting edge of applied genetics and immunology than others, and practitioners must master multiple modalities of care from chemotherapy to surgery, radiation therapy, and transplants; and increasingly, biological, immunologic, and elegant genetically-based treatments.

Oncologists hold a very special position in the eyes of those they treat, in no small part owing to the nature of the enemy they fight. They are not magnificent demagogues (MDs) parsing out secret poisons to patients indifferent to the gravity of their daily toils. Nonetheless, they can find themselves often and appropriately playing the role of parish priest, psychologist, father confessor, coach, confidant, and counselor; it goes with the turf. In addition, as what little research there is suggests, they may not always be strong on emotional or psychological communication or expressing empathy.

Oncologists are human; we hurt with our patients and families. Ironically, though, there is not a lot of structured support out there for cancer doctors. The data is scarce, but what is there regarding burnout and psychological pain in oncologists is, not surprisingly, sad and sobering.

Although a cardinal rule is to always remember that the patient is the one with the disease, there is no doubt that the more informed we all are regarding the whole enterprise, from rumor to advanced tumor and the weight and impact and role each diagnosis has on all the players on the team, the better the outcome—in significant ways.

This book thus looks at why some oncologists chose such a sobering field and offers to practitioners different insights into managing the whole patient and, in part, themselves during a difficult emotional journey for all.

Oncologists inhabit a world of words, wonders, hospital wards, and clinics that are foreign to the patient. This book looks into the front and back office staff as well as the rules of the road while an inpatient. The more each patient understands where he or she will spend so much time, the better the experience will be for all.

Most family and friends experience considerable discomfort when interacting with a seriously ill or perhaps dying friend or loved one. They wonder, *But what do I say?* Although the singular moment of death is experienced alone, the journey need not be. In the section "But what do I say?" I offer some help and observe that we are in this boat of life together.

When it is time to dock for some, we must hold fast to the loved one's hand and help him or her lovingly ashore.

We close by sharing some true stories of remarkable patients and their journeys.

This is not a medical text on the treatment of malignancy, per se, or prevention, screening, or cancer survivorship. This book describes what happens and what works best for the whole team when the possible diagnosis becomes the proven and potentially fatal diagnosis. A major aim of this book is the goal of reducing anxiety and helping those confronted with this disease to marshal their internal resources to conquer their natural fears and ultimately learn to become cancer survivors. I hope to address many of the often unspoken truths that, now found in one place, can act as a guide for what is for many the most frightening time of their lives. I hope to return that crucial sense of control.

Why do it this way? In large part, it is because little other published work does so. This book highlights the gift that improved patient–physician communication can be, especially when the patient and family are fully informed. There is never enough time in today's practices to fill all those gaps; this work will help. This is big-picture thinking with the picture being you and how it all can be decipherable—instead of it being a transaction of doing as advised, but doing so not as fully educated as you might have been.

Embracing that overarching concept is of incredible assistance when we see this as a journey with many well-known milestones and probable adventures along the way, with common waypoints for most. Think of it as understanding in more depth the nature of what largely happens to and for all. In explaining a professional sport, one needs to have context and overview in addition to the details of how the game inevitably proceeds and who does what when. That requires time and careful organization. Having such a continuum of understanding not only engages all those in the fight but also steels them to do their part as best they can and prepares them for what is next.

This book is needed because medicine is enveloped and cloaked in mystery. It is replete with magic decoder rings and secret handshakes. Irrespective of Hollywood's latest or greatest umpteenth version of a real doctor show, society is largely ignorant of the mysterious and frightening world of cancer medicine. Cracking that code and empowering the patient with knowledge will undoubtedly lead to healthier lives and happier journeys for all.

This book is about teamwork. Patients are experts in teaching us physicians to be *complete* clinical oncologists. There is plenty of angst and agony to go around when pursuing diagnosis and committing to do battle against a malignancy. Wise physicians in many regards embrace patients on the journey as partners whose informed engagement is crucial to success. We ideally want them informed, forewarned, and feeling that although they are the one with the disease, and although their autonomy is first and foremost, this journey is a team effort. The more we all know about the terrain, the better.

Superb cancer care is only possible with teamwork. The enemy is the cancer and, many times, the anxiety the cancer and its treatment fosters. Everyone brings different skills, needs, agendas, perspectives, and languages to the fight.

Thus, the audience of this book is everyone on the team. It is an enormous responsibility and burden to care for cancer patients. It is no less an enormous burden and responsibility to be a patient with cancer or a family member of someone who has been diagnosed. There is the rub: the knife cuts both ways. Patients and families have a responsibility to learn as much as they can and participate in their disease as much as possible. Furthermore, using all manner of techniques, health-care providers have a responsibility to share their perspective on the burdens and responsibilities of their role on the cancer-care team and express appropriate empathy—a surefire way to increase trust.

Musician Roy Clark penned some great lines in his tune "Yesterday, When I Was Young": "I ran so fast that time and youth at last ran out. I never stopped to think what life was all about ... And only I am left on stage to end the play." I hope that this book will help you gather more tomorrows and realize you are not alone.

Now, read the directions first.

READ THE DIRECTIONS FIRST

La Dolce Vita
(A Recipe) for the Sweet Life

Over our lives, we develop quite a palette for the bountiful buffet of personalities out there. We learn what seems to taste good and pretty much agree on what or who seems to leave a bad taste in our mouths. We learn that in the kitchen of life, where we concoct recipes for how to deal with everyday reality, no true surprises are produced.

This is as it should be, as the ingredients for life's sweetest and most nourishing and sustaining meals are not that mysterious. We all have access to them. If there is any magic, it is in remembering the tried-and-true recipes. As is so often the case with us mere mortals, we forget them fastest when we need them most, such as when tumor is the rumor and cancer is the answer.

Certainly, when we suspect or are diagnosed with cancer, all hell can break loose emotionally and in other ways. Granted, it is tough to start thinking about poetic notions like recipes for the sweet life. It may seem like whimsical pabulum or the stuff of nice-sounding adolescent romance novels.

Fair enough. Most cancer patients are not adolescents, and cancer is not a romantic novel. We all know that if ever there is a time to get it right, put on your game face, follow the rules, and pay attention to what Momma taught you and "get religion," it is when you are in one of the foxholes handed out randomly by fate.

Equally true is that the mindset, the lifestyle with which you embrace the disease, has immense impact. Repeatedly, I have seen families and patients have meaningful improvement in handling the gamut of emotions that occur from rumor of tumor to cancer as the answer when they affect a simple yet profound attitude. Namely, they remember what works best in frightening times. In my thirty years of watching this transition from fear to fortune, the remembering of the recipe for a sweet, fulfilling, and enriching life is a practical part of the battle gear when putting on armor and engaging the beast.

There is good news. The best recipes always taste better when you are famished or when tough times hit the cupboard of our lives. Similarly, there is nothing quite like good ole home cooking. Remember times when Gramps had a little GI indiscretion, Dad quipped about stepping on a frog, and your little brother shot peas through his nose from laughing so hard while Mom acted utterly disgusted, muttering, "When in God's name can we ever have a nice family dinner?" Of course you do, in some manner or another. Being with those you love and loving every moment when the main thing on the menu was not pretentious made it easy to digest heaping helpings of love. There is nothing more nutritious.

Therefore, as regards recipes for living when first hit with the diagnosis, the more you can nourish and sustain yourself in the company and care of those who love you and whom you love, the better the meal.

Now let us look at how God made us to be nourished and how to sustain ourselves with calories that can build more than just courage. Let us read the directions we came with for a sweet life in the midst of not-so-sweet news.

Beware, pretenders and offenders to common sense, when it comes to nutritious lifestyles, just as you would beware of magical promises of cancer cures. Mothers are rarely wrong. So, for starters, do just like Momma said and pay attention when better judgment tells you, "Don't eat that; it's not good for you!" Stay away from the too-pretty packaging. Be wary of the have-I-got-a-deal-for-you, empty-calorie garbage that will seem to pop out of everywhere from the Internet to the airwaves to late-night TV, as well as the trendy quick-fix self-help books with titles that seductively seem to talk just to you—yes, only you! Of course, there are many well-intentioned and indeed very helpful things out there in the world. However, if it seems too good to be true, if it goes against common sense, or if it does not pass the mommy test ("where did you hear that nonsense?"), go back to the basics that have been there since man first sought to alleviate suffering and live the good life.

The best recipes come from seasoned chefs who have tossed quite a lot of salad in their lives. These are folks, as you and I, who have made many meals in tough times. They have burnt some and undercooked others, but they know what really works. Here is what seems to top the list of appetizing aptitudes and attitudes that make a great recipe for a sweet life during tough times.

We said in the dedication and introduction, and it will echo repeatedly throughout the book, that you are not alone and there is a shared nature to humanity. Nothing makes you incomprehensible or unlovable. The same is true for recipes for life; they nourish all.

From Plato to Charles Schultz's Peanuts, thoughtful Thoreau to inane Inspector Clouseau, Gandhi or Christ to whomever your sage best model for life may be, the recipe is unchanged. Certain ingredients just keep popping up. They are all readily available in the cupboards of your heart and the pantry of your minds. They are all essential for a substantial, nourishing life. They will all keep meat on your bones and sizzle in your soul when the tough times, like the diagnosis of cancer, come calling. Best of all, the only criterion to enter the kitchen to cook up your own concoction is a pulse.

Start with a pound of *purpose.* Load up on plenty of this. No matter how dark, dismal, or desperate things are, with purpose there is a path and ample provision for your heart and soul.

Add a pinch of *productivity.* Just get your hands dirty and make something—anything—more than it was to start with. Dirty hands can clean minds just as fuel treatments blow the carbon out of our engines.

Then stir in *cream of creativity.* Remember, this singular gift marks you as the most wondrous of all creations. Only humans have that divine spark, the ability to create. It may be a ship in a bottle, a new whatchamacallit patent, or a smile on someone's face. Your creativity is not about scope and grandeur; it is about keeping the flame alive. It is about the ability to affect the world around you in a manner that, no matter how infinitesimally, leaves it with more and better than how it found you.

Then simmer. Some folks called this ciphering, chewing it over, or sleeping on it. It never means dwelling or getting ready to boil or blow up. It means having a gentle patience with your endeavors, remembering you already met the only criterion to enter the kitchen in the first place—a pulse. In addition, remember that there is no egg timer for hatching goodness.

Take time and have faith that your endeavors will bear fruit, and soon the sweet aroma of creative productivity will fill you up. Productivity and creativity are seemingly separate, but they are mutually wonderful and intimately intertwined, and together they make for magic. Sort of like life, eh? The stew of life is always better than the sum of its parts.

Next, lightly flour this meal with *forgiveness.* Always have some on hand. Moreover, it only works if you give more of it away than you recently got—darndest thing how that works! Even better, opportunities to use it are never in short supply.

Add two—no, add three heaping helpings of *humor.* In the final analysis, you will never laugh so deeply as when your favorite comedian is yourself. Granted, it is a tough gig, and phew, what a hard audience, but when you get the auto-giggle going, look out, it's life-sustaining and infectious.

Caramelize the entire concoction with *kindness*. The best way to do that is blindly and almost randomly. Just like forgiveness, have it ready to add a little loving crust to seal in the sweetness. You will know when; you always do.

Of course, you have to have tunes. Start to sing, hum, whistle—do whatever you do that makes the melody of your mind, the rhythm of your walk, or your own little "idiotsymphony" come to life. Moreover, never miss a chance to invite others to join the band. Giggling, chortling, guffaws, and hearty ho-hos count; they are always in key.

Now, as soon as you can, run around the kitchen twice. Wow the world that you are animated and alive. Toss a tomato, juggle a jujube, and assault the pits: cherry, avocado, or life. No matter what, do it with flair and keep moving to your groove.

Now close your eyes and savor smells. Seek out the scent of a woman, a man, puppy breath, New England autumn leaves, or your mama's lasagna. Repeat every time the stink of suffering or worry tweaks your nose.

Remember, if you do not cut yourself every now and then, singe a few hairs, or get burned a time or two, this recipe for life just will not turn out right. Every master chef experiences pain, so be prepared. The pain-free kitchen is not worth cooking in, and mama was right—the pain of the fear of pain can be twice as disabling as the real thing.

Finally, find a window—any window—and look to the sky. Look for the glow of others enriched by passing through the tale and tail of your comet, as well as theirs.

Bon Appétit! Mangiare Bene! Enjoy!

READ THIS SECOND, BUT LEARN IT FIRST

Autonomy

"Autonomy" is the single most important word and concept the reader of this book must grasp. Philosophically, it refers to the fundamental principle that all humans are independent moral agents with the personal capacity to make moral decisions and act on them. To the largest extent, life is about choice—your choices.

The word derives from the Greek "*autonomia*," meaning "self-rule." In modern days, autonomy most often equates with the phrase "self-determination." Individuals are autonomous when their actions are truly their own without coercion or inappropriate influence.

Sometimes when judges hand down decisions, they really hit the spot. Sometimes their words are not too legalistic, and they nail the beauty, power, and scope of their decisions in terms most can understand.

Certainly one would think all legal decisions are important. However, one of the core principles in Western thought and law, one of the guiding lights of our constitution, and absolutely one of the most anchoring truths in both caring for cancer patients and being cared for is patient autonomy.

Often in this book, I express that the patient is the one with the disease. In the final analysis, after all the health-care system can do to make information and access to care available, the final decision belongs to the competent adult. That is how it should be, and physicians, families, and patients must never forget it.

Listen to how beautifully American judges state this: "No right is held more sacred, or is more carefully guarded, by the common law, than the right of every individual to the possession **and control of his own person,** free from all restraint or interference of others, unless by clear and unquestionable authority of law" (Union Pacific R. Co. vs. Botsford, 141 U.S. 250 [1891]).

Here is another ruling that clearly distills it down to the issue of medical decision-making: "Every human being of adult years and sound mind has a right to determine what shall be done with his own body; and a surgeon who performs an operation without his patient's consent commits assault, for which he is liable in damages" [Schloendorff vs. Society of New York Hospital, 105 N.W. 92 [1914]). Thus, patient autonomy refers to the capability and right of patients to control the course of their own medical treatment and participate in the treatment decision-making process.

Indeed! That is also a core guiding principle of this book. Repeatedly in this book, you will see that physicians and their teams must fully inform their patients to the best their ability and the best of the patients' ability to understand. Health-care providers lead the patient to intelligence. However, it is the patient's job, once led, to think. As you will hear repeatedly, the patient is the one with the disease.

Why keep hammering this home? God gave you the gift of choice and the greater gift of sufficient intelligence to make those choices *if* you are sufficiently informed. That is exactly what this book is attempting to do: inform. That is why this section appears early on. Patients must know the power they rightfully can claim. So empowered, they will be able to transform the pain of anxiety, which is fear of the unknown, into the hero-producing powers behind fear, which are a God-given hardwired set of emotional, physical, and intellectual responses that can and do lead us to wise, autonomous, personal decisions.

Therefore, once one is an autonomous patient, one must inform oneself about some of the key players and passions and emotions and events as one moves from tumor being the rumor to cancer being the answer that will be dealt with by one's personal health-care team.

Furthermore, we will now look at the nature of anxiety versus fear;

the persona of cancer, so to speak; some operational details of the world of oncology; and, finally, the persona of your major ally in the fight, your oncologist. Then we can jump in together, arm in arm, with hearts, heads, and minds aligned, and learn what to do when tumor is the rumor and cancer is the answer.

ANXIETY AND FEAR

It is *anxiety* that is the killer. We humans suffer most when not knowing all that needs to be known, especially when there is so much to fear. I choose, as do many dictionaries and as have countless great religious leaders and philosophers, to define "anxiety" as "fear of the unknown."

I frequently relate a parable to my patients on this crucial subject. Let us travel back in time to the clan of the proverbial caveman. In one cave, somewhat safe from the elements and huddled about a fire, is a family fraught with anxiety toward the savage carnivores outside. These beasts only know this clan as prey. The clan shrinks under the weight of this knowledge, convinced that the predators will most assuredly find and devour them. The clan huddles all the closer, shaken by every foreign sound and every dimming of the fire. They dare not move. They are not ready to battle for their next meal or to survive. That is the primordial example of paralysis by analysis; it is as old as man. That is anxiety.

In the hillside just to the east, another clan of warriors huddle. They know well the dangers that lurk and are ready to pounce as the fire dims and the sounds draw near. Fearful of what they know, and *armed,* they set forth into what will now be the *known*. History has shown us that this clan will survive. That is the liberating power of fear inciting action.

Both anxiety and fear evoke the same visceral and pressing emotional urgings. However, for the first clan, the *unknown* fuels their feelings. That is anxiety, and that is the end of that clan. However, the second clan knows that the bigger enemy is anxiety, fear of the unknown. It is fear of anxiety that drives them to action. Anxiety is the road to paralysis. Fear can ignite action without guarantee of success, but action nevertheless.

Anxiety disorders in patients and their relationship to the quality of life have been the subject of legions of studies in the medical literature. Their conclusion is universal. Anxiety is as much a killer as is living in constant bodily pain. What is life worth, one wonders, when the icy soul-sucking grip of the never-and-forever lie holds you tight to its bosom. This lie screams into your psyche, saying, "It will never change, and it will forever be the same."

Anxiety is not abnormal and may, in fact, be an emotion that leads to a positive outcome. Nonetheless, it is almost the kiss of death when it too easily evolves into the loosely defined term "morbid anxiety," causing panic, irrationality, and paralysis. There is little doubt that morbid anxiety has negative consequences in many regards for the cancer patient as well as his or her family.

Granted, some malignancies with a less ominous prognosis will not elicit as much morbid anxiety. Once again, the key is that the patient *knows* that the prognosis is less ominous. It is *knowledge* that is the oncologist's first and most precious gift to the patient. It is *knowledge* that the patient and family must demand. Knowledge delivered through teaching must be thorough, comprehensible, and empathetic. The flow of information must never stop. Physicians must teach patients how to deal with family, friends, sources on the Internet, the staging procedures and their meaning, the treatment, and the value of second opinions. Patients must learn well that they will not be alone, that thousands have handled this and that others were no less anxious and no braver.

Physicians must speak to their patients of the odds of cure, remission and durability of remission. They must not shy away from discussing spirituality, life's goals, and the effects of treatment on normal bodily function. Common anxiety-laden patient questions, such as "What functions or abilities will I lose?" and "What functions or abilities will I keep?" are essential front-burner issues. Discussions must be frank regarding the specter that pain, nausea, and vomiting often represent to patients. Moreover, physicians will find that the more empathetic time they spend with a patient, the greater the patient's trust and quality of life will be.

Patients need to know if research studies hold out a realistic promise.

Oncologists must explain the amazing armamentarium of medications they have, the psychological assistance patients will be given, and, potentially, the beautiful role that hospice may play. Most of all, *patients* must be put in charge by being given repeated, slow, but thorough helpings of knowledge. That is the key to killing anxiety. Caretakers must indeed take great care to embrace the God-given, hero-making emotion of fear, break the paralyzing bonds of anxiety, and guide patients and families onward to face the future.

THE ENEMY

First, a parable. Winter was coming early to the western Cordillera range of the Sierra Nevada, and the mountain man knew it was time to head down to safer ground. While packing his mule, he heard from behind a cold, craggy granite precipice the unmistakable hissing and eerie rattle of the deadly western diamondback. Then, strange as it seemed, the snake spoke and began pleading with the rugged frontiersman: "Pleasssse, oh Pleassse," it begged while hissing. "Winter has come early, and I will ssssurely freesssse if you do not put me in your pack and take me down to ssssafer, warmer ground."

Hard-won experience told the mountain man to be wary. He declined, stating firmly, "You will surely bite me before the trail is through." The snake assured him he would never do such a thing if the man would save him. Thus, reckoning back to lessons from his ma and pa—long since dead after hard labor on the rocky western Kentucky soil—the cautious but kindly outdoorsman took pity on one of God's creatures. Carefully, against his gut instincts, he placed the viper in his pack and headed to lower, warmer ground.

At the end of the journey, as promised, the mountain man reached into the pack to release the viper. Of course, the snake struck, injecting the outdoorsman with blindingly painful venom and the near certainty of an ugly and lonely demise. The Good Samaritan of the frontier was enraged, and while still lucid, he reminded the snake of his promise.

The snake replied, slowly and sincerely, "But you knew I wassss a sssnake when you helped me; I just did what sssnakes do."

And so it is with the enemy, cancer.

"They're toast." That is not a rare expression uttered by some physicians in private when hearing of a severely threatening diagnosis. I have heard this common irreverent comment and similar ones uttered by my colleagues and young residents when referring to those newly diagnosed with cancer. Curiously, these flippant declarations do not always follow a diagnosis of advanced or terminal disease. These insensitive quips have even popped out at the mere confirmation of the mere diagnosis before any determination of stage or degree of severity. Why? It is because cancer is the ultimate terrorist, the perfect enemy.

Cancer: the anathema, the incubus—nothing evokes more fear. There is no greater pariah to caretaker, clinician, or patient. Indeed, the very origin of the word "cancer," from the Latin word for "crab," speaks legions regarding the dread with which we regard the word. Why is this?

Perhaps we fear cancer's amazing talent for infernal mimicry of the norm. Cancer cells imitate normal cells, but perversely. Perhaps we detest the macabre brilliance by which cancer cells systematically unravel the elegant mysteries of normal cells. Cancer cells, regarded by some scientists intellectually as little medical miracles, take their cue from normalcy but with a deviant twist. They grow constantly, irrepressibly.

Their mere presence conjures up visions of evil humors reminiscent of those alluded to by Galen, the ancient Greek founding father of medicine, as they swarm over the unsuspecting patient. They are admirably ingenious rogues with innumerable deceptions cloaking them from our immune systems' elegant surveillance and intelligence network. They have amazing techniques that protect them from detection and eradication.

Cancer cells will also not stay put. They marshal innocent patients' wondrous blood vessel factories and command those factories to build an evil network of canals and thoroughfares of new vessels that bring the malignant little monsters nourishment and usher them on journeys to distant organs to wreak havoc. These princes of parasitism suck essential nutrients from us, decimating our defenses. Some cause local mayhem, blocking critical passageways, bowel and bladder alike. Some make us weep blood. Some sneak off to the otherwise pristine recesses of the brain, confounding movement and sensation while causing neurological crises. Malignant and malevolent, it is no wonder we hate cancer with unbridled passion.

Cancer is so poignant that in our battle against it we employ potent poisons in a sort of chemical and biological warfare. These therapies frequently count on the "good guys," our normal tissues, to hang in there despite the sometimes enormous toll they exact on our body. The quest is rather daunting—to kill a cancer cell and still leave normal cells and tissues largely undisturbed and surviving normally. For some, successful surgical removal of the cancer holds a pivotal place in the armamentarium. For others, blasting away with radiation is the treatment. Others receive chemical, biological, or combined assaults.

Cancer can be, and often is, killed. However, biologically resistant and insolent to the last, this enemy will not die without a fight; but without a fight, the patient often will die.

BROAD OVERVIEW OF THE NUTS AND BOLTS OF ONCOLOGY

In this section, I present an overview of the structure of the field of oncology and some critical terms and aspects all patients will encounter. This sets the stage by being less in-depth than an individual might find in some textbooks for professionals on the matter, and it covers some material that will appear again in different formats later on.

You will also see the tone change just a bit when we get to the direct and dry science. The material is going to be in-depth and perhaps of no interest to many of you. Nonetheless, I urge you to take a good look at it all, even if you only understand it notionally. The reason is this: cancer is damn frightening and profoundly complex. The more you understand, even notionally, the tools we use to describe it and classify it and its treatments as well as its origin, *the more you can control the experience.* The more you comprehend its "mindset" physiologically on a cellular level and the tools we have to image it and eradicate it, the more you can engage in outside reading that is focused and appropriate. Facts are your fodder and fuel to go from a leap of faith in your treatment to informed conviction, and I suspect the material is not so dry as to not be worth a run-though.

The more you understand putting all the pieces together, the more peace you will have. If only it serves as reference for loved ones or perhaps not at all, you still have the comfort of knowing it is there for you to understand more. It is not essential that you know all of this, but the more you master, the more you will master the anxiety that seeks to direct you, preventing you from being in the director's chair.

Thus, the book can serve readily as a reference, taking you wherever you need to go to learn more about the journey you are on or are about to undertake. Take advantage of that structure; peruse the table of contents, selecting easily what you need, and jump right in.

In this section, you will learn enough to become familiar with the road and major signposts starting from your first rumor of tumor until you actually begin therapy because cancer was the answer.

Overview of Specialty

Let us first look at what is required to become a medical oncologist.

Training requirements:

- university (BS or BA) — 4 years
- medical school (MD) — 4 years*
- internship — 1 year
- internal medicine residency — 2 years
- oncology fellowship — 2 years
- (or) hematology fellowship — 2 years
- (or) hematology/oncology — 3 years (combined)

The above is needed to sit for the exam for board certification in hematology or oncology (separate boards).

Training falls under the auspices of the American Board of Internal Medicine. You must be board certified in internal medicine and complete the training of the above fellowships to be eligible to sit for oncology or hematology written exams. Essentially all those completing the fellowships sit for the medical oncology exam, and about 50% sit for the hematology board. My advice is that one should never be treated by a non–board certified (in medical oncology or hematology) physician, with a few exceptions. (Leukemia and lymphoma are often treated expertly by both.) The board pass rate is 58–65%, with board certification being good for only ten years; board members must pass a new exam each decade. As

*Osteopathy degree is also acceptable in place of MD

mentioned, many do not sit for the hematology board and remain "board eligible" until their first request to sit for the exam, and then eligibility is good for six years. This system is under review.

Specific and Related Fields

Medical oncology involves the management of most cancers in adults and is one of the younger internal medicine subspecialties. The need for a "cancer specialist" did not arise until the early 1970s, with the advent of sophisticated chemotherapy regimens. This required specific training for delivery of drugs and follow-up of unique, life-threatening side effects, as well as much more in-depth understanding of the natural history of a disease, promulgating the need for a "quarterback" for cancer care. Patients are usually referred to us *after* the diagnosis. There is significant overlap with hematological cancers of the blood system, such as leukemia and lymphoma, as mentioned above. Our role has largely evolved to being deeply involved behind the scenes when the diagnosis is suspected but not made.

Pediatric oncology involves cancers of children and young adults (up to eighteen years old). The above training is similar, with a pediatric residency instead of internal medicine.

Gynecologic oncology treats ovarian, cervical, and uterine cancers. An obstetrics and gynecology residency followed by a two-year fellowship is required, with formalized board certification.

Urology involves the primary surgical approach, but not the chemotherapy, if any, of bladder, kidney, and prostate cancer. There is a significant degree of chemotherapy treatment performed by the urologist directly into the bladder for the more superficial bladder cancers. There is some extent of treatment of recurrent or even preoperative and immediately postoperative hormonal manipulation of prostate cancer being increasingly done in this field. Training is four years after a one-year surgical internship.

Otolaryngology, also known as ENT, involves primarily surgery only on cancers of the head and neck. There is a four-year residency after internship.

Surgical oncology largely concentrates on breast, colon, melanoma, and other solid tumors; some have training sufficient to credential them to give chemotherapy. This entails a five-year residency followed by a one-to-two-year fellowship.

Neurosurgeons deal largely with the removal and/or biopsy of tumors of the brain or spinal cord tumors. This entails a seven-year residency.

Thoracic surgery concentrates on early-stage lung cancers and occasional open biopsies of the lining of the heart or other chest structures. This entails a five-year residency followed by fellowship.

Orthopedic surgery deals with the primary surgery of bone cancers or metastases, as well as the surgical removal and stabilization (via rods and pins) of bones weakened by cancers.

Radiation oncology entails a one-year general internship. After a three-to-four-year residency, radiation oncologists administer radiation as primary treatment to different types of cancer, such as brain tumors, lung cancers, and some lymphomas (cancer of lymphocytes); or as treatment after surgery (such as to the breast after removal of breast cancer) or treatment along with chemotherapy (synergism)for cancers of the head and neck, rectum, anus, and lungs, or treatment of local, painful, bony areas of tumor that have spread.

The Scope Of The Problem

Perhaps not obvious to some, and certainly not meant to be clever, age is the greatest single factor worldwide for developing malignancy. Think of it. Assaults of whatever nature from the outside are constant (to varying degrees) and continuous. Our own aging argues for how our major mechanisms to fend off the various external causes of cancer are not what they used to be in our youth. Think of sun-caused skin changes and cancers.

Cancer may one day replace heart disease as the number-one cause of death worldwide, with a growing burden in poor countries thanks to more cigarette smoking and other factors. Globally, over thirteen million people are diagnosed with some form of cancer yearly, with eight million deaths. This represents a global cancer burden doubling in the last thirty years of the twentieth century, doubling again between 2000 and 2020, and nearly tripling by 2030. By 2030, over twenty-five million people a year may be diagnosed with cancer, with two-thirds dying from it.

In men, lung cancer is the most common form in terms of new cases and deaths, while breast cancer is the most common type among women in new cases and deaths. More men than women get cancer and die from it, with cancer currently accounting for about one in eight deaths worldwide.

Trends that will contribute to rising cancer cases and deaths include the aging of populations in many countries, as cancer is more common in the elderly and cigarette-smoking rates are increasing in poor countries. Some countries have made progress in curbing cigarette smoking, which causes most cases of lung cancer as well as many other illnesses. In the United States, the most recent figures show that for the first time since records have been kept, less than 20% of adults were smokers in 2007. However, cigarette companies are finding new customers in developing countries. About 40% of the world's smokers live in just two nations—China and India.

Decades ago, cancer was considered largely a problem of Westernized, rich, industrialized countries. However, much of the global burden now rests in poor and medium-income countries. Many of these countries have limited health budgets and high rates of communicable diseases, while cancer treatment facilities are out of reach for many and life-saving treatments are not widely available.

At the same time, progress against cancer is occurring in such places as the United States and Europe. For example, health authorities in the United States report that cancer diagnosis rates are now dropping for the first time in both men and women, and previous declines in cancer death rates are accelerating. They attribute the progress to factors such as regular screening for breast and colorectal cancer, declining smoking rates, and improved treatments.

Let's look a little more specifically at the numbers in the United States. Cancer causes about 25% of all deaths and appears to be on track to replace cardiovascular disease as the number-one cause of death. One cancer alone, lung cancer, causes 30% of all deaths. Prostate cancer is second in men, responsible for 25% of deaths. Prostate cancer is also the most commonly occurring cancer in men, with breast cancer just ahead of lung cancer in women.

Cancer is uncommon in adolescents and children, with only about 150 cases per million in the United States, with leukemia being the most common. If we put all ages and both sexes together, the odds of getting cancer are about 460 in 100,000. This disease is not rare.

Cancer in the first year of life has an incidence of about 230 per million in the United States, with the most common cancer being neuroblastoma.

In the United Kingdom, cancer is in the lead over cardiovascular disease, yet it appears much less frequently in third-world countries, most likely owing to much higher rates of death due to infectious diseases, such as malaria and TB, and accidents.

Nonetheless, cancer remains a major public health problem worldwide, with skin, lung, prostate, breast, colorectal, and urinary/bladder representing the majority of types.

Scope of Chemotherapy

The word "chemotherapy" in this book, when used without any modifying terms, will refer to drugs used to fight malignant cells. Obviously, this sounds as though it could refer to drugs we use in the treatment of any ailment, but that would bring in all of infectious disease, cardiovascular disease, bone and joint maladies, and so on. So, for our purposes, let us stick with its adopted typical meaning in most minds and hearts. Typically, these drugs are given in some kind of standardized regimen, either alone or in some well-thought-out, rationally designed, and previously tested and developed manner to fight cancer.

Sadly and fascinatingly, the field owes a lot to the observed effects and understood chemistry of the lethal mustard gas used in World War I. Without too profound a modification, so-called nitrogen mustard became one of the first successful agents in human malignancy. The US Food and Drug Administration (FDA), National Institutes of Health, and National Cancer Institute for all intents rose to master the method of safe and expedient development and testing of new drugs.

The observation of the effect of mustard gas on the bone marrow in patients with cancers of cells of part of the immune system, known as lymphomas, led in December 1942 to several patients with advanced lymphomas receiving the compound by vein. These patients experienced massive improvement that was dramatic but short-lived. After the war records were declassified, the race to exploit these drugs and use them against cancer was underway. Soon mustine, the first chemotherapy drug, was developed. Afterward, many other drugs were used in combination, and remissions with cures of some lymphomas—one in particular known as Hodgkin's disease—were being tentatively reported. After that, drug development exploded into a multibillion-dollar industry, although the principles and limitations of chemotherapy discovered by the early researchers still apply.

Cancer cells not only tend to divide and have children or daughter cells more often than their normal counterparts, but they keep doing so. Your liver does not keep growing; it knows when it has reached just the right size. If it is injured and the injury is not too bad, it will regenerate to just right size. This is not so with malignancy.

Chemotherapy can try to take advantage of the nonstop division of cancer cells, but this means one may see effects on other tissues made of rapidly dividing cells, such as bone marrow, digestive tract tissue, and hair follicles. Obviously, and particularly in the case of bone marrow, decrease in normal cell counts can occur. In the case of bone marrow, this is known as "myelosuppression"; this can be dangerous and require careful monitoring and support if red cell counts fall into the range of serious anemia; platelets fall, increasing the risk of bleeding; or certain types of white blood cells fall, dramatically increasing the risk of infection.

Notionally, the overarching purpose of cancer chemotherapy may in some cases be expressed as palliative, which means there is no hope of cure. In such cases, the treatment is intended to alleviate symptoms and perhaps prolong life and do so in a manner the patient agrees is worth the effort, as it is often not free from toxicities that must be weighed against benefits.

Then there is therapy clearly planned as a regimen intended for cure. This is an all-out attack against all the cancer cells with or without surgery or radiation or other therapies as part of the plan. The oncologist will tend to give doses known to have the power to kill cancer cells and support the patient through the dangers and toxicities, possibly requiring hospitalizations, transfusions, or other support, as the goal of cure is possible. Full doses administered on time are used consistently in this course of treatment.

Then there is the use of chemotherapy before a primary modality of therapy, which might be radiation or surgery, to reduce the burden of cancer cells and eradicate nonlocal metastasis, as well as make surgery more feasible with a better result. This is called neoadjuvant chemotherapy, and it may have cure as its intent.

In contrast to neoadjuvant therapy, adjuvant chemotherapy is a post–primary treatment (typically radiation or surgery) modality used to mop up supposed remaining local and distant cancer cells. This therapy is done based on the understanding for a particular cancer that both local and, especially, distant development of cancer is at risk to occur after original therapy but may not ever occur or may rather take a long symptom-free time to do so, with the adjuvant therapy being given after local therapy.

There are about 450 drugs approved and mainly used for the treatment of, or directly in principal support of, the treatment of human cancer. Broadly, chemotherapy is the treatment of cancer with drugs that can destroy cancer cells by impeding their growth, reproduction, and rate of spread. Thus we can broadly classify drugs by names that are meaningless to many but will ring bells for anyone one who has taken a few chemistry courses.

Amazingly, many of these come from stumbled-upon observations in the plant and animal kingdom. Others are products of so-called rational drug design. The National Cancer Institute (NCI) has played an active role in the development of drugs for cancer treatment, with over half of those drugs currently used coming from their drug development program. Consider this: over four hundred thousand compounds have gone through NCI screening and are in its drug repository, of which eighty thousand have been screened since 1990. Drugs can enter any level of this program, depending on how much is already known regarding them. Thus, it is a system designed to not waste time. The NCI supports the majority of clinical trials in the world, with over 1,500 ongoing at one time that have some major NCI connection. Then there are some private foundation-funded trials, university trials, and trials in other nations, bringing the total to over 2,000 ongoing per year in the United States, representing well over 70% of all trials worldwide.

The sales of cancer drugs will grow at nearly double the rate of the global pharmaceutical market and may pass $80 billion by 2012, according to IMS Health, the leading provider of information services for the healthcare industry who covers markets in more than one hundred countries around the world. Expensive new treatments, an increasing number of patients on chemotherapy in major markets and evidence that more people in emerging markets are gaining access to modern targeted therapies will contribute to sales of cancer drugs growing at a compound rate of 12 to 15%, IMS said.

In 2008, US sales of oncology products exceeded $50 billion. This comprises nearly 17% of all of worldwide pharmaceutical sales growth for that year. As techniques to diagnose disease earlier, as well as detect metastatic disease earlier, develop, and the understanding on a genetic and immunologic basis of each patient's cancer cells abound, much more elegant and specific therapies will rapidly shuttle their way through the FDA's drug-approval pipeline. This will not slow down.

In 2007, Titus Plattel, IMS vice-president for oncology showed laser-accurate vision when correctly predicting that "double-digit sales growth in oncology drugs [would be] fueled by increased use of targeted therapeutic agents introduced over the past 10 years ... [in addition to] first-time innovations coming to the market and longer treatment periods for growing numbers of patients." Indeed, since 2007, over forty new and important chemical entities were released as safe and effective either alone or in combination with other drugs or types of therapies, contributing to the exploding cost of treatment.

The more we learn of the *why* of the development of malignant cells that escape or overcome immunologic surveillance and destruction and the *how* of their potential and timing for spread on a basic scientific, genetic, immunological, and clinical level, the more that knowledge will be exploited. The distance from laboratory bench to patient's bedside will continue to shrink as not only new drug classes with mechanisms of action helpful to many sufficiently similar patients will be proven safe and effective, but also the more tailor-made therapies for specific cancers become a reality.

"Ten years ago it was all about chemo," said Dr. Kim Lyerly, director of the Duke University Comprehensive Cancer Center at the 2007 American Society Of Clinical Oncology annual meeting (the largest cancer-care meeting in the world). "This time you walk down the convention center and it's all about new targets. And we can get more mileage out of these drugs if we can predict who will respond."

Here is a brief explanation of the *how* of present anticancer chemotherapy.

Chemotherapy is the use of powerful medicines to kill cancer cells. However, not all chemotherapy agents act the same way. Some of the newer therapy is aimed at specific targets within cells and not principally at highly dividing (multiplying) cells. Nonetheless, the idea is either to try to exploit some level of an Achilles' heel present in the malignant cell that is either absent or not crucial for cell survival in healthy cells. This can be done directly or by means of a cascade of events.

Some chemotherapy drugs affect the behavior of cancer cells without directly attacking them, and some directly attack the DNA of the cells, preventing them from multiplying or triggering their ultimate demise. Others do not act directly; they target the molecular abnormality in certain types of cancer. Depending on their biochemical mode of action, chemotherapy drugs (also called an antineoplastic or cytotoxic drug, meaning "toxic to cells" or "cell killing," respectively) are grouped into different therapeutic classes, listed below. You may find it useful to have a deeper understanding of just what drugs are being used and why. Feel free to talk with your treating physician regarding these drugs and their combinations. This may also be of great help when looking on the web for new clinical trials and treatments with combinations different from those you have seen. It will also help you understand the differing spectra of toxicities that may occur with these drugs.

Alkylating agents (also called DNA-damaging agents): Alkylating agents form chemical bonds with the DNA of cells of all kinds but more so with those that are more actively dividing (more target available). The drugs incorrectly link rungs on the ladderlike structure that DNA can be envisioned as—a ladder of two legs of what are called nucleotides that match up only one complementary base pair at their ladder rungs. At the rung area, the pair called A always matches up with T, and G always matches with C. Then the whole ladder is twisted and folded. The explicit pattern of those "rung-connected pairs" with nonsense spaces and other fillers and such, is your DNA. That code, when read through unzipping and sending a messenger of the unsoiled code to protein factories of the cell, contains instructions for the production of proteins that are necessary for all the functions of your body. If the code is wrong or unreadable, all manner of havoc can break loose in this intricate system. Alkylating agents can stop tumor growth and set the stage for tumor cell death directly or in time by creating cross-links of chemical bonds in the ladder of the two complementary strands that should not be there. So linked, cells cannot go through the normal cycle of cell division, repair, and production of daughter cells, as they are unable to reproduce their DNA—an essential step to cell division. Alkylating agents include several drugs; the most common are: cisplatin, carboplatin (Paraplatin), ifosfamide, chlorambucil, busulfan, and thiotepa.

Antimetabolites: These anticancer agents work by inhibiting the synthesis of nucleic acids (DNA, RNA), which are essential in cell division and the making of daughter cells. So, while they do not make alkyl bonds as the drugs above, the outcome is very similar. Normal cells that divide rapidly will be adversely affected. The benefit comes from the fact that unless and until cancer cells show resistance specifically (unusually) or generally to these drugs, they are often initially more sensitive to the effects of these drugs than normal cells during the necessary processes of cell multiplication. In nature, cancer cells divide more frequently than normal cells, and therefore any halt in cell division affects cancer cells more than healthy cells.

The antimetabolites are among the oldest chemical agents used in chemotherapy and are broadly divided into three groups, depending on their therapeutic action.

- **Pyrimidine analogues:** These molecules are found mainly in nitrogen-containing bases that mimic the essential building blocks, the nucleotides, of DNA and RNA, which hold the source code and further directions for everything in a cell and made by that cell. One of the antipyrimidine agents is {5}-fluorouracil (5FU), a drug used in the treatment of many cancers, principally colorectal cancer and pancreatic cancer.

- **Purine analogues:** These are substances that inhibit enzymes that are crucial for the assembly, maintenance, duplication, and tying together of DNA: DNA polymerase, DNA primase and DNA ligase. One powerful common example is fludarabine, a chemotherapeutic drug used to treat chronic lymphocytic leukemia.

- **Antifolates:** These are drugs that, through direct competition, interfere with the synthesis of a crucial vitamin used in many levels of mammalian cells—folate. One of the most common of antifolates is methotrexate; it acts by inhibiting dihydrofolate reductase, an enzyme essential for synthesis of purines and pyrimidines.

- **Plant alkaloids and terpenoids:** These are alkaloids of vegetable origin that have therapeutic properties. They prevent the formation of what is known as "the spindle," an egg-shaped structure similar to devices used to shake dice in some betting games. During cell division, the spindles run the long axis of an egg-shaped device and are what chromosomes need to guide themselves along when the mother cell divides into two daughter cells and takes a full complement of chromosomes to each of the two cells. Cancer cells are more sensitive, to a degree, than normal cells prevention of spindle formation causes the cells to remain blocked at the cell division stage and unable to divide, and thus multiply in number. The most common alkaloids that affect the spindlelike tracks include vincristine, vinblastine, vinorelbine, paclitaxel and docetaxel.

- **Taxanes:** The taxanes also halt cell division and were originally found in the English Yew tree. Tumors find it difficult to grow. Although they can be used in the treatment of many tumor types' cancerous conditions, the taxanes are used mainly to treat advanced stages of breast cancer, lung cancer, and metastatic ovarian cancers. The taxanes include paclitaxel and docetaxel.

- **Topoisomerase inhibitors:** DNA topoisomerases are essential enzymes that maintain the highly specific and elegant coiling, twisting, and orientation in three-dimensional space of DNA. This is not only not random, but its integrity must also be maintained for accurate functions such as copying, reading of the DNA code, and then recombining when DNA unzips, reads itself, and makes perfect complementary strands of itself for each daughter cell. Among this class of chemotherapy drugs are amsacrine, anthracyclines, camptothecin derivatives (irinotecan), and epipodophyllotoxin derivatives (etoposide and teniposide). The topoisomerase inhibitors are used to treat several types of cancers.

Antitumor antibiotics: antitumor antibiotics are a class of chemotherapy drugs used to treat many malignancies, such as acute myeloid leukemia, breast cancer, and non-small-cell lung cancer. These drugs act by preventing cell division in both cancerous cells and healthy cells that multiply rapidly, so the therapeutic index—or margin of safety between where they seriously impair normal cells versus irreversibly damage cancer cells—is very narrow. The most common antitumor antibiotics include the following:

- aclarubicin
- bleomycin
- dactinomycin
- daunorubicin
- doxorubicin
- epirubicin

- mythramycin
- mitomycin
- zorubicin

Hormones: Some cancers are either hormone-dependent or hormone sensitive cancers (such as some breast and prostate cancers). This can be both a positive or negative sensitivity, and drugs are used to exploit this. Hormone therapy can be used to block hormonal stimulation by acting at various aspects of their metabolism, thus stopping or slowing tumor growth. For example, some drugs manipulate circulating testosterone's effect on prostate cancer; other drugs interfere with the ability of hormone-responsive breast cancer cells to reproduce and thrive in a progesterone- or estrogen-rich environment. Some drugs work at local cancer cell receptors, and some work distantly in aspects of the endocrine system, including the brain in areas such as the pituitary gland and elsewhere. It is really rather marvelous the ways that these cells mimic and try to exploit the norm as well as the ways science has uncovered this and exploited their doing so.

Monoclonal antibodies: All of us are equipped with an amazingly intricate immune surveillance system in a liquid containing antibodies, cytokines, interleukins, interferon, and more, and a cellular system somewhat analogous to a complete army of intelligence cells—short-lived marines, cannibal cells: the metaphor really does go on and on. The immune system is wonderfully connected and communicates rapidly with all of its aspects. We fight bacteria, cancers, viruses—anything we sense as foreign, such as transplanted organs and, of course, tumors. The Nobel Prize in Physiology or Medicine in 1975 went to scientists who discovered we can engineer antibodies highly specifically for just one foreign entity. The race was then on to make these antibodies fight against cancers and perhaps even attach to them payloads of radiation, biologic toxins, or chemotherapy, as well as to try to deliver cancer cell–specific therapy. Think of this as being somewhat like a silver bullet. In some cases, the antibody alone does the trick. The whole point is specifically leaving healthy tissues and cells alone while trying to target something very unique about the cancer cells, thus addressing the Achilles' heel notion that was raised earlier. This is now a multibillion-dollar industry and is growing rapidly.

Of course, one must never underestimate the workarounds cancer cells can develop; but overall, the direction of research and therapy with this notional type of approach to monoclonal antibodies is positive. A common bottom line of therapy is that the antibody singles out the cancer cells and deprives them of something essential, blocks some important pathway, or delivers a payload of something toxic. In many cases, this triggers the cancer cells to commit suicide. In the beginning, these antibodies used mouse cells to make the antibodies, and humans reacted with anti-mouse human antibodies. I was on the first team to publish the building of techniques to humanize these antibodies. In so doing we "saw," by tacking radioactive light to the antibody, breast cancer metastasis in a patient that other scans could not see. In short order, a billion-dollar industry was thriving, principally involving non-Hodgkin's lymphomas. Soon other cancers joined these lymphomas on a large scale. Drugs classed as monoclonal antibodies include the following:

- Herceptin, used in the treatment of breast cancer
- rituximab, used to treat lymphoma and other similar malignancies

Podophyllotoxin: Podophyllotoxin is a plant-derived (American and endangered Himalayan mayapple) compound from which we get two drugs. These make cells get hung up and unable to multiply just before the life-cycle phase called G1. This is the phase in which they start doubling up their DNA prior to dividing. These drugs also block cells past G1 trying to actually make the double DNA (to give half to each daughter cell). We see what these drugs (etoposide and teniposide) do, but we still cannot clearly state exactly how they work. The mechanisms of their action is not yet known. Owing to the rarity of their plant of origin, scientists are trying to find the genes of their DNA codes (just like forensic scientists do in solving crimes) to be able to make the chemicals in the lab by teaching certain cells to be factories for the chemical.

Nanoparticles: These particles fall in the size between atoms and small molecules and can be designed to be identical to each other. They are finding increasing use in biomedicine. For example, some of our drugs are very insoluble using conventional techniques. Getting the essential active agents into the size of nanoparticles allows a highly concentrated delivery of drugs. Nanoparticles made of magnetic material can be used to concentrate agents at tumor sites in the body that have been first identified by monoclonal antibodies with a few atoms of iron attached. You now have a tumor sitting vulnerable to agents affiliated with external magnetic fields. This is a novel way to localize, at the near atomic level, a highly toxic therapy that might well leave otherwise unengaged (magnetically speaking) tissues alone. Think of as a laser sight with a focus as tight as a few molecules.

Electrochemotherapy: This is the idea of somehow giving a physical chemistry or immunologic or biochemical fingerprint to that which you want to singularly find and eliminate. Imagine injecting a chemotherapeutic drug that is then followed by an application of high-voltage electric pulses locally to the tumor that facilitates the passage of some drugs that normally cannot get transported across the cancer cell wall's defenses and into its interior. Early work with the antitumor antibiotic bleomycin and the alkylating agent cisplatin is showing some benefit in combination for treatment of skin cancers or those just under the skin, no matter what the original tumor type may be. Using this as a cue, endoscospists (clinicians using flexible fiber-optic scopes to look into tubular structures, such as the GI tract) are combining these lessons to catch tumors at extremely early phases, avoiding more invasive surgery later. The idea is to minimize impact on surrounding normally functioning cells by specifically targeting and then eliminating the tumor cells. This can be done either by identifying the cancer cells easily or using techniques to which they are uniquely vulnerable. This should result in an increased tumor kill and/or reduced toxicity.

Specially targeted delivery vehicles are given a differentially higher affinity for tumor cells by interacting with tumor-specific or tumor-associated antigens. In addition to their targeting component, they also carry a payload, whether this is a traditional chemotherapeutic agent, a radioisotope, or an immune-stimulating factor. These vehicles will vary in stability, selectivity, and targeting motif, but they all have the same aim of increasing the maximum effective dose that can be delivered to the tumor cells. Reduced systemic toxicity means that they can also be used in sicker patients, and that they can carry new chemotherapeutic agents that would have been far too toxic to deliver via traditional systemic approaches. Think of the drone technology we now have in warfare that is designed to allow the drone to single out a vehicle with a specific license plate or some other highly specific trait with laser accuracy and spare all bystanders while delivering a payload.

More non-DNA- and antigen-targeted therapies: Some cancers have a well-defined defect. One in particular, chronic myelogenous leukemia, has a defect known as the Philadelphia chromosome, wherein one portion of genes or DNA material have a highly specific deletion and movement to other sections of DNA strands, making a chromosome known as the Philadelphia chromosome (named after the city it was discovered in). This leads to the bone marrow cells getting a message to code for a category of gene family known as a type of tyrosine kinase, which leads to out-of-control and overtime bone marrow activity. At one time, the disease was only curable by a bone marrow transplant with well-matched donors and recipients. The death rate from therapy was high, with death more likely for patients who waited too long to try the risky transplant. In time, rational drug design and targeted drug therapy led to an almost nontoxic pill that blocks the aberrant type of tyrosine kinase seen in the disease. Now most patients have high-quality remissions, if not cures.

Other targeted therapies: In one form of acute leukemia, a class of drugs known as the retinoids were discovered to force the arrested maturity of one type of adult leukemia into maturation and eventual control. The following retinoid drugs are being looked at in multiple malignancies: bexarotene, isotretinoin, tretinoin, and ATRA. In addition, we now see exciting work with the following:

- **Vaccines**: The well-known example is used to prevent a large proportion of cervical cancers.

- **Targeted therapies against cellular enzymes or products.**

- **Genetic manipulation:** This is achieved by inserting specific workhorse pieces of DNA that help single out malignant cells or program them to self-destruct selectively.

- **High-dose chemotherapy with stem-cell rescue:** This includes auotologous (yourself) or allogeneic (other humans) peripheral blood or bone marrow transplantation.

- **Biologic response modifiers**: This involves substances such as interferon and interleukins, which use the body's own immune system to fight cancer and to reduce treatment-related side effects.

- **Ultrasound and cryotherapy:** Ultrasound therapy uses high-frequency microwaves to try to break apart tumor cells; cryotherapy freezes tumor cells using inserted probes.

- **Radiation sensitizers:** These are drugs that increase the sensitivity of just cancer cells, allowing for less damage to surrounding cells and more targeted treatment.

- **Antiangiogenesis inhibitors**: These are drugs that, when delivered, inhibit the tendency of some cancers to cause the blood vessel system to be stolen, so to speak, in a manner that brings more nutrients to the cancer, giving it a growth advantage as well as providing highways that facilitate the cancer's ability to access more remote areas of the body.

In sum, the more we understand about that which confers malignant behavior to malignant cells, as well as all the special tricks and traits malignant cells use, the more we single out those seeming advantages as targets for the design of increasingly specific therapies with decreasing toxicity. The same holds true for finding the vulnerabilities some of these cancers have separately from or in excess of their normal counterparts.

Thus we see how the word "chemotherapy" is not only complex and colorful but also not at all necessarily a bad thing. Furthermore, the search for new and more specific agents from the plant and animal kingdom for rational drug design and tailored therapy have brought us over 450 approved effective compounds. More on the types of therapy and beauty of the rationally designed clinical trials comes later.

Scope of Lay Knowledge of Malignancy

Numerous studies have assessed, not only in Western nations but also worldwide, the extent of knowledge and understanding of cancer by the nonprofessional. It matters little if one is asking about the diagnosis; biological behaviors; types, effects, and benefits of therapies; causes; or odds of response and long-term effects—the fund of knowledge by the layman is abysmally low. This underscores the argument supporting the need for books such as this, and it reminds us of the enormous power anxiety has in this disease. The gap of fact versus fiction existing in the nonprofessional population is a jumbled mishmash with lack of clarity and discernment on all fronts. It is driven by fear of the unknown.

People in rich and poor nations alike have faulty understandings of the causes of cancer and need further education as to how to fend off the disease. Studies have shown that in all parts of the world there is a greater tendency to believe that factors out of our individual control, as opposed to lifestyle choices, are the main cause. The sentiment that we are tossed to the winds of fate or bad luck from genes is largely present—and, of course, wrong.

A 2007 report, based on a survey sponsored by the International Union against Cancer (UICC) of nearly thirty thousand people in twenty-nine countries was released at the start of a four-day world cancer congress in Geneva. In high-income countries like Australia, Britain, Canada, Greece, Spain, and the United States, as well as low-income nations, the survey found that the refusal to recognize that alcohol consumption increases cancer risk ran at 30% to 50% of the population. Of course, cancer risk does rise as alcohol consumption rises. There was overall denial that obesity is a cancer risk factor and a greater belief that an increase in the consumption of fruits and vegetables in the standard

Western diet will have a more powerful impact than moderation of alcohol and cessation of smoking. This is, of course, wrong. Strikingly, there was an unfounded perception that stress posed an ominous proven danger as regards developing cancer, similar to the common understanding of the credible data regarding stress as a contributing factor to heart disease. Air pollution was also incorrectly held as a major cause of cancer. “In general, people in all countries are more ready to accept that things outside of their control might cause cancer, like air pollution, than things that are within their own control, such as being overweight which is a well-established cancer risk factor,” declared the UICC.

The survey showed that in low- and middle-income countries, people were more pessimistic about the chances of treatment curing cancer. In the poorest countries, 48%felt not much could be done once the disease had taken hold. In middle-income countries, 39% had the same view, but in the richest countries, pessimists totaled only 17%. The problem with the fatalistic view, said the UICC, was that it could deter people not only from seeking treatment but also from participating in cancer-screening programs that can save many lives.

This is only a snapshot of studies that echo the same point. The fund of knowledge of nonprofessionals and the accuracy of that knowledge regarding causes, methods of diagnosis, treatment modalities and odds of response, morbidity of treatments, and, frankly, most of the relevant aspects of human malignancy are archaic and a poor reflection of reality. Why? Because it is the very nature of a beast with so many frightening faces.

Cancer is a disease not always externally seen that can affect anyone in any organ and spread at will, causing all manners of havoc; its therapies, without guidance and correct counseling, are held by many to be worse than the disease. It is a disease that can cause inexplicable wasting and distant effects from only local tumors and alter quality of life in dizzying arrays. This is why the profound anxiety exists. Imagine a process wherein a few cells somehow imitate their benign counterpart organ on a genetic level. Then add in their selective growth advantage—not stopping, not staying put, tricking and fooling the defenses of the body, escaping detection and eradication, and using the body’s own building blocks to spread. Then they require typically difficult, intense therapies to eradicate them, and those therapies may not be sufficiently cancer specific to spare normal functions and tissues so that not only the disease causes all manner of impairment of health quality issues and risks, but so also may the therapy. Imagine the problems that arise when the scope of accurate, sufficiently detailed knowledge of the enemy is sparse and largely incorrect. Thus, again, the need for this book.

Scope of Adult Oncology Practice

Our patient population involves treatment of those over eighteen, with two-thirds of patients being over sixty-five. The diagnosis of a primary (first-time) cancer process is usually initiated by the primary care physician. Often, a radiographic study (plain film, chest X-ray, mammogram, etc.) is ordered to evaluate a symptom (pain in bone, cough, lump in breast, etc.) or abnormality (lesion, "hole" in bone, mass in lung, microscopic calcifications on mammogram, etc.) Tissue diagnosis is then made. Radiologists may use a fluoroscopic device to biopsy bone, or needle localization to biopsy breast masses; pulmonologists may use fiber-optic bronchoscopy to look into and biopsy the lung. Then the pathologist reads the biopsy sample as cancer, not cancer, or suspicious and perhaps gives a level or grade of severity, depending on the cancer type, and then calls the physician that sent him biopsy tissue to inform him of the diagnosis.

Special stains of cell-tumor-associated products or fingerprinting of the traits of the material follow. These can include Her-2/neu, estrogen, and progesterone testing in breast cancer and many more immunologic, hormonal, or genetic markers or assays of the actual biopsy material. Thus, getting enough tissue is crucial. Also being sure to get clear margins is often very important; if this is not done at the biopsy phase, it should be done later. There is a phrase, intended to be a bit rough, that I drill into the heads of all of my students. It makes a crucial point and completes the mantra of the title of the book: "Although tumor is the rumor and cancer is the answer, tissue is the issue; no meat, no treat." Getting to the meat of a diagnosis requires specific and *adequate* tissue.

This is not said to be cute; it is said to be memorable. "Meat" means you need to be sure you obtain enough of the right specimen from the right spot (often assisted in the OR by various scopes and scanners), and have the right labeling of orientation (where exactly the specimen came from). Submitted in the right way, fresh Vs must be fixed in the right amount. Most importantly, the specimen needs to be submitted by the right people who not only know all of this but also do so as a team. Discuss your case before biopsy and at every decision point along the way in conference as a team.

When there is a team approach,

- your pain and suffering are guaranteed to go down;
- your odds of remission, its quality and durability, and even the chance of cure go way up;
- you recuperation at home is much better;
- your family is closer and more supportive;
- your insights into the less-than-optimal management of the most frightening diagnoses are greater, improving your ability to take and give in support groups; and
- you will live and love more.

If you read this book, I guarantee that with YOU at the helm, your odds are best. This time YOU is an abbreviation for Your Oncology Universe. All orbits around you, the patient!

Treatment Setting

Patients are treated primarily in the outpatient clinic setting. There has been a large evolution from the inpatient setting to the outpatient (clinic) setting, largely pushed by medical advances and health-care reform that has decreased inpatient stays. New drugs are introduced specifically for the clinic setting more often than not.

There are also oncologist reimbursement issues. Outpatient care is often more lucrative, with occasional, uncommon inpatient episodes as a consequence of treatment (e.g., immediate complications, such as allergic reaction to chemotherapy during infusion or chemotherapy leakage out of veins and into tissues, causing tissue damage (necrosis) and leaving skin ulcers). There are also delayed (days to weeks) complications: infections, which can be life-threatening; diarrhea with subsequent dehydration; nausea and vomiting, which very uncommonly can be relentless and delayed (weeks to months); and neurological complications, as well as blood counts requiring blood-replacement products.

Prevention

This book has a focus on those individuals that engage cancer when tumor is the rumor or cancer is the answer. Thus, the massive and crucial field of prevention, cancer surveillance, and screening is intentionally not addressed in any depth. Nonetheless, this book is also designed as a reference that can be read in logical order from start to finish, with each section also being able to stand up on its own, complete unto itself for quick referral as needed. This means that there is background information about the nature of cancer that better prepares you to fully participate in your care and exercise your autonomy. Thus, some comments about prevention and screening are included.

Without the intent of being macabre, there is also an understandable fascination with and attraction to the science of oncology, as it represents conditions that broadly encompass all aspects of the human condition—psychosocial, ethereal, and of the flesh. It does so as a mimic of the normal tissues on the most fundamental genetic and macro, or gross anatomic, levels. Cancer is a respecter of no one. Its understanding and treatment involve all aspects of medicine more deeply than perhaps any other field. More research dollars are poured into it than perhaps even cardiovascular disease. More drugs are rationally screened and designed for its treatment and management each year than any other disease, and discoveries in its basic science routinely open more doors into the nature of what life is and the tools that tell us so. An invader of anywhere, its story is one of the stories of the progress of modern medicine in all of its aspects—drug therapy, radiation treatment, and surgery, as well as combinations of all three.

Thus, we know some of its causes, but not nearly enough; and we know some ways to screen for it, but nowhere near well enough to profoundly impact the disease yet (with some exceptions). Thus, physicians are responsible to counsel all patients and family members regarding what we do know about diet, alcohol, sexual behavior, obesity, exercise, self-examination, overexposure to sunlight, Pap smears, mammograms, fecal occult blood, and sigmoidoscopy. There are numerous sources the physician can refer the patient to, such as the American Cancer Society, The American College of Surgeons, The National Cancer Institute, and many more. A simple call to 1-800-4-CANCER will do it all.

There is *no* proof yet that the patient without symptoms or high risk factors benefits from routine scans of the body (whole-body CAT, MRI, ultrasound, and such). As we will discuss later, avoid reasoning by the anecdote wherein some singular episode of something having occurred in the past is incorrectly taken to mean those results apply to you and that you should thus be tested despite having neither signs nor symptoms of proven high risk factors. Tests cost money and emotions. Many tests done in this screening manner are neither sensitive nor specific (no false positives or false negatives); nor are they worth the test cost, safe, or effective as a screen. Another exception is the patient with a clear family pedigree of a number of cancers, such as breast, various colon cancers, and other rare genetically based syndromes, as well as clinical presentations highly suggestive of an underlying malignancy. In addition, it has been shown that in the appropriate age groups, mammograms and colonoscopies performed in patients with no known risks does make sense. This is also true of routine Pap smears with exams, and is possibly true for routine blood testing in specific age groups for a specific protein related to prostate cancer with a well-done physical exam for prostate cancer.

An overview of the top five areas of progress from the standpoint of diet, nutrition, and weight management and cancer were recently the subject of a poll of the American Institute of Cancer Research. They concluded that (1) excess body fat is a major cause of cancer, (2) the scientific study of who survives and why is now fully underway in our research and university centers, (3) technology is making the evidence on causes much clearer and out of the realm of unsubstantiated claims, (4) a growing connection between diet and genes seems to be taking shape, and (5) the same connection is present between diet and cancer links in general.

However, once a cancer is clinically established, it is not clear that any radical change in diet will have a direct impact on that cancer, while not removing the possibility that it may impact development of a second cancer that has not yet taken hold (this is theoretic and nearly impossible to prove). Mega diet changes or, frankly, any dietary change radically different from those recommend by the National Institutes of Health has simply not yet been shown to be capable of stopping tumor growth, cause sustained remissions or cures, or prevent spread once a tumor is clinically visible with routine tools, such as physical exams and scans.

Cancer prevention means taking active steps intended to decrease an individual's, or a whole population's, risk of developing cancer. Most cancers have environmental issues as causes (other than aging) and lifestyle issues at their core, meaning to some degree that they may be controllable. Thus, there is some reality to stating that certain aspects of cancer can be considered preventable. For example, lung cancer does occur in people with no risk factors, directly or otherwise, but they are a small minority. Thus, never smoking or being around it (secondhand smoke), never being chronically exposed to significant levels of radiation or certain chemicals, and a few other lesser factors are steps one can take to markedly diminish, but not totally remove, the risk of developing lung cancer.

Most experts say that about 30% of cancer risk can be diminished by improving exercise, decreasing alcohol intake, not being obese, avoiding tobacco products, eating an adequate diet, avoiding of sexually transmitted disease, and, to a modest degree, avoiding severe air pollution, as well as avoiding exposure to naturally occurring background radiation.

Dietary recommendations that may decrease cancer risk are (1) reducing energy-dense highly processed foods and high-corn-syrup sugary drinks, (2) increasing plant-origin foods, (3) decreasing processed meat and high proportion of red meats, and (4) limiting consumption of alcohol, salt, and mold-risky cereals.

The data for each of these recommendations ranges from clear and strong to highly suggestive. Studies carefully looking at these observations show diminished colon cancer rates as well as pancreatic, stomach, and breast cancer rates in populations of patients who markedly differ in these risk factors.

The notion that some form of medication readily available to all can limit our risk of all cancers is very attractive but unproven and is often the source of great sorcery against unsuspecting patients' souls, and quackery. In certain circumstances, there is some suggestive data. For example, aspirin has been found to reduce the risk of death from cancer overall, but it is not a risk-free drug. Teasing out how much of the effect is due to decreased cardiovascular disease is tough, but the slight suggestion remains. The hormone-blocking drugs tamoxifen and raloxifine can reduce the risk of breast cancer in high-risk women by 50%. Finasteride may decrease the risk of prostatic low-grade cancers in men. The nonsteroidal anti-inflammatory drug celecoxib and a relative have shown in cases of familial adenomatous polyposis that they may decrease the risk of developing malignant polyps; this is possibly also true in normal people (with polyp tendency). However, this benefit comes at a price of increased cardiovascular risk.

Vitamins have not been found to be effective at preventing cancer, but low levels of vitamin D are associated with increased risk; the nature of this observation is unclear. Beta carotene supplementation may actually minimally increase lung cancer risk, and folic acid not only does not decrease colon polyps, but it may also increase them. Vitamin C definitely does not diminish cancer risk, and it is dangerous, just as is Laetrile, when given in large doses.

There are vaccines, recently developed, that prevent infection by some viruses that are associated with cancer, and therapeutic vaccines are in development to boost our immune response against certain types of tumors. Two vaccines against certain strains of human papilloma virus that together cause 70% of cervical cancer decrease later development of cervical cancer in infected patients. These vaccines also have a role in protection of males from later development of anal cancer in those chronically infected with HPV viruses.

Screening

Cancer screening involves efforts to detect cancer before it is noticeable in terms of signs or symptoms. Screens could be as simple as tests on stool for nonvisible blood, tests of the sputum, urine, and multiple blood assays for proteins or blood markers associated with cancer, and various types of medical imaging.

Universal screening means applying the tests without disqualifiers to all people. Selective screening means limiting the test to specific people who, for any number of reasons, increase the odds of a true positive result and decrease the odds of a false negative result (which is when we wrongly state all is well based on the test but in reality cancer is present).

One has to balance factors that affect test outcome before applying a screen in either case. There may be harms, clinically as well as psychologically, from the test. There may be unnecessary radiation exposure, allergic reactions to dyes, and so on. A test with such risks should be suggested only when the risk of failure to screen a high-risk patient is higher.

Sensitivity and specificity are covered a number of times in this book, and it is well worth the time to gain some basic grasp of the concepts. If a test is not sensitive, it will miss cancers when they are there. If it is not specific, it will wrongly claim cancer is there when it is not.

All tests can produce false positives and false negatives, with false positives being more commonly produced. Experts look at all of this and come up with the positive predictive value of a test, which is a wise calculation based on collected data that a test claiming to show cancer in an individual has whatever power or accuracy to reveal true, positive results.

If a cancer is rare, there is not much rationale for screening tests; nor is it often helpful in young people, as cancer is mostly found in people over the age of fifty. There are some exceptions, but not many that stand up. There may be cultural differences: in the United States, we screen for colon cancer far more than stomach cancer, but in Japan, stomach cancer screening is commonplace because stomach cancer is commonplace there.

Positive screens may mean a lot more people undergoing invasive biopsies. If a test produces many false positives, you may have bad outcomes if the biopsies hold some risk. The same holds true when screening for diseases for which treatment may not be suitable or available. If treatment is not available, then diagnosis of a fatal disease may produce significant mental and emotional harms and must be weighed in an informed manner.

Even when treatment is available, finding cancer early may have no impact on outcome. The only thing, then, that screening does (if positive) is make it appear the patient lived longer, when in fact the added time was at discovery, not at the end of his or her life. Furthermore, the only length of time increased is a period of the patient knowing they have cancer, for which there may or may not be effective therapy. This is also true if the treatment result from screening is the same as without screening. All this is the notion of lead-time bias, where one knows the diagnosis earlier, making it appear he or she lived longer.

A powerful screening program reduces years of potential life *lost* and disability-adjusted lives (it increases healthy lives). It truly catches diseases earlier and makes a difference in doing so.

In our zeal as scientists, we can over diagnose. There are some cancers for which no treatment may ever be necessary. One can see this in the elderly with slow-growing cancers. Prostate cancers and hormonally receptive breast cancer in the elderly come to mind where perhaps no harm is done to watch and treat symptomatically, in select cases, if and when therapy might be poorly tolerated and not affect quality of life or survival.

Remember, the patient is the one with the disease. Physicians and their patients should look at the logistical burdens the testing proposes and decide if it will take too much time for little reward. For cultural reasons, patients may not wish to participate. The law of patient autonomy must be respected.

Of course, there is the issue of the cost of screening. The US Preventive Services Task Force recommendations ignored the issue of money. However, most good tests and the studies that evaluated them include a cost-effective analysis. Obviously, all else being equal, the less expensive test is the one supported. Such analyses do not just compare two tests to each other; they look at all the detailed costs associated with the test from development to interpretation and follow-on biopsies. However, the costs to the individual are often hard to quantify and may not be included, such as time away from work.

The US Preventive Services Task Force (USPSTF) recommends cervical cancer screening until age sixty-five for women with a cervix who are sexually active. They advise annual stool blood testing and less frequent sigmoidoscopy or colonoscopy starting at age fifty until age seventy-five (every five to fifteen and ten years, respectively). Routine screening for other cancers is not recommended. There is some disagreement regarding screening for prostate cancer. There is also some controversy on when to start mammograms in women with no family history. Presently the consensus is every two years for those fifty to seventy-four years of age. Some researchers feel strongly that yearly mammography does more harm than good. As mentioned, Japan screens for gastric cancer, and they use photofluorography to enhance sensitivity. (That is, they use a dye to assist the human eye in looking for cell changes.)

Genetic testing for certain high-risk patients is recommended, as certain cancer syndromes are known to exist. The BRCA1 and BRCA2 genes are looked for in breast, ovarian, and pancreatic cancers. A number of other genetic tests are now suggested in certain GI and GU tumors for patients in families with multiple prior cancers. Patients showing as positive for these gene mutations then undergo more frequent other tests, such as mammograms, various scopes, and perhaps even preventative surgery or a trial at chemoprevention.

Again, the scope of this book is not screening. Far more detailed information can be found at the National Cancer Institute site for patients and at 1-800-4-CANCER.

Cause

This is not a book centering on the cause of cancer, its prevention, or its survivorship. Those topics and perspectives are covered in droves. However, this work relates to patients suspected of having cancer who are found, in fact, to have it and find themselves awash in a sea of anxiety with almost no life buoys of knowledge to keep them and their families afloat until reaching a safer shore.

Entire careers have been devoted to the cause of cancer. For the perspective this book strives toward, it suffices to say that most cancers find their cause in an environmental basis. Large-scale monozygotic (identical) twin studies have shown that about 80% of adult cancers are not primarily due to inheritance. You are not predestined to develop cancer—with some notable exceptions of well-studied examples and family syndromes. Cancer is part of the aging process in many of us. For example, the majority of all elderly males have slow-growing prostate cancer.

Malignant transformation and growth of a cancer is a genetic event, but there must also be a breakdown, overwhelming or effectively hiding from the patient's immune surveillance system, that accompanies the early malignant events, allowing or facilitating their survival. Once again, this too is an acquired event and not something inborn or preprogrammed to happen (a common misconception). Of course, as we age, the constancy of the spontaneous rising up of cells with malignant potential can eventually overload us as part of the normal process of aging. Nonetheless, it is not true that old age simply means you will definitely develop aggressive malignancy; it is more complex than that.

The cascade of events leading to the malignant transformation of cells and their subsequent ability or tendency to grow and spread is possibly the most active field of all clinical and basic cancer research. Your inherited genetic makeup does clearly have a role, but it is not usually deterministic. There are unknown acquired genetic defects. Smoking is a major cause. Other causes are a high-fat and low-fiber diet, and viruses, such as is seen in AIDS and more rarely in the virus of mononucleosis. And certainly alcohol and radiation exposure in excess increase risk.

The causes of cancer, while not a particular subject of this book, are nonetheless heavily related to our goal, in that false beliefs in causes are often the battleground of numerous rumors, where incorrect and damaging viewpoints and opinions can run amok. For example, to some an honest answer regarding "why me?" can seem flippant and almost irreverent because the response is, "why not?" Cancer is not a rare phenomenon, and the longer you live, the greater the odds you will contract it. Of course, for some patients, some strong singular risk factors are a familial relationship risk (inborn increased odds for a specific cancer). But, to the largest extent, the answer is that it is a common disease whose risk increases with age and some lifestyle choice factors and that there is no one single cause most of the time. For example, although cigarette smoking is a singular factor, the type of tobacco and the manner of the exposure is important, and some (most) people escape development of both the small-cell (solely related to tobacco products) and the more common non-small-cell cancers of the lung.

I will review the major categories of cause without delving into sophisticated data, as that would take us off target too long and too far for too little reward.

It is usually impossible to prove exactly what caused a cancer in any individual, because most cancers have multiple possible causes. For example, if a person who uses tobacco heavily develops lung cancer, then it was very probably caused by the tobacco use. But since everyone has a small chance of developing lung cancer as a result of air pollution or radiation, there then is a tiny chance that the smoker's lung cancer actually developed because of air pollution or radiation. In some cases, we simply do not know why a person develops cancer.

Cancers are primarily an environmental disease, with 90–95% of cases attributed to environmental factors (if we include age) and 5–10% due to genetics. ("Environmental" means being of nongenetic cause.) The common causative agents are tobacco exposure (25%), obesity and diet (30%), chronic infections (30%), radiation—meaning both nonionizing (think suntans) and ionizing (think radon, x rays) (10%), and lack of physical exercise and environmental pollutants. Stress is not clearly related to the cause of cancer in humans, although this is chronically debated.

Lung cancers are highly related to tobacco smoking. Tobacco smoke has substances in it known as mutagens, which cause DNA mutations, which impact cell growth and increase the likelihood of metastasis. Mutagens that specifically cause cancer are known as carcinogens. Various carcinogens can cause various cancers, such as cancers of the head and neck, bladder, esophagus, pancreas, larynx, and kidneys. Tobacco carcinogens are related to 90% of lung cancers, and tobacco smoke contains over fifty carcinogens. Lung cancer causes about a third of deaths in the developed world and one in five deaths worldwide.

Many mutagens are carcinogens, but not all, and not all carcinogens are mutagens. Alcohol is like that; about 10% of male cancers in Western Europe are related to alcohol, whereas about 4% of female cancers are.

Cancer related to one's occupation may represent between 2% and 20% of all cases. Every year, at least two hundred thousand people die worldwide from cancer related to their workplace. Millions of workers run the risk of developing cancers like lung cancer and mesothelioma, from inhaling asbestos, and leukemia, from exposure to benzene.

Diet, physical activity, obesity, and the overall adverse impact of obesity on immunity and the endocrine system play a cooperative role in many cancers. Poor diets low in balance of whole grains, fruits, physical activities, and obesity are related to approximately 30–35% of cancer cases. In the United States, excess body weight is associated with the development of many types of cancer and is a factor in 14–20% of all cancer deaths. Physical inactivity is believed to contribute to cancer risk not only through its effect on body weight but also through negative effects on immune system function and through the endocrine system.

Diets that are low in vegetables, fruits, and whole grains and high in processed or red meats are linked with a number of cancers previously discussed. In addition, a high–salt diet is linked to stomach cancer. The frequent third-world food contaminant aflatoxin is associated with liver cancer, and betel-nut chewing with oral cancer. Thus, you will see cultural differences that shift when populations move into a new country of residence and do or do not continue their diet or origin culture.

We previously discussed infection, with perhaps as many as 18% of cancers worldwide being related to infections. These infections were largely previously addressed, but it is worthy to note that both viruses and bacteria have been implicated. Viruses that can cause cancer are called oncoviruses. There are also viruses that cause forms of rare leukemia. In polluted third-world rivers, parasites, such as *Schistosoma haematobium* and the liver fluke *Opisthorchis,* can cause can cause bladder cancer and cancer of the gall balder and liver ducts. This is not an all-inclusive list, but it rather stresses the point that chronic irritation from infectious causes can lead to malignancy.

Radiation can cause all types of cancer after typically long periods of exposure and duration of radiation. Large doses have effects more immediately, while most exposure has a long latency period between total lifetime dose and the development of malignancy. The young are most vulnerable to the bone marrow toxicities of radiation, and the elderly to skin cancer due to lifetimes of exposure. The jury is in on tanning beds; skin is damaged, and the risks for all types of cancer are increased. Children and adolescents are twice as likely to develop radiation-induced leukemia as adults are, with radiation exposure before birth having ten times the effect. Ionizing radiation is not a particularly strong mutagen. Residential exposure to radon gas, for example, has similar cancer risks to secondhand smoke.

Living near a nuclear power plant or power lines does not impact your cancer risk. The steps involved with chronic ionizing radiation in forming cancer are well known and are cumulative. Radiation is a more potent source of cancer when it is combined with other cancer-causing agents, such as radon gas exposure plus smoking tobacco.

The familial syndromes were briefly touched on previously. Members of these families can have increased risk of specific cancers, such as breast, ovarian, and colon, as well as cancer in general. Adding to the prior list are individuals who inherited a defective gene for repair of routine damage. The gene for controlling cell growth in these people is a mutation of gene *p53*. They run the risk of a number of cancers, especially soft-tissue cancer and brain cancer. Mutations in the retinoblastoma gene lead to the same-named cancer in children. Those with well-known genetic syndromes in general tend to have a generally increased risk of cancer (for example, Down syndrome, a condition in which three copies of chromosome 21 are present).

Some substances cause cancer primarily through their physical, rather than chemical, effects on cells. Asbestos and other naturally occurring as well as synthetic fibers can lead to mesothelioma when inhaled. Physical trauma as a cause of cancer has been debunked, with the sole possible exception of chronically drinking scalding-hot tea, causing inflammatory defensive repairs similar to what is seen in people with chronic reflux of gastric contents. It is the repair, not the trauma, that is the culprit.

Hormones were also previously addressed, and the general mechanism is their stimulation of the growth of hormone-dependent cells, which may become uncontrolled and malignant.

Cancer is not a transmissible disease. It is not infectious other than the rare possibility of transfer of cells during pregnancy and the extremely rare transfer of cells during organ transplant (the most common of that rare event is melanoma).

Pathophysiology of Cancer: How Do They Do the Voodoo They Do?

A normal cell transforming into a cancer cell requires those genes regulating cell growth and maturation to be altered. There are two broad divisions of genes at this point. There are oncogenes, which support and promote cell growth and reproduction, and tumor-suppressor genes, which inhibit cell division to a normal survival rate.

The gain or loss of an entire chromosome can occur, or more commonly, there can be spontaneous mutations of the nucleotide sequences we discussed previously. This can occur on a large or small scale, thus amplifying the gain or loss of the original blueprint for normalcy in the cells. Sometimes this material shifts on the chromosome or moves completely to another with or without loss where it moved to. Sometimes it repeats or is simply deleted.

A well-known example that we previously mentioned is the Philadelphia chromosome, or translocation of chromosomes 9 and 22. This occurs in a chronic leukemia where a bcr-abl fusion protein is the new product, made because of the movement and shifting or translocation of chromosomal material, causing a cancer-producing type of enzyme, a tyrosine kinase, to be made.

Anywhere along this magnificent blueprint code of DNA, on any of the chromosomes, small-scale mutations—including point mutations, deletions, and insertions—can occur. These mutations might occur near an area known as the promoter area of a gene, making it more likely for its product to actually be expressed or made with altered function of the protein that it is now coded for.

DNA material might even get inserted when a foreign virus, such as a retrovirus, gets put in the DNA and its code for viral oncogene may be turned on. And if these defective alterations in the code persist, daughter cells may proliferate with the defect, and the rumor of tumor then becomes the answer of cancer. Native normal DNA seems to have some ability to detect these types of errors, and even the ability, to a degree, to not only find them but correct them to safeguard the cell against cancer. If significant error occurs, the damaged cell can "self-destruct" through programmed cell death, termed "apoptosis." If the error-control processes fail, then the mutations will survive and be passed along to daughter cells. Moreover, as said, rumor then becomes answer.

Thus, this constant tension is set in motion wherein the DNA code remains under assault and self-repair. With enough adverse pressures, cancers can be born, and the cell, under more stress, might promote the chance of that rumor becoming tumor, and the chain reaction of daughter cells into full-fledged cancer can then get underway. Alternatively, a further mutation may cause loss of a tumor-suppressor gene, disrupting the apoptosis-signaling pathway and resulting in the cell becoming immortal.

A further mutation in signaling machinery of the cell might send error-causing signals to nearby cells, soon progressively allowing the cell to escape the controls that limit normal tissue growth. This rebellion-like scenario against self can soon become like a Darwinian struggle of survival of those most fit to live. If the clone of malignant daughter cells is most fit, a nasty process called clonal evolution gets underway. This drives progression from a single cell to a clone to tumor large enough to detect. These cells then metastasize and invade as treasonous enemies in your own midst.

Life Cycle of Cancer

Cells may move on to make daughter cells—cells that for all intents and purposes are identical (unless damaged in the process) to the parent cells. The basic ideas apply differently to cells that have a nucleus (eukaryotic cells) and those that do not (prokaryotic cells). The latter cells are in the plant family and divide by a pinching sort of mechanism know as binary fission, but the eukaryotic cells go through a magical, delicate dance filled with precision and wonder.

In these cell division cycles, the more the cells do, the shorter the cycles, or dividing or doubling time, and the greater the threat of a defect. The intent is to make enough of everything so each daughter cells will have all it needs. The nucleus is where the entire DNA needed for the instruction of the cell doing all of what it does resides. In order to have daughter cells, it must make exact copies of its DNA, and then these duplicate pairs of chromosomes pull apart—one in one direction and one 180 degrees away.

These eukaryotic cells have three basic phases: interphase, in which the cell grows, accumulating nutrients needed for division and doubling its DNA; the M phase, which is the actual division; and the final phase, called cytokinesis, which starts once the two new daughter cells are formed. This is repeated, following the pattern of intricate instruction in each sequence of paired nucleotides that are specific (genes), for making a specific protein for specific functions that builds—in time, with billions of other proteins and molecules—you.

Multiple steps lead to a malignant cell that multiplies and defies the usual restraints on the growth time it takes normal cells to replicate, as discussed in "The Enemy." One measure of the aggressiveness of a tumor, remembering it can vary from patient to patient and within the life of a patient, is the time it takes to double in mass or number of cells—the so-called doubling time. It can range from three hundred to six hundred days for colon, rectal, or prostate carcinoma, to sixty-six hours for high-grade lymphomas and leukemia.

Very broadly, similar to a factory producing a final product, cancer cells individually go through a life cycle where they are in varying stages of vulnerability as they are preparing building blocks to make the daughter cells.

Some forms of chemotherapy are, by their nature, very specific and impair these crucial steps; others are not what is called cancer cell–cycle specific. Some can affect cells at more than one stage. Research has become rather elegant in trying to understand and exploit both the somewhat generic vulnerabilities that occur during the process of cell division as well as the more specific individual cancer cell needs that might occur, wherein only the more rapidly dividing cancer cells might be injured in excess and irreparably, compared to their normal counterparts.

Tumor Growth Characteristics

Tumor cell growth largely depends upon its microenvironments—the neighborhoods, so to speak, of vascular supply—to bring nutrients in to sustain cells and nourish them during multiplication, and for transportation of garbage and toxic byproducts away from the cell. It also is dependent on the oxygen content being sufficient to complete successful cell division. All the while, successful growth is affected by the degree to which the host's (your) immune system can suppress, impair, or perhaps eradicate some portion of cells trying to multiply. In addition, other cells seem more destined to spread after various triggers and thresholds are met locally. They seem to home in on distant organs as if they were programmed to not only seek out the blood or lymphatic vessels to travel in (as opposed to direct extension and invasion), but also to stop and set up shop once arriving at specific organs or regions (lymph nodes, liver, spleen, lung, brain, and so on). These cells that have metastasized (spread) then continue to grow. They somehow survive, for all intents and purposes being invisible to the host's immune surveillance, and thus they progressively increase the burden and impair overall "performance status" of the host, as well decrease the function of whatever organ(s) they have invaded.

Thus, the portion of cells dividing or able to successfully divide and spread is not a constant. This type of phased growth curve seen in many cancer cell models is common but not always the rule and is named Gompertzian after its main describer. Understanding the nature of these growth spurts, just like those in humans from infant to toddler to adolescent to adult, helps enormously in understanding times of maximum vulnerability and gives clues as to what sort of intervention may work It can also show how vulnerable those cells may be compared to a mature and self-replenishing normal adult cell.

There are numerous variations on these themes, and they are broadly unique for each cancer. Some cancer remains somewhat dormant for a long time. The span of time from the development of the first colon polyp cancer cell until the formation of the first detectable malignant polyp can be from three to as many as ten years. Some are aggressive and relentless. Some lymphomas and leukemias are more like a science fiction nightmare in their speed of growth and in size, locally invading and spreading through the vascular conduits of the body, wherein they can block and paralyze normal function or literally replace the previously healthier organ. For example, ureters from the kidneys can be blocked by local bilateral cancer-engorged lymph nodes, causing obstructive kidney failure. Bone marrow can fail from rapid replacement of the marrow by actively dividing tumor cells.

Clinicians use the known tendencies of the growth-curve characteristics of tumors they are treating to develop treatments that work not only because they are directly toxic, per se, but also because they have some advantage of hurting the tumor rather than the host because of differences in cell growth cycles.

Although well beyond the scope of this text, some human cancers can double from a theoretical initial "mother cell" and divide into daughters to the level of 10 grams, or 0.35 ounces, in two weeks. That amount is about our level of detection on physical examination or CXR, CT, or MRI scans. However, with more sophisticated molecular, immunological, and even genetic tools, alone or coupled with various markers, dyes, or radiation, the detection rate is increasing as smaller and smaller depots can be found.

It usually takes thirty doublings to reach clinical detection. For our slowest cancer, a patient may have had a tumor for years before detection.

Once a tumor reaches about 10^{12} cells (1 kg), it usually represents such destructive local cancer, widespread cancer, or deterioration of the patient that death is imminent. Other than for specific research assays, we do not generally attempt to count cancer cells, but we use various clinical laboratory and radiological, immunologic, and magnetic-imaging tools to find malignancy and approximate its volume. Where it is, how fast it is growing, and what dysfunction it is causing are all much more to the point than cell counts. As mentioned previously, there are some scenarios (leukemia) where we do need our best assays to tell us, as close to reality as possible, that no individual circulating malignant cells remain.

In other solid tumors, counting cells is neither possible nor necessary, as typically, once all detectable cells or markers for the cancer are gone for a long periods with close surveillance, the odds of calling that remission a probable cure increase. In some cases, all we have, based on collections of a lot of clinical and laboratory data, are probable odds of recurrence over time. In most of those scenarios where we cannot see any more tumor using all our imaging techniques, the odds are very low for recurrence and high for relapse-free survival. But again, close watching is needed, as odds are people-less numbers and your cancer is very personal indeed.

Rational Naming of Cancers

The cell type that the tumor resembles microscopically, and is therefore presumed to be the origin of the tumor, helps us classify cancers. These types include the following:

- **Carcinomas**: These are cancers derived from cells of organ linings and skin—epithelial cells. This group includes many of the most common cancers, particularly those often found in the aged. Most of these develop in the breasts, lungs, prostate, colon, and esophagus.

- **Sarcomas**: These are cancers arising from what is called connective tissue, such as bone, cartilage, muscle, nerve, and fat, as well as supportive cells both in marrow and out of marrow.

- **Leukemia and Lymphomas**: These two classes of cancer arise from the blood-forming cells that leave the marrow and mature in the blood and the lymph nodes, respectively.

- **Germ-cell cancers**: These cancers most often present in the ovaries or testicles and derive from the specific cells most closely related to stem cells or pluripotent (capable of being almost anything) cells.

- (**[prefix]blastoma**): Cancers in this category are derived from immature "precursor" cells or embryonic tissue. These are also most common in children.

We more specifically name cancers by using the above names as a suffix and the organ of *origin—not* the organ where a tumor has spread to—as the prefix. Some examples of full names are breast carcinoma, bone sarcoma, chronic lymphocytic leukemia, and so on. Even when we name a cancer of origin and the amount at the origin is minuscule and the spread to a location is massive, we still name it by its place of origin, because that is what confers most of its personality for treatment choices. One may have a tiny primary breast carcinoma with massive lung metastases, for example. Regardless of the location, this carcinoma would be treated as breast carcinoma.

When a mass or masses are benign (a decision based on clinical microscopic and genetics criteria, not size or growth) they are named using "-oma" as a suffix with the organ name as the root. For example, a benign tumor of smooth muscle cells is called a leiomyoma. (The common name of this frequently occurring benign tumor in the uterus is "fibroid.") There is some unfortunate confusing naming overlap with melanoma and seminoma; both are always malignant.

Some types of cancer are named for the size and shape of the cells under a microscope, such as small-cell or spindle-cell or giant-cell carcinomas, and then further criteria delineate more precision.

Pathological Diagnosis

Pathological diagnosis means the diagnosis arrived at from looking at the biopsy material under the microscope and applying whatever compendium of studies, stains, tests, or consultations are needed to be sure its name is correct.

The following rules must never be broken: Never confuse the ability to name a tumor with the ability to understand it. Never accept a tissue diagnosis (biopsy result) as unequivocal until it clearly is. Never act on verbal reports from anyone on anything. Be sure the pathologist has adequate samples, especially when clinical and tissue data do not make sense together. Never hesitate to get another pathology opinion from outside in any nonroutine or nonobvious situations.

There are conditions that are very early stage, very low level, and of uncertain odds to progress to cancer of their organ of origin. Arguments have been made to not call them cancer, and perhaps this has some merit. However, the majority of those conditions are precancerous if left alone. Thus, you may have names for cervical intraepithelial neoplasm—angry cells that do mark a patient for risk of evolution to cervical cancer but at present can be treated with curative intent. The diagnosis is a pathological one.

Similarly, in breast cancer there is a condition called ductal carcinoma in situ. This refers to cells with malignant potential (or actually "malignant cells" is more accurate) that have stayed within their microscopic tissue boundaries. Studies so far show that although patients with this condition will probably not need chemotherapy, they will need further surgery, possibly with radiation, to follow limited surgery, and if they are candidates, possible oral tamoxifen to follow.

The prostate can exhibit a low-grade neoplasia, which is probably the slowest growing of all prostate cancers. Patients with this condition should have regular close follow-up for years, and with signs of change it is wise to consider a full evaluation for possible surgery more aggressive than biopsy.

Bladder cancer can exhibit a similar situation of cancerous cells in situ (no invasion). However, patients with this condition are at grave risk without further therapy (not removal of the bladder, though). Similar to breast cancer, these malignant cells are staying within a limited and important area, but they have a definite risk of progression. There are those who suggest, using these examples, that we should not call these cancers at all to assuage patient anxiety. I disagree. We should do as this book does and take the time to fully educate the patients in reasonable depth as to what we know about these early cancers or cancer-prone marker situations.

One must always, when possible, have the specimen obtained the ideal way and studied in the ideal manner before ever declaring a diagnosis of malignancy or being cancer free. Sometimes one has to go back for more biopsy material or better clear margins. The point is clarity using the nomenclature the clinical world has agreed upon so that decisions are made in uniform manners.

Signs and Symptoms of Cancer

The location of the cancer may explain the presentation of symptoms. However, cancers can affect distant organs, be small, exude significant symptoms, and be relatively large and unknown. Without growth, they may make you lose appetite and lose a great deal of weight. They can cause fluid retention or diarrhea, facial flushing, and headaches without being in the brain.

There may be seizures and arrhythmias without tumor being in the central nervous system or touching any cardiac structures. Tumors may cause leg swelling with muscle wasting. Some may dramatically increase the odds of venous-side blood clots, which can be dangerous and spread to the lungs as pulmonary emboli.

Some syndromes have names and characteristic tumors causing them. Paraneoplastic syndromes are the constellation of signs and symptoms and laboratory or other clinical findings associated with the presence of a specific few embryological-related underlying malignancies, such as high calcium seen in breast cancer, head and neck cancer, and multiple myeloma even without tumor in the bone. Increased clotting can be seen in adenocarcinomas (glandlike) that produce excess mucous, which triggers the clotting factor cascade.

Obviously, some symptoms can depend on the location of the tumor. Signs and symptoms of central nervous system malfunction may well be caused by tumor that has spread to or started in the brain. Signs and symptoms of obstruction can occur based on the cancer blocking nearby channels and conduits. For example, cancers in the back of the abdomen, such as cancers of some lymph nodes and cancer of the urinary bladder or pancreas, can cause ureter or bladder obstruction. Higher up they can cause obstruction of parts of the intestine and ducts around the pancreas. Colon cancers can cause, in very late stages, obstruction of the lower GI tract. Cancer of the liver or the ducts around the liver can cause bile-flow obstruction.

Cancers can ulcerate on the skin, such as some skin cancers or melanoma, with changes in borders and color and easy bleeding; or they can cause odd rashes and skin changes. A lot of the swellings of cancer can be painless. Cancers can cause bizarre neurological symptoms that are widespread and do not fit any one pathway. That is the often the clue for an underlying, unapparent malignancy.

Organs may silently grow enlarged because tumor is either obstructing flow from them or is directly invading them. There may be a general feeling of enormous fatigue or night sweats in characteristic patterns. There may be unexplainable psychiatric symptoms or depression. There may be anemia without the bone marrow being affected, or there may be advanced invasion of the bone marrow with low white blood cell counts and risk of serious infection, anemia, and low platelet counts, creating serous risk for easy bruising or bleeding.

The point is that there may be highly suggestive syndromes, local or distant effects, and considerable overlap as to possible causes, as well as curious but highly suggestive and almost specific syndromes suggesting only one or two possible diagnoses even though initial tests may not show the primary tumor. There may also be pain from stretching of organ capsules or pressing on organs or conduits and passageways or spread of tumor to bone with fracture or impending fracture.

Thus we can see that there are many ways for tumor to be the rumor and cancer to be the underlying answer.

Stage of the Cancer and Prognosis

Extent of disease, organ of origin, cell type and grade (angriness), local invasion, regional and distant spread, functional status of the patient, and the first detectable changes of early cancer provide a basis for treatment. Knowing which organs are most likely to be involved can spare needless suffering and save dollars and emotions. Knowing exactly where the cancer is and is not, how invasive and how advanced it is, and using specific and explicit internationally agreed-to staging criteria is crucial to learning what works and what does not, stage by stage. Multi-institution, let alone international, collaboration is impossible without us all speaking exactly the same language when referring to the impact of treatment regimens on various stages. Knowing how specific treatment regimens alter the course of untreated cancer prevents the selection of therapy that offers little or no advantage over no treatment. Knowing how often the cancer in question produces the observed clinical pattern permits the recognition of an atypical pattern that may herald an unrelated treatable benign condition. Knowing how the tumor produces symptoms and death enables the physician to provide optimal palliative care.

Broad Concepts of Goals and Timing of Treatment

It is essential that all are clear as to what outcomes are probable and possible. Are they cure, prevention, prolongation of life without cure, relief of symptoms, or urgency vs. buying time? *It is hard to make a patient without symptoms feel better,* except perhaps emotionally, but treatment given to prevent recurrence of disease in such patients is very common. Thus, it must be clear to all as to what the intent is: curative, adjuvant (treatment given after primary treatment to prevent recurrence), neoadjuvant (treatment given before primary treatment to improve the effect on the primary tumor, such as giving chemotherapy before breast cancer surgery to shrink the tumor), or palliative.

As a general medical legal guideline, the medical oncologist should provide comprehensive care and not a narrow focus. Decisions should be logically based on the best data available and evidence known to date without subjecting the patient to every available test. Life is to be prolonged at a functional level that the patient defines and that the thorough oncologist can state as a possible goal after adequate staging and testing has been done. Therapy can be individualized, taking into consideration age and life goals; patients should neither be threatened nor coerced into choices or deserted consequent to the choice they made.

However, the patient's right to swing his or her fist ends at the oncologist's nose. Physician and patient must both be clear on this early on in the therapeutic relationship. There is always a positive role for the physician in oncology, especially with the terminally ill. This is often very hard for providers, as our training is not adequate in such areas as emotional, psychosocial support, and therapy, and burnout of purely clinical oncologists is not rare. Remember, the empathetic physician walks on a very tight rope, and the cold-hearted (or so it seems) walk alone.

Vocabulary of Survival

The language of the oncologist needs to be clear to the patient and family. Physicians need to be very clear from a legal standpoint that "cure" is a statistical term. It applies to groups rather than individuals in that it means a patient is free from cancer for a duration equal to the survival expectancy of age-matched controls without cancer. Time tells us if you are cured, with increasing certainty. Comparisons to known odds tell us your probable odds at any point in time, assuming adequate continuing evaluation is being done. Some patients' survival curves never really reach 100%, as there are still patients at years ten to twenty and beyond who relapse and die. This is seen in breast cancer in some settings, for example. Of course, the cooperation of international scientists for decades in building those survival curves also tells us that such an outcome is rare, but not unheard of.

The survival rate refers to how many patients are alive (if that is stated), or disease-free and alive, over specified periods. These may be stated as actuarial, which means they are compared to a control group without the disease, or stated as the median-adjusted survival, meaning that half are alive or disease-free and half are not.

A complete response is just that—no detectable disease by ever increasing highly sensitive tests, some at the genetic level. The tests necessary to declare invisibility are fairly well standardized and unique for each cancer.

A partial remission means there is a 50% reduction in the tumor's bi-dimensional measurable mathematical product. This is calculated by simply looking at the measurements of the tumor, such as height, width, and, if possible, depth, before and after treatments or over time, calculating the total volume of the tumor, and then comparing those two results to each other.

Anything less than a partial remission without progression is stable disease.

THE ONCOLOGIST

Why Oncology?

The roads chosen for a career in oncology are diverse. Some choose research; some enjoy a mixture of the laboratory bench and bedside. Others choose full-time private practice as opposed to academics, while others go into the big business of biotechnology research and have a path marked by brilliant entrepreneurial zeal. Owing to the military paying for medical school, I had my road chosen for me as a largely clinical route with significant exposure to all of the others—especially clinical research and teaching.

While oncologists are not all the same, most cancer clinicians are quite similar in their heart of hearts, their thought processes, and (I think), in many ways, their spiritual view of all of this. I have found that most of my colleagues share an immense sense of purpose and meaning in their practices and research.

The most frequently asked question I have received from trainees and colleagues alike is "How can you do it, and why do you do it?" This is usually followed by "I could never do oncology."

This is the best answer I have been able to muster.

There is an indefinable but unmistakable nature to being human. It is unique to the species, reproducible, and immensely sensitive. The human mind and heart connect as a somewhat huge spiderweb of the finest silken threads, capturing and suspending every experience of life in the chambers of consciousness. Life-threatening situations, such as the diagnosis of cancer, pull upon all of those threads, thus bringing one's world into unparalleled focus.

I have never seen this nature more vividly than when my patients have faced the enormous fear malignancy evokes. I have seen the diagnosis cement the realization that we are all connected and, in a practical sense, underscore the insight that we are and always can be truly knowable. In the practice of oncology, patients and providers alike quickly accede to the marvelously hidden plot—the master illusion whereby we appear to differ.

Cancer respects no organ or person. Furthermore, the oncologist must have intimate knowledge of all the fields of medicine, radiology, and pathology, as well as a finger on the pulse of breakthroughs in basic science. They have an armamentarium of diagnostic tools unmatched in depth and elegance, and the field is perhaps better organized than many internationally in terms of asking the next best clinical question through cooperative research and clinical trials.

Once the team of caretakers and cared-for coalesces, a dance begins. It is a dance whose rhythm is the beat of the patients' trek to garner knowledge and quell anxiety by doing so. It can be hero-making.

Cancer unravels, mocks, and challenges the norm more than any other malady. The wonderfully divine plan of human existence at the cellular level is never clearer than in the thick of the battle of fighting cells that mimic the norm.

When tumor is the rumor and cancer is the answer, the sweetness of the privilege of simply being alive is immediate. The solace and comfort offered by the health-care team, family, and loved ones is more pressing than usual. In facing the possibility of premature death, the pulse and zeal for life, as well as perhaps redefining it, beats more soundly. What truly matters can become transparent. There is also a sense of camaraderie in fighting a war of great and personal consequence and not having to do it alone with both people and science as allies. Oncologists have a ringside seat as the heroes and the health-care team "box with God." More than once, although frequently bruised, battered and stunned, the team wins a round—and, with increasing frequency, the match. *That* is part of the answer to "Why oncology?" for me.

MD: What Is In a Name?

Since the beginning of time, the world has set physicians apart as magnificent demagogues (MDs) for many understandable reasons. I am not talking about arrogance, per se. The enormity of knowledge acquired, the responsibility, and the immense emotions entailed lead to a very circumspect world for the physician. It is a world that patients really cannot understand easily. Enhancing this is the reality that patients often lean more toward being a patient than a *participant*. Although understandable, other than when the competency of the patient is in question, it is best for all if the patient and family deeply participate in their cancer care. There is *always* a better outcome when the other "MD" is exposed—the magic decoder ring. Becoming the master of our journeys occurs when we all share in the secret handshakes of what initially is overwhelming information, and in time *everybody* gets in the boat, grabs an oar, and pulls hard.

However, many physicians are not that eager or aware of the necessity to crack the code and share the secret handshake. There is considerable variance in this regard depending upon medical specialty. It should come as no surprise that some fields attract abstract thinkers more than immediate-action, black-and-white problem solvers. Some fields of medicine attract urgent "fix it" types; some attract urgent "find it" types. Some medical specialties appeal to hand-holders, and some physicians prefer a practice more removed from patient contact, let alone in-depth emotional engagement.

What About Oncologists?

Oncology is a mixed bag. It tends to attract deep thinkers, but certainly not to the exclusion of all other fields of medicine. Oncologists tend to be folks who like to box with God. They are intellectual problem solvers who love to master immense and diverse amounts of knowledge and who live to ask the next best question. Although it has improved and there are many notable exceptions, oncologists' strongest suit tends not to be in-depth personal, emotional, or spiritual engagement with their patients.

Frequently, oncology support staff, nurses, and front-office personnel alike soar like angels in this regard. By no means am I implying that oncologists do not feel deeply or fail to understand the profound emotional aspects of their practice. In fact, I think they do both of these things. Rather, owing to time constraints, frequently pressing urgency in diagnosis and treatment, self-protection, and an appropriate need to remain somewhat distant emotionally, the in-depth engagement of patients in manners discussed in this book is not overwhelmingly preeminent.

Oncologists are not only not immune to stress, but they are also magnets for it, as are many other physicians. In oncology, however, one faces terrorism of the highest and most clever degree every day, as discussed in the chapter "The Enemy." Accrual of new patients to an oncology practice usually occurs for ominous and frightening reasons. Patients do not become cancer patients for routine, typically reversible diagnoses. It is not largely about some surgical procedure or therapy in which everyone always turns out just fine. New patients become a lifelong affair, and interactions with family and support systems are intense and long-term. Loss of patients is often owing to death. Fear, both physical and spiritual, is commonplace. Thus, stress is frequently a disease that affects the patient, his or her loved ones and supporters, *and* the oncologist and his or her staff.

Let us just pull back the protective white coat on this phenomenon of stress for a moment. Hans Selye spent almost five decades studying stress since the 1930s. A noted psychologist, Herman Feifel, observed the intense enmity and perhaps fear physicians characteristically have of death. Sociologist Renee Fox's work echoed similar conclusions when it focused on those physicians conducting pioneering work. As discussed in the section "Clinical Trials," research and implementation of research results are the hallmark and mainstay of this field of medicine more routinely than many others. The tempo of moving information from the laboratory bench to the bedside is high, and the intensity enormous.

Stress is essential for life. Without the eternal struggle between tension and release, joy is muted, passion is subdued, biological and personal growth are stunted, and life becomes a bore. However, out of balance, stress can be damaging. Today's oncologist must deal with insurance companies and HMOs exerting various levels of control regarding patient treatments owing to reimbursement issues. Oncologists typically work very long hours, and the demands for rigorous documentation can be pressing. (Fortunately, technology is beginning to ease that burden with digital patient records.) Compounding this is some natural professional disgust with the everyday business pressure foisted upon the oncologist unlike ever before.

Thus, there are sufficient ingredients in the mix that do not foster an environment allowing lengthy visits with patients. The sheer patient volume necessary to maintain a practice can be overwhelming, simply not affording sufficient time to meet the entire emotional, psychological, spiritual, and, at times, educational needs of the patient and family. All the while, the oncologist is the authority, the mentor, the captain of the ship. To whom do they talk? Other physicians? This is not likely, and what little data is out there confirms it.

The intellectual orientation of a physician starts to form early. Medical school is a culture that reinforces the concept of immensely delayed gratification. Loyalty to the guild takes on almost priestlike proportions. The sheer level of physical and mental labors is staggering. The mind is often governed by way of an addictive technocracy whereby dependence on data, tests, and technology tends to supplant other more creative and less didactic techniques of collecting information and solving problems. All of this combines seductively and may lead physicians in training to be unaware of and underestimate personal needs and the power and promise of human relationships. Medical school sentiments of privilege, honorable responsibility, and excitement quickly mellow.

Although these notions have broad applicability among many physicians' groups, a primary source of tension in oncology is the physician's changing role from "curer" to "life-prolonging champion of the fight against the disease," and then to "sustainer," when active therapy is no longer useful. This is difficult, heady stuff. Most surveys to date note that "not enough time" is right at the top of challenges and easily competes with the need to keep up with new medical information, difficult patients or family members, the number of patients who don't get better, and the paperwork.

In 1991, one survey reported burnout in over 50% of the more than one thousand long-term clinical practice oncologists who responded. The incidence of burnout was lower among university-based oncologists. University oncologists' time is somewhat protected, as their practice entails a large portion of teaching, and competent residents and fellows often assist with research and physician load. Three of the major stressors identified by the respondents were dealing with dying patients, reimbursement issues, and a heavy workload. The researchers suggested that the lack of preparation for dealing with the emotional aspects of oncology contributed to job stress and burnout.

In a subsequent similarly sized study of British oncologists, the prevalence of psychiatric disorders was 28%. Clinicians who felt insufficiently trained in communication and management skills had significantly higher levels of stress than those who felt sufficiently trained. The authors concluded that improved training in communication skills might provide a useful tool to lessen the stress of practice.

As is intuitively obvious, being in the captains' chair and dealing with repetitive human suffering and frequent losses takes its toll. Just as one cannot deny his or her creativity, one cannot escape the pressure of simple human sorrow. The first response of oncologists is to detach in order to remain effective. However, too often this means this means they become disaffected, unengaged, and non-communicative as regards the issues addressed in this book. In time, everyone loses.

When physicians detach, they may lose some of the quiet comfort of knowing they have been effective in alleviating suffering, which they may have sought out in pursuing a career in medicine. One is on sacred ground when intimately involved with the sufferer and taking action to alleviate suffering. Here is the rub: Chemotherapy, potions, and pain meds may enormously mitigate distressing symptoms, but anxiety and emotional anguish are insidious tormenters not as easily diagnosed or treated by formula. Physicians can have an enormous impact in these areas.

I am not inventing any new ideas. There are no truly new lessons to life or truly original emotions. There are variations on universal themes. Pain, whether it is psychic, emotional or physical, is the same in any language. Effective and broad-reaching communication, sympathy, and empathy, coupled with dispensation of in-depth information, are benign opiates patients and families are happy to depend on.

Studies have shown that a lack of formal training in communication skills heightens physicians' daily stress. Every day, oncologists are bringing bad news; discussing prognoses, complicated therapies, treatments of pain and suffering; and dealing with a dizzying array of future pitfalls and milestones. So what to do? It starts with enhancing communication skills to decrease stress for all. The key is to engage the patient and family. The time spent reaps immense rewards for all and, in effect, maximizes the quality life not only for family and patient but also for physician and staff. In the final analysis, it actually saves time to invest time.

However, enhancing these skills starts with dissecting and discovering all that needs talking about. Data are easy for the oncologist. Analysis of data comes as quickly to the oncologist as does fear to patients and families. One first must know what to talk about before teaching how to talk about it. This book informs the patient and presents a wealth of information to help him or her participate more fully in the journey and perhaps more deeply develop appropriate relationships with his or her health-care team.

Doctors are hardwired to keep up with the latest advancements through reading and continuing medical education. Perhaps many can view this book as a form of critical reading and continuing medical education. The syllabus was suggested by excellent experts—a few thousand patients.

Enormously successful politicians, pundits, and prophets all know that we can enhance our sense of competence and lessen our feelings of anxiety when we feel understood and understand. Doctors must impart a wealth of information to their patients and families. In like manner, there is an enormous amount of needs and knowledge that the patient wants the doctor to address. What the patient does not know to ask yet can be a source of even greater anxiety.

Let us be reminded that *it is hard to feel overwhelmed when you are in familiar territory.* It is easy to be overwhelmed when you are on unfamiliar ground no one wants to traverse. This cuts both ways for patients, families, and physicians. When there is a canyon of uncovered ground, conflicts and crises can grow; sadly, these rarely are brought into the open, let alone the examining room. Fear, time constraints, lack of information on the part of the patient and family, and lack of eager engagement and pursuit of patient and family intellectual involvement by the health-care team top the list of usual culprits.

Certainly, there is a wealth of information routinely disseminated by the health-care team in most encounters. Rather, it is the depth, the intimacy, the focus, and the scope that have the greatest positive impact. Granted, there is often simply not enough time to time to engage everything by even the most enterprising, experienced, and engaging health-care teams (and there are plenty of these). Thus, this book may help. Consider it a field manual, survival guide, and reference.

Patients should never feel abandoned. However, *abandonment usually carries a realistic component of personal responsibility.* The traveler who refuses to seek direction, the motorist leaving for a journey low on gas, the camper without basic overnight survival gear, and the homeowner who leaves the doors unlocked invite problems. Patients and families alike must minister somewhat to their own needs. Self-care begins with self-esteem. It is empowered by knowledge—knowledge of needs versus wants and knowledge of enemies versus allies. Patients must have the knowledge of resources that are available, and they must also have the lessons of history from those sufficiently similar to themselves, so that they may apply those lessons to themselves. Others have walked a similar road before, and patients must know and truly understand that. Thus, this book.

The past generation has seen enormous advances in technology. Generic medical school training has continued to progress with more in-depth education and attention to the nuances of patient and family communication. More attention to interfacing with those who are enormously frightened is the norm. Internal medicine residencies are also moving forward in this regard. Lastly, fellowship training in oncology has begun to pick up the cue of improved communication with families and patients as well as with oneself as the (often) captain of the health-care team. But there is a lot of ground to cover. When one looks in the oncology world at all the presentations from the podium; abstracts presented and published; poster, plenary, and "meet the professor" sessions; and published articles, one finds a slowly growing but still small body of work, such as this book.

So is this really such a big deal? Yes! Cancer is one of the great anathemas. Not too many utterances can whip up a faster frenzy of emotion, thought, and agitation other than "You have cancer." Knowledge is our greatest asset—patient knowledge.

Cancer is both incubus and pariah. The mere mention of the word strikes fear in the hearts, minds, and souls of millions of patients and families per year. These souls are awash in a tumultuous sea of blinding anxiety and pounding waves of enormous ignorance. The vast majority of non-oncology providers avert from its care and quickly defer to the too-few medical oncologists whose job it is to fight this sort of terrorism on its most personal and persistent level. The patients are not the only ones who carry a burden in the battle. Perhaps if we all understand this, we can pull the oars together and share the journey.

Selected References

(In alphabetical order)

Agrawal, M. and E. J. Emanuel. "Attending to Psychological Symptoms and Palliative Care." J. Clin. Oncol. 20, no. 3 (February 1, 2002): 624–626.

Baile W. F., R. Buckman, R. Lenzi, G. Glober, E. A. Beale, and A. P. Kudelka *SPIKES—A Six-Step Protocol for Delivering Bad News: Application to the Patient with Cancer* Oncologist, August 1, 2000; 5(4): 302–311.

Einhorn LH. ASCO 2001 *Presidential address.* J Clin Oncol. 2001; 19(suppl 18):1S–5S.

Fallowfield LJ, Lipkin M, Hall A. *Teaching senior oncologists communication skills: results from phase I of a comprehensive longitudinal program in the United Kingdom.* J Clin Oncol. 1998; 16(5):1961–1968.

Freudenberger H. *Staff burn-out.* J Soc Issues. 1974;30:159-165.

Gundersen L. *Physician burnout.* Ann Intern Med. 2001;135(2):145-148. J. Clin. Oncol., May 1, 2003; 21(90090): 57s–60

Jackson V. A., A. M. Sullivan, N. M. Gadmer, D. Seltzer, A. M. Mitchell, M. D. Lakoma, R. M. Arnold, and S. D. Block"It was haunting ... ": *Physicians' Descriptions of Emotionally Powerful Patient Deaths* Acad. Med., July 1, 2005; 80(7): 648–656.

Jenkins V, Fallowfield L. *Can communication skills training alter physicians' beliefs and behavior in the Clinics?* J Clin Oncol. 2002;20(3):765–769.

Lee, S. J., A. L. Back, S. D. Block, and S. K. Stewart. *Enhancing Physician-Patient Communication* Hematology, January 1, 2002; 2002(1): 464–483.

Maguire P, Booth K, Elliot C, Jones B. *Helping health professionals involved in cancer care acquire key interviewing skills - the impact of workshops.* Eur J Cancer. 1996;32A(9):1486-1489.

Meier DE, Back AL, Morrison S. *The inner life of physicians and care of the seriously ill.* JAMA. 2001;286(23):3007–3014.

Mount BM. *Dealing with our losses.* J Clin Oncol. 1986;4(7):1127–1134.

Papadatou D, Anagnostopoulos F, Monos D. *Factors contributing to the development of burnout in oncology nursing.* Br J Med Psychol. 1994 Jun;67 (Pt 2):187–99.

Penson R. T., F. L. Dignan, G. P. Canellos, C. L. Picard, and T. J. Lynch Jr. *Burnout: Caring for the Caregivers* Oncologist, October 1, 2000; 5(5): 425–434.

Ramirez AJ, Graham J, Richards MA, et al. *Burnout and psychiatric disorder among cancer clinicians.* Br J Cancer. 1995;71:1263–1269.

Remen RN. *Recapturing the soul of medicine.* West J Med. 2001;174:4–5.

Roter D, Fallowfield L. *Principles of Training Medical Staff in Psychosocial Communication Skills.* In: Holland JC, Breitbart W, eds. Psycho-Oncology. Oxford, England: Oxford University Press; 1999:1074–1082.

Shanafelt, A. Adjei, and F.L. Meyskens. *When Your Favorite Patient Relapses: Physician Grief and Well-Being in the Practice of Oncology* J. Clin. Oncol., July 1, 2003; 21(13): 2616–2619

Steensma D. P. *The Narrow Path* J. Clin. Oncol., April 1, 2001; 19(7): 2102–2105.

Tulsky, et al. *Enhancing Communication Between Oncologists and Patients With a Computer Based Program.* Ann Int Med, 2011;155255: 53–601

Vachon MLS. *Stress and Burnout in Oncology.* In: Berger A, Portenoy RK, eds. Principles and Practice of Supportive Oncology. Philadelphia, Pa: Lipincott Williams & Wilkins; 1998.

Whippen DA, Canellos GP. *Burnout syndrome in the practice of oncology: results of a random survey of 1,000 oncologists.* J Clin Oncol. 1991;9: 1916–1920.

Wolpin B. M., B. A. Chabner, T. J. Lynch Jr., and R. T. Penson. *Learning to Cope: How Far Is Too Close?* Oncologist, June 1, 2005; 10(6): 449–456.

SUSPECT THE DIAGNOSIS

As said in "The Enemy" and will be reiterated later in "The Telling," few things other than the diagnosis and treatment of cancer can take a patient on a psychological and emotional rollercoaster of conjuring fear and loathing as well as becoming embraced in love, deep understanding, and insights.

Each of the major steps of the journey from when tumor is the rumor until cancer is the answer will hold this to be true. The lymph node found on physical exam, the new skin growth, the not-so-routine clinical complaint, or the everyday "Oh, it's nothing" becomes something, and with it comes anxiety. For millions each year, the stage is set that something needs further examination. Eventually some type of biopsy for tissue will be needed, and in short time your nothing may become the something that puts your heart in your hand and a lump in your throat on the journey to the oncologist.

The oncologist may first enter the picture when the diagnosis is suspect but not confirmed. This is a tricky situation dealt with case-by-case on the fly, in a careful manner customized for the individual patient and family. To be sure, there are some fundamental and universal ground rules when approaching that point where suspicions of a cancer diagnosis are dismissed or founded. Perhaps the most important of rules is the time-proven adage, "Although tumor is the rumor and cancer may be the answer, tissue is the issue; no meat, no treat." Yes, it is crude, but right on target.

Oncologists *never* label a patient with a diagnosis of malignancy without absolute certainty and as much evidence as time and safety allow.

They always have tissue confirmation from a biopsy of some manner unless it is simply too dangerous or not possible to get to the area of concern. Usually, the broad array of tools and superb clinical skills make obtaining tissue safe and quick with little lasting discomfort. It logically follows that one *never* pronounces a recurrence without the same degree of certainty. It is important to note, however, that not all recurrences need to or can be biopsied.

In most situations, the notion of a clinical presentation consistent with recurrence by a patient with known malignancy being very apparent is common and does not require invasive techniques. Nonetheless, when the odds of recurrence are low, owing to the typical personality or original early stage of the primary tumor or the passage of a long time since treatment or a remission, biopsy may be needed. Rarely, in some cancers, a second biopsy is needed, because some cancers actually change, needing a different approach than the original treatment.

When we suspect the diagnosis, oncologists often have to work quickly behind the scenes. Not only do we not wish to step on the toes of the primary physician while nonetheless guiding the primary physician as to what the best diagnostic route may be for those for whom tumor is the rumor, but we also want to avoid missteps or erroneous statements being made by those who go before us. Thus, a delicate balance must be struck, as the entrance of the oncologist prior to the diagnosis being certain can understandably be quite evocative of enormous anxiety for the patient and family. Thus, it is essential for the primary, or soon-to-be referring, physician to identify for the patient and family what roles the many future consultants have. An individual who serves as the "quarterback" must be identified quickly with full consensus and understanding of their role by all.

This concept of focusing the attention on the right professionals applies to the family as well. *It is the patient, not the family, who has the disease.* The role of the family is enormously important. However, family and friends, the Internet, and media, as well as other health care providers, frequently inadvertently or overtly inundate the patient with stories that are either inappropriate or way off base. Their influence must be anticipated and never underestimated.

This is a time of reinforcing the message of the autonomy and individual nature of the patient. A good analogy is the vehicle identification number of cars of the same make and model. These vehicles may have enormous similarities but run differently based on age and other factors. This is precisely the situation with each patient. Patients are individuals with a disease; *they are* not *their diseases.* It is never just another case of non-small-cell lung cancer. The philosophic point raised above has enormous practical applications. Oncology is not a one-size-fits-all endeavor.

The health-care team must decide early whether the oncologist will lead or initially remain behind the scenes. Sometimes the oncologist does not take over until there is definitive diagnosis or a diagnostic dilemma evolves, at which point he or she steps forward. Once again, one must never underestimate the importance of timing the oncologist's entrance into the world of the patient and family. The comfort zone of the referring provider, of course, will largely affect this. There is great variability in this regard. Some primary referring providers remain very involved, and others wish to pass the reins on to the oncologist as rapidly as possible.

Once it is clear that sufficient information exists to state the diagnosis and begin to put antianxiety lassos around the beast, some insights may be enormously helpful for patients and their supporters:

- **The first few days being a daze** is to be expected. Confusion, upheaval, immense sadness and disbelief, anger, and crisis of faith are common. Faith can be challenged and thought lost, or in some cases, galvanized.

- **A powerful sense of loss of control** and even greater fear of that ensuing is commonplace. This is something oncologists may assume up front and address directly with the facts as they become evident and their reasoning behind diagnostic or treatment algorithms in advance of crossing those bridges.

- **Empathy builds trust and greater patient engagement** in the process. It must be real, not feigned and not delegated to clinical staff (the norm), as the emotional bond of therapeutic alliance is best with the physician as well as the treatment-administering oncology nurses. Patients trust less empathetic providers less than more empathetic ones, and without full trust, not being capable of being their own doctor, they can be left to themselves—not a satisfactory situation for anyone.

- Patients may think it is the **worst thing to have ever happened to them**. It may not be. But anxiety paralyzing a patient from action would be the worst. It is very therapeutic to have anger, and it is very therapeutic to fight. However, it is soul sucking to roll over before fully informed and well-reasoned decisions can be made. Patients would be wise to transform anxiety into fear—fear of the known—through knowledge and never stop learning all they can, as that knowledge is power in the fight. God has hardwired us for heroics—unbelievably so, as it may seem. I have not seen a cowering cancer patient yet who totally collapsed, refusing to being informed when information was offered to him or her.

- It is a myth that in life or oncology any meaningful portion of your decision must be made spontaneously with no time **for reasoned reflection** and rational thought.

- It is not a myth that it is unhealthy to **rant, rave, and react angrily.** I see plenty of reason to be very angry, whether it be at altered life plans, unhealthy personal behaviors leading to cancer, or sheer damn bad luck, as in "Why me?" You have my permission—and, I am confident, God's—to be simply initially angry.

- **It is very real to be shocked,** and when one has been smacked in the face, reeling from the blow is natural, normal, and expected. Retreating from life or retreating from the fight before receiving all the information needed to make wise decisions once calm, or just giving up the ghost, is not okay. Your life is your own, and your anxiety is to be honored, not discarded when you are frightened most. Even if you seem most alone, and rarely anyone is, let knowledge be your friend and counsel. You also must eat, exercise if possible, and attend to the activities of daily living, as you are very much alive and the journey has barely begun. You need not go right back to work unless you know you cannot; there is no rule about this. If you need a little time, take it. If you need family, get them involved right away, and if you need alone time, take it.

- **Own the disease and your reaction.** Do not become the caretaker of others who swoon or swing into inappropriate and certainly not helpful reactions over *your* news. This is your news and your life. This is your trauma and trek; own it. For now, you are the star of this show. Believe me as to the necessity of my stressing this. You do not live or die for others. If you want to handle all communications with others, that is fine. If you wish to delegate, that is fine as well. It is your call. This is a time in your life during which the most frightening of all scenarios has dropped on your doorstep. For the moment, you are not as in control of your destiny as you were before. Understand and fight the overwhelming panic of the diagnosis and your morbid imagination trying to rip the helm from your hands. You have barely set sail, and your disease is not—and shall not—be you. Your diagnosis may try to direct the show. You must not rest until you wrest from every opportunity the control God intended you to have over these moments. Get knowledge. Demand information and experience your feelings, but do not let your feelings define you. This book will help; I promise.

- You have likely heard this before: **"The next step is knowledge. It is the best anti-anxiety medicine in the world."**

- Although knowledge will be your greatest pal, if you can, **muster up an army of at least one other to form an allegiance with you** to conquer ignorance and face fear. There will be personal business issues that you will need to attend to, as well as the new administrative and secretarial assistance needed to stay on top of all the tests and appointments and their results and the inevitable questions they will engender. I often encourage that either a small handheld recording device, or better yet a trusted friend or family member, act as a scribe to objectively write what was said, not felt, and what needs remembering, not fearing. This is wise to do with every consultant, including your primary oncologist and, of course, your original referring primary care provider, if that is how all this started. Such scribes must understand that this is not about their feelings or interpretations; they are robotic scribes capturing all that was said in context, without error or asking from the source until it is correct. Even in our aggressive American culture, there is still too much reluctance of patients to take such an initiative.

Avoid blind trust. The relationship you want most, initially, is with the truth. The facts and figures, expressed in detail in context, and their relationship to your diagnosis will help you understand what your disease is, what it means, what can be done, and what decisions are next.

- **Never surrender autonomy**. Your scribe is a partner there to assist you so that, through the frenzied fog of anxiety, you can muster yourself for the fight and have your facts straight.

- Author Jessie Gruyman, president of the Center for the Advancement of Health and survivor of many a life-threatening diagnosis, wrote *AfterShock: What to Do When the Doctor Gives You—Or Someone You Love—A Devastating Diagnosis.* She offers the concept of a contract of sorts with a partner. I support the notion, and I have used it in my practice for years. Key issues Jessie covers are for partners to agree to attend appointments, confirm in advance of their attendance, always reevaluate and check in with the one diagnosed as to what role they have and should play, and address in detail whether one is a passive listener or authorized to ask tough questions. Make sure the duties of scribe are clearly outlined, from the practicalities of paper and pen or laptop all the way to details such as whether a summary transcript would be useful. Partners must always remember that the patient is the one with the disease as they become familiar with laws regarding privacy of medical information and learn to keep their opinions to themselves unless specifically asked. To those who understandably and naively feel this is a waste of precious time and too intense an endeavor, I say think again.

- The anxiety mitigating impact alone on a now engaged and in-control patient is God sent. Literature suggests the **diminishing stress gained though being engaged may diminish overall suffering and positively impact quality of life.** The more aware and in-tune patient will bring any new signs or symptoms to their team with greater precision and speed, and that is always good.

- The patient and the health-care team **are enmeshed in an intricate and not always predictable dance.** Suggesting the patient should have no record of emotions, moments, and meanings that give them context in the greater therapeutic meaning borders on cruelty. Listen, learn, and engage, and if you cannot understand, bring in that specially selected scribe to help.

DIAGNOSIS

The Opening Pitch

The actual or impending moment of rendering the diagnosis is a critical and unforgettable time for every patient. Physicians would be wise to know the personal space the patient needs and adhere to it. It is also wise to tune in to whom the patient wants to have there when the moment comes. The cancer team should be quick to evaluate the level of support available and offered by family, friends, church, social groups, and employer. Patients must be oriented to reality to avoid "calamitizing" as soon as possible. This may or may not have been the worst that has happened to an individual, but it will not go away on its own, and retreat is usually not a reasonable option. Your physician will be wise to use sympathetic listening coupled with a thorough emotional inventory to screen for any coexistent psychological disease, such as depression or anxiety disorders, as these will invariably not only need to be treated but will also be magnified under the duress of the cancer diagnosis. The more your doctor knows, the more he or she can help.

Patients will often recall who was there, who said what, body positions, tone of voice, and the like. Doctors must always place prime emphasis on patient autonomy. A doctor can lead patients to intelligence but cannot make them think. It follows that the right of a patient to swing his or her proverbial fist ends just before the doctor's nose. Those are key parts of the contract.

It should be stressed to patients that they can handle the journey, as thousands before them have done so. Patients should hear their doctors telling them that intense feelings are the norm. Once again, anxiety is fear of the unknown and of what has not yet happened but what may happen. It will paralyze. Fear of the known is something that most patients can handle remarkably well.

The key is to turn anxiety into fear through information, facts, knowledge, and kindness. Both anxiety and fear can be destructive; they are not in a contest with each other as to which is worse. Fear will force responses or reactions to be sure, and it will do so quickly in oncology, as events will move rapidly. Anxiety, such as fear of recurrence, requires some acceptance as well as distraction and engagement in other activities until the anxiousness passes (such as major anniversaries being cancer-free, for example). Nonetheless, both are bears that can be battled appropriately. Time and events eventually eclipse anxiety wherein you have a choice of replacing them with healthier thoughts or not. Fear is present and real, and one way or the other, it will have its moment or engagement, as it is concerned with reality rather than what may be.

How You Say It

Style of communication is critical. It is easy to fall into paternalism. This is where, similar to the dad in *Leave It to Beaver,* the oncologist parses out packets of information regarding the diagnosis. That should stay in 1960s TV Land. Rather, the issue is for oncologists to individualize each "big talk," as I call them, with each family. This is a sacred time and a private time.

There are practical concerns as well. The patient, and whomever they choose to be there with, must be able to hear and *remain uninterrupted.* Personal space and cultural and socioeconomic differences can be quite relevant. Delay and procrastination are irreparable mistakes. Once the diagnosis is certain or the urgency of the situation warrants it, the talk should occur. Doctors must maintain, and patients should demand, personal eye contact. The greater the doctor's candor, the more trust will be engendered. The attitude of the informing physician is immediately transparent to patients in fear, and the doctor's perceived attitude is enormously influential in how patients begin the journey. Our mothers were right; you get only one chance to make a first impression. The rest is gravy or damage repair. It is important that further staging procedures or consultations are seen as a positive approach to the disease rather than simply more physical or emotional experiences to be feared.

Lies, Damn Lies, and Statistics

Statistics are tools used to describe the behavior of populations of similar patients based upon looking at how they did—not how you are doing—for the purpose of trying to predict and inform how you will do. You are a not a number; you are an individual. Understand that statistics try to inform you how patients sufficiently similar to you have fared.

Remember, though, that the answer that comes out of applying statistics will tell you with what degree of certainty groups of patients like each other in all relevant ways will likely perform with a certain level of certainty. Although this is intended to be a guide for the individual, the statistics are still presenting the *odds* of what or how an individual will do as a member of a group with a given stage or treatment regime. *Statistics are not a magical prescription* that cannot be avoided. People do beat the odds, so to speak. It is the odds of beating them that we can calculate compared to the larger group if you are to be an exception.

Statistics is an elegant science in which one can know (1) the predictive powers of tests, which is the ability of a test's yes to be yes and no to be no with great certainty; (2) whether you can compare two patients or two groups of patients with confidence that they are highly similar in all relevant ways and thus know that any difference in outcome is due largely to them being treated differently; (3) whether an outcome was more by chance or was truly a prediction of what will happen, almost always while stating what "almost always" means (for example, the odds of heads or tails is pretty much 50% with a penny, but the odds of any particular dice number always coming up are no better than one in six); (5) the number of patients needed to be treated in a trial of a hypothesis to be able to even have a chance of knowing whether you can discern a true difference between one treatment and another; (6) if trials of different treatments have the power to give you an answer before you run them and not just after they are done; (7) what factors are the most important individually or as a group in determining possible outcomes (for instance, how high a penny is flipped, who flipped it, the temperature, any wind present, or the fact that the head side weighs a tiny bit more that the tail side); (8) how powerful conclusions can or cannot be drawn when one groups multiple trials done at different times by different people on very similar patients;(9) how strong the evidence is for us to support one or more conclusions, on a range from absolute certainty to mere chance; (10) if there is no realistic way to know certain answers because of the nature of the factors that determine the outcome, such as when there is just not enough data at hand to make a comparison or enough patients who can be similarly described; and (11) the difference between opinion versus heavily held opinion, which can be, when understood, more powerful than a surgeon's scalpel in cutting out truthful pieces of reality.

Physicians often use the acronym GIGO (garbage in, garbage out). This is an important concept that refers to the folly in trying to reach or give a conclusion if you have poor study design or a poorly constructed method to ask for odds of a patient taking one particular treatment (or odds from not taking treatment). Not only can good statistics point out that you have muddied the water in trying to come up with an answer, but they can also bring clarity as to how you have done so.

Think of it like this: Let us ask what the best route to school is. To answer, you need to be sure you know and keep constant everything that can affect the answer, such as time of day, weather, mode of transportation, driver, air pressure in the tires, amount of traffic, day of week, and more, before you run the test many times. If you have poor control of all the variables and put "garbage" into the study, you will get garbage for answers. If, however, multiple studies have consistently shown a direction or choices for you to take and what the outcomes for groups of similar patients have been, your physician can tell you that and do so with some degree of certainty or define the lack of certainty.

Finally, statistics can tell you if there are biases in the treatment studies that can inappropriately influence the results. For example, when asking a new question of one treatment versus another in highly similar patients, it is important that we know before treatment that either treatment may work with the same degree of chance.

The bottom line is that physicians will offer treatments to patients based on either many or few experiences of similar patients, and because of the elegant and competent statistical analysis done on those patients, physicians can offer treatments that are indeed at least the standard of care. Statistics, when properly used and understood, can highly inform intelligent choices.

Listening for Those Whispering in the Patient's Ear

Physicians must first listen to what their patients think they know. Physicians must know what *the patients* know, fear, suspect, have heard, or, God forbid, have overheard, as is all too common. They need to know what *patients* have in their head about cancer and what the diagnosis means to *them*. Only then can physicians understand where a patient is starting both emotionally and intellectually. This also clears the air and affords the doctor an excellent opportunity to customize the game plan of imparting information to the individual. We experience cancer individually. One size does not fit all.

It is imperative to realize that none of us arrives at the diagnosis of "cancer" without morbid preconceived ideas. Then there is the insufferable onslaught of the media, the assemblage of well-intentioned relatives, and the thoughtless, groundless declarations from well-meaning, often misguided friends.

Frequently in life, whenever *it* hits the proverbial fan, newly minted experts fly off the fan blades. These are folks, good intentions aside, who act as if they have graduate training in advanced cancer care and are all too eager to deluge you with their newfound genius. Articles, media, and all manner of experts who seem to explode out of the woodwork may soon be assailing the newly diagnosed patient and family. Family and friends may seem to ooze from every nook and cranny with some anecdote of a friend with cancer (frequently not even the same disease) and will recommend some wild remedies.

The best approach is to deal with these issues head-on and use the *Physicians' Desk Reference* (PDR) and web sites discussed later as a guide regarding various potions and pills—and always tell everything to your physician. If you feel you cannot do this, share it with the family member you know would "take over" if you could not speak for yourself. If that trust is still not there, get another physician and explain why tactfully.

The cancer team should take a polite stand and not denigrate or humiliate when perhaps well-meaning others light upon vulnerable prey. There is usually no shortage of well-meant outrageous advice and stories seeking to compare your unique situation to all others. This is dangerous stuff, and the best advice is to focus on mastering facts first. Get data, turn it into information and knowledge, and then, with the help of your cancer-care team, go to reputable outside sources and gain wisdom.

Another bane or boon is the media. Despite the harm they do with half stories and hype, let us remember that the enormous harm to society caused by censorship and restraint is far more insidious, permanent, and far-reaching.

The vast majority of *accurate* and *personally relevant* knowledge of a medical illness for most people comes strictly from a physician. Thus, it is up to physicians to have their facts straight as well as very up to date. Physicians need to be aware of what patients can find on the web from rumors mills, blogs, irresponsible inside-scoop publications, and other less reputable sources. Physicians should become familiar with some of the superb web sites for cancer patients that do exist, starting with the one your taxes pays for at the National Cancer Institute, www.cancer.gov/. A well-informed patient is frequently indeed a much healthier patient. Certainly, family group involvement in reading, perhaps starting with this book, should be encouraged.

A medical journalist's job is not to be a doctor but rather to write the news as best as is provided to him or her. We have a saying in the military that one of the most dangerous weapons is a brand-spanking-new second lieutenant with a pencil. The point is that the journalists may journal or write well, but they are not clinicians, and even while many understand that, the holes in their coverage reinforce the risks of simple reading and believing. They also write for the masses. You are not the masses, and the *you* that is not in their article is the one with *your* disease and all its unique characteristics.

Patients are usually not critical readers and should practice checking out the latest breakthrough against what their physician tells them. The sheer ignorance and frank misuse of medical vocabulary and grammar that leads to wildly erroneous conclusions is amazing. Using one instance that seems related to you to more deeply understand your situation and prognosis has profound limits. Time spent guiding patients to reputable sources to develop a bond of honest and patient communication is always worth it.

There is also an enormous temptation of disreputable sources that make outrageous unsubstantiated claims to generalize. It is often difficult for patients to grasp that they are individuals and that the articles they read are not necessarily specifically about them. Furthermore, patients should beware the frequent whiff of sensationalism about a new technology that may have little or no bearing on their situation.

Also beware the media junkie who might as well be sitting on the medical or research campus stoops or hanging about biotech cafeterias. These are folks addicted to "breakthrough" technology, and they sing its praises every time the slightest whiff of something new is in the air. Remember, there is distance and time from bench (laboratory) to your bedside, and thank God for it. It is there for patient safety. News is often mistaken for information and the starter gun to begin therapy, which it usually is not. Even when it opens new and wonderful avenues of investigation and perhaps trials of treatments, let the system do what is does and is profoundly motivated to do—prove if it is safe and effective and how it compares in all manners to other patients with the disease. The devil is always in the details as to whether every new glove is a handy right fit for you.

There are breakthroughs. Some do apply to large groups, and they are glorious. However, nothing comes easy. Nonetheless, with uncommon exception, when patients gain access just in time to some new, highly promising treatment, we must remember the rules about nothing being a payment-free cure. It may be only (and I use that word with caution) a psychological or financial wild goose chase since it is new, with no indication of just how durable responses or remissions may be. Our bodies usually do not easily fly into a fairyland where all are cured and none fall sick to other effects of the new breakthrough. Although exceptions are uncommon, they have happened, such as the superbly well tolerated and revolutionary Gleevec in chronic myelogenous leukemia.

Finally, patients should never be embarrassed if they do not know of the latest heralded wonder treatment that hits the streets. Physicians should be honest, lending their critical mind but not necessarily their vote of credibility when miraculous new cures are brought into the discussion.

Preconceived Ideas

They are unavoidable, have variable life spans, and are frequently dangerous. Get the facts, read this book and numerous other sources, and give yourself a break from preconceived ideas. Do not try to build bulwarks around preconceived ideas to authenticate them as powerful when, in fact, they are biases and opinion that are not necessarily true. Do not buy batteries for the bogeyman. Rather, introduce these ogres of your imagination to your team without prejudice or embarrassment and let your team help you with sorting fact from fiction. Even if all is true, turning on the lights and swinging at those bats in the belfry of your unfound biases, especially when not alone and in the light of the physician's office, is often wise.

Never preconceive how weak your will is for the journey. Of course you are afraid, but trust me, you are amazing. Cowardice or the sheer inability to handle the diagnosis and treatment is rare. People are remarkably brave. Your oncologist and their team, survivors and in-treatment supporters whom you will be immediately pointed toward, and in-treatment professionally moderated groups can all help. There are many resources, and the best is guaranteed to be the shortest distance away—yourself.

Use *When Tumor Is the Rumor* to fuel your hopes that you, too, can excel in the journey no matter where the fight may lead. You will be deeply touched and will touch in return. Become informed and fully engaged, a never-ending process in the journey.

In life we are rarely assaulted by true emergencies, the sort of thing for which instant action is the only reaction possible. Think about it; they are not that common. I am an oncologist and a retired colonel telling you this is so. Your team is where you place your confidence and pledge your allegiance to reflection and response, not just reaction. I assure you your cancer hates the measured, coordinated, comprehensive response, never having enough time to regroup. Your health team will flourish with it.

Information and a competent team who view teaching you as one of the many first steps to action is what you need. If you do not see that, speak up. If they do not hear you, go elsewhere quickly. When selecting therapy with your team, place high value in high-level trials supported by the National Institutes of Health and major cancer centers in major cooperative groups. This is how we know so much today, and such therapies are often available with nonacademic physicians as well. Chances are high that treatments as part of a national protocol known to be a good standard are being compared to others also known to be a standard. Ask about that after reading the clinical trials section.

Assess Patient Goals

It is generally wise, after informing the patient of possible and probable outcomes and *confirming that the patient understands,* to determine the specific goals and their practicality for the individual. Cure may or may not be an option. However, many diseases can have a very long course marked without serious suffering. Return of prior functioning may or may not be reasonably attainable. Therapies to achieve particular goals can have markedly differing intensities and place dramatically different demands on the patient and family. Flexibility with treatment options and further diagnostic evaluations is essential. There needs to be a truthful mixture of just the right measure of certainty and hope.

Psychological Issues

We all bring our own set of coping and interpreting skills, or lack thereof, to the diagnosis. These may or may not mature and evolve in time. The oncologist needs to sort these out straightaway. Moreover, preexistent psychological issues will come into play at this time, and clinicians need to be exquisitely sensitive to this. These can become intensified in general or even magnified and directed largely on their health-care team. Although the experience of a cancer diagnosis may have permanent personality-altering effects, it is silliness to expect all patients to instantly mature or evolve into an enormously effective coping style. People will do what they do; not what one may wish them to do. Furthermore, if patients are not being real and genuinely themselves when initially dealing with the disease, they may never be able to evolve into a more effective coping style. One can lose more than time by running away from a diagnosis.

The losses patients feel are both real and perceived, and even if not shattering they may be life-altering. Issues such as whether there will be a loss of health and physical integrity, a loss of friends and loved ones through rejection, and an inability to perform the duties of daily living, hobbies, and self-care will arise. The very important impacts on job and finances, self-esteem, and the all-too-pervasive guilt of "What did I do to deserve this?" may come flooding at the patient. The loss of control can be overwhelming.

Fundamental initial emotional reactions are actually quite reproducible and common in our culture. After decades of practice, I have observed that anxiety, sometimes veiled as hostility and anger, leads the pack.

The oncologist may see sleep problems, compulsive behavior, and an inability to concentrate. Guilt and petulance may follow, with "What could I have done or should have done?" An entitlement-based demanding demeanor may rarely arise. Once again, the goal is to impart knowledge that can bring the patient toward informed and willing choices and compliance with what is known to be true. Teamwork is then possible.

There are two *D*s worth mentioning that some patients may fall into: depression and dependency. I am not referring to the clinical diagnosis of major depression, although certainly cancer patients may experience this. I am referring to a reactive, transient depression. A newly diagnosed patient may experience blunted emotions, insomnia, lack of appetite, withdrawal, and literal slowing down. Depression can often be mistaken for dementia; thus, establishing the diagnosis expertly is crucial.

Dependency can be particularly severe. Although it is uncommon, I have seen patients immobilized in advanced cases of dependency. This is as simple as it sounds. The patient surrenders all sense of autonomy and self-initiated behavior with also handing over control of his or her life to someone else. This is typically some family member, but I have had a few patients wish to pass it all to the savior in the white coat with MD after his or her name. As dependency and depression in this setting are both reactive phenomena, it is critical to know the patient's temperament and level of functioning *before* the diagnosis. Treatment, including medications and talk therapy, can be extremely effective, and most patients respond. This is not to say that patients with unrealistic post-diagnosis behaviors cannot respond as well without them. They can, but it poorly prepares the patient for the reality of making future decisions as well as encouraging a realistic, aggressive approach to rehabilitation. Regain of physical as well as psychological and emotional strength when doing so will be the hallmark of return to normalcy.

Some physicians, usually unwittingly and often as a reflection of their own underlying personality, elicit and reward the dependency of patients. This is obviously not wise, as no one's shoulders are broad or strong enough to carry the burdens of others' cares in crisis. Less commonly, in my opinion, some oncologists are very passive about patients' nonengagement and seeming willingness to go along with whatever is offered without question. As mentioned, this could be fear and undue or misplaced respect for the physician, or it could be echoing of their pretreatment personality. I have seen such individuals who were hiding and cowering under the tyranny of "What if," "Maybe," "So what," "Who cares," and "If only I had ..." also do quite well.

The personality, per se, of the patient is not deterministic of survival, and oncologists are not in the business of personality diagnosis or changing—nor would they be even if such changes were in their little black bag of wonders. Rather, the journey will elicit prior coping skills. They must be recognized, and if problematic, they must be dealt with by the entire team, as they do affect the treatment team on some level.

Positive interactions are more honest and revealing, as silent suffering is often reduced. The notion of a positive outcome from a "pay it forward" attitude and seeking and finding joy in the teeth of suffering and despair is not hogwash or Hollywood pabulum. It does make a material difference on life's quality. It can also be breathtakingly beautiful to be touched by patients who find this path.

Facing your mortality can either serve the team well or, if not, sentence one inappropriately to some sort of hell that simply need not be. Fear- and anxiety-driven bad behaviors and "stinking thinking" cannibalize hope. Although past behaviors will not guarantee future responses, they are often a clue. Thus, physicians must welcome input and insight into how patients have handled prior stresses. Oncologists must also look for coexistent stresses and be especially attentive to the behavior of the patients' loved ones.

Although possible, blind denial of the diagnosis, severity, or probable prognosis by patient and family is rare. It is usually transient and recognizable early. Once again, information, sympathy and emotional engagement are highly effective ways for one to break through. More severe, disabling and dangerous denial is actually quite rare. Patients and families virtually always want to know what is happening and what may transpire. I have had only two patients severely injure themselves because of complete withdrawal from reality after diagnosis.

The exceptionally quiet patient can be vexing. The patient's reticence may be a manifestation of outright denial or stoicism. It will slowly kill the family. It may be depression, or rarely some manner of spiritual acceptance from the start. When it happens, it requires either prior experience or carefully matched counselors to help manage the situation when the line the patient straddles moves from seeming acceptance to acquiescence. I have seen this with not only treatable but also curable diseases. It happens that the rare patient gives up even before getting in the starting blocks.

The patient is the one with the disease, not a well-meaning loved one. It is rarely acceptable to fail to divulge to the patient all information because of doubt in the patient's ability to cope with the revelation of the diagnosis. In such rare cases, one must always seek professional and documented psychiatric opinion. Incompetent patients are rare, and they are virtually the only case where the rule of total confidentiality and total disclosure to the patient do not apply. Families may oppose complete revelation. I have seen that happen. However, the rule is sacred. Failure to obey it is a sure road to disaster and creates emotionally impotent patients and emotionally paralyzed loved ones.

Sex and Significant Others

Oncologists are often amazed that they need to stress that cancer is not contagious and that sexual activities are helpful for cancer patients, not harmful. I have some great anecdotes of this. Patients and their lovers need intimate contact. Patients may feel they are no longer desirable, and lovers may fear to cause harm. Physicians should address this basic and essential means of human expression and contact and encourage it. One must look to the healthy spouse for veiled depression and exhaustion through a misplaced sense of self-mortifying duty. The data on spouses of those diagnosed with cancer suffering strokes and heart attacks in the heat of the battle against their beloveds' cancer is very clear; they are at high risk to fall ill themselves.

Spirituality

Spirituality is a very real issue and comes to the fore at the time of diagnosis. Spirituality, religion, and theology are not synonymous. We humans are more than mere flesh. A soul can and does ache deeply as cancer burrows into our lives. "Existential" is not a fancy word one bandies about in sophomore college classes or self-help books. The diagnosis of cancer evokes thoughts, feelings, ideas, dreams, experiences, and aspirations that are crucial in shaping individual destiny and vital to the form, texture, and flavor of a patient's self-chosen style of existence and personal stance. The experience of cancer is fundamentally on an existential level.

Doctors do not have to evangelize, but they do have to inquire and find the appropriate level of assistance. Personal touch is also an important issue at the time of the diagnosis. All patients want some level of touch, from a mere handshake to an embrace or a good cry. All patients have their boundaries, and it is wise for providers to seek them out and meet them there. Touch is not just physical but also emotional, spiritual, and intellectual; it may simply be the provider's body language and words. I implore physicians, touch your patient; it could well be you someday.

This is a time to solidify faith and not question it. The answer to the question of your shaking faith is "Believe." You already know the "Why me?" question is not answerable. It is not a fair world and cancer is no respecter of persons. Disease is unimpressed, for the most part, by us; maintaining your health helps enormously, but never enough. You came in alone, and you will leave alone, but you are not alone now.

Hear me when I tell you that faith can move mountains. It may be the healing of personal emotions and family emotions. I think believing in miracles is miraculous enough, and I never go looking for them; however, I have seen the unexplainable twice in thirty years.

The one mountaintop experience we must claim together with the patient is Mt. Understanding. We are not in this alone to live on Mt. Solitude, where the torrent of tears flood down and fear erodes hope.

Read, listen, learn, and reach out. Let this be a season where the weightiness of worry is diminished as we engage as a team.

The Role of the Family

Family conferences are wise, as families usually wish to be involved. Oncologists must ally with them, but the patient must always be the center of everything. Family leaders will evolve. It will be clear soon enough who the family leaders are. However, knowledge of state laws regarding next of kin is essential.

When it becomes necessary, families can have an immense burden lifted by recognizing and understanding the fundamental right of patient autonomy. Families should learn that when asked to make serious decisions on behalf of the loved one who can no longer decide for himself or herself, they are being asked to be the patient, not themselves in the patient's shoes. This is so-called substituted judgment.

When patients cannot speak for themselves, or when family conflict arises, there should be a spokesperson armed with a pencil and paper. A spokesperson can be a great help to avoid painful and time-wasting repeated conversations. I try to get a note-taker assigned right from the start. Often, this is the patient or the patient's spouse. They decide. I encourage recordings, but I prefer practicing the more active role of note-taking. After the first meeting, I generally ask the note-taker to relay the gist, the big picture, of what he or she heard. This can save a great deal of heartache and save the day. As a practical issue, patients and families need plenty of paper, as well as encouragement to interrupt and ask questions. I often tell them they can bring a tape recorder if it will help them, although I usually do not do that in families who will rely only on that and thus not fully engage. It is a judgment call with the goal being having everyone on the same page.

As is practicable, I try to schedule family conferences in advance. If families wish to record a conversation, I simply turn on my own pocket digital recorder for the obvious legal documentation reasons. It only takes a few seconds to download it onto a PC in a secure manner.

Patients need a realistic sense of control as soon as possible in the process of receiving the diagnosis. Thus, this is not a time for tap-dancing around issues. Everyone must strive to reach a working, mutually understood grasp of the diagnosis and its implications. As with all active listening, everyone must check in with one another so that all are mutually clear. I have known clinicians (myself included) to leave a room, swelled with pride and comfort that they, as great communicators, had done a marvelous job. In some cases, that is far from true. It is not about fault. It is about everyone working hard to get the facts in the open and be clear on what those facts mean and how they relate in an understandable manner to the patient so the patient can make informed decisions.

Patients can be victims of some families, and some patients' care can suffer owing to satisfying the guilt or panic of such families. I have more than once facilitated the patient taking charge and telling such unhelpful members to "cut the crap". Those are times to have a recorder running. Disagreements will come, and this is not a contest. The goal is everyone being on the same team and the patient winning, especially as the definition of a win may change over time from cure to quality-of-life issues or smaller, specific bucket-list goals.

The common family conflicts are usually variations on a theme. A common example is where one family member wants the patient left alone to "die with dignity" while others want to fight to the end. In such cases, the mantra that the patient is the one with the disease has been left at the wayside. Family members might be working out their own issues of redemption, salvation, or resurrection of old hurts now again made acute by the present crisis and possible impending loss of a second chance. Once again, the key is communication. Everyone must discuss all the reasonable options while making it clear that it is the patient's final decision. Having reached a decision, everybody needs to get on board or get out of the boat. It really is as simple as that. It is imperative that patients state their wishes to clearly-worded questions in the presence of the family while *both* the doctor and family, other than asking appropriate questions and assuring clarity, hold their tongue.

There should never be private conferences with individual family members or groups of family to the exclusion of others. Dogmatism is a another disaster waiting to happen. Physicians are neither God's messenger nor the patients' messiah. Another admonition is that patients and doctors can be sure that engaging in historical criticisms of past providers will not rewrite history and may incite hysteria. It is far wiser for oncologists to reassure about past care or, when unsure, to simply say nothing and urge a focus on the present.

The difficult family is another breed entirely. There are usually private agendas among these family members riddled with guilt and fear that will color all interactions. There is the "translator from hell" phenomenon, in which what the oncologist clearly means does not get across. There are occasionally family members that are inappropriately demanding of time to suit their convenience. They may also be individuals whose overpowering fear or need to control simply prevents them from assuming the role of the student who, without bias, accurately transmits—not translates—information. Disease is not convenient and does not use a time clock; clinicians will have to help such individuals face that. Doctors must also look out for those family members who flatter inappropriately and criticize former physicians. This is invariably an alligator pit. Typically, such folks will in time demand excessive consultations and question every treatment method. Once limits are set, clinicians sadly must be ready for repercussions ranging from accusations of insensitivity to outright litigation. Thus, it is wise to invest a reasonable amount of time in the beginning to build and buttress a bridge for the enormously difficult canyon cancer patients and their families must cross.

Teach Your Children Well

It is my opinion that families should keep the younger members of the family informed. Families usually have a realistic idea, on an objective level, of what each child *can* comprehend. The error, if made, tends to be in assuming what the child *should* comprehend. Remember, children may fantasize that they caused the illness, especially if they are kept away from the patient. In addition, children are not stupid. They know something is wrong, and game playing is often transparent and misunderstood. It can potentially teach a very wrong lesson regarding how to face difficult times and the reality of pain and suffering in an unfair world. Emotional instability of children may manifest as regressive behavior that ranges from infantile to greater dependency to even lack of toilet training. Most importantly, it is a dangerous thing to leave the child ill-equipped to handle the trauma as well as kept away from a loved one that may be dying. This does not help the child, and it damages both the child and those who are suffering. Frequent hospital visits are important for both the child and the patient. If needed, the oncologist can assist the family with getting professional help for children.

Cultural Differences

Doctors must pay attention to cultural differences. People from different backgrounds and parts of the world have very different ways of relating to the physician. This may range from deification, rarely some level of disdain, and even total acquiescence and deference. Despite the variability, it always remains wise for doctors to treat their patients as the folks in charge and engage them as the expert consultant who will not allow avoidable errors in decision-making. Patient autonomy is pivotal to a successful treatment road. Providers must stress who is and is not God and make it clear that it is *not* the doctor. This is, at times, unnerving, but it is usually surprisingly very well received.

Focus on Symptomatic Relief

A difficult scenario arises when, in rendering the diagnosis, it is also made clear that only symptomatic care, or so-called palliative care, is available. Sometimes diseases are so advanced or resistant to treatment that the discussion may need a predominant focus on relief of symptoms. Sometimes the patient's general medical condition makes it reasonable to have such a focus. On occasion, a well-informed, competent patient may choose only symptomatic relief for any number of reasons. Thus, discussing the option of symptomatic care is always germane.

The patient and physician must be mutually clear as to what the odds are for a response, its duration, the odds and nature of relapse or progression, and the costs—psychologically, physically, and financially. The first step is making it clear that such care refers to improvements in symptoms, irrespective of temporary changes in blood tests or other diagnostic studies. Otherwise, expenses and anxiety can grow exponentially and perhaps unnecessarily while temporarily inflated hopes die on the rocks of reality.

Introducing Clinical Trials

Although I cover clinical trials separately later, the issues initially arise when explaining either the diagnosis or the rationale for proposed treatment. Trials are a perfect match for some personalities, but the whole idea of experimentation or randomization (explained later), no matter how carefully couched, can be frightening. This is a major dilemma for medicine in general, as clearly this is a major way in which treatments are developed, yet less than 5% of all eligible patients enroll in clinical trials. This is particularly sad when considering that these trials are the only valid means of determining a treatment's effectiveness.

When there is an opportunity to offer a patient a trial, it is wise to follow a commonsense rule: be sure the patient knows exactly what is happening at all times, and always provide one copy to the patient, provide another to the patient's primary care provider, and place one in the patient's chart. One cannot predict who will volunteer for trials. The ethical rule is straightforward, as all ethical rules should be. Physicians should present the trial in terms of a balance of what other therapy is available and its possible results—the goods that the trial may offer and the harms that the patient may experience from either the trial or other therapy. Secondly, the patient must give fully informed consent after significant time has been provided for him or her to reflect and have his or her questions answered.

The trials have to go through all manner of review boards and must be among the next best questions to ask. Your credentialed physician may not have a trial for which you are qualified, and you may not be qualified for a trial anywhere near you. No worries; the issue is to receive at least the standard of care, and happily essentially all US-trained, US-board-certified oncologists deliver it. Sadly, fewer than 15% of those who could be on a trial enroll, but that number is getting better. You get all manners of scrutiny from being on one, for obvious reasons, and if they are level three or higher, you are guaranteed to receive a treatment as good as the standard of care. Trials ask if there is something we can do better.

Introduction to Complementary and Alternative Medicine

It is imperative that physicians explain, using every form of metaphor, simile, parable, analogy, or allegory, how medicine has learned what it has about a disease over the years and that this usually occurs because of carefully planned research. There are notable unplanned observations leading to breakthroughs, but in cancer care, they are the exception. Patients need to understand certainty based on vast data versus only suggestive information. Successful clinical trials involve many patients and show how groups similar to an individual patient fared. However, individual patients, although likely to behave like the ones in a similar group, are still individuals.

Sadly, largely owing to desperation, unapproved (non-FDA, non–National Cancer Institute) treatment regimens can find an easy mark in the cancer patient owing to unscrupulous practitioners offering savory hints of wondrous results. Patients are often easy prey for quackery. That is why I have included a special section on Complementary and Alternative Medicine (CAM). Patients and families spend billions on unproven therapies every year. Significant portions of cancer patients try CAM, while most at least listen to, if not solicit, information regarding it. There are rarely corroborated results of success that can withstand scientific scrutiny. The reason for this is simple: there is no financial or political/legal pressure to do so. The claims that do exist regarding wondrous results from CAM raise more questions than answers. The questions these claims raise are of massive importance. Each must be addressed at the time of rendering the diagnosis to a patient or shortly thereafter, as the issue of trying CAM will undoubtedly arise.

Quackery always has a pitch that many cancer patients will struggle with if left on their own. For example: "Medicine is hiding the real cure because of profit and bad pharmaceutical companies," "We have the secret," "You can do this only by fresh air, diet, and exercise; there is no need for 'bad,' nasty, poisonous medicine or radiation." That is sheer nonsense; this can be seen if one calmly reads through both this section and the one that follows. I also refer the reader to the NCI site, the Mayo Clinic's cancer site, and www.QuackWatch.org.

The major issues CAM raises are these: How do we know if responses that are real are due to the alleged CAM therapy? How do we know if these alleged responses are durable and reproducible in most patients and can be applied to a given patient's situation? What monitoring is necessary? What are the toxicities of these therapies, and are they compatible with conventional therapy? How do these CAM therapies truly compare to conventional therapy? Well-done head-to-head comparisons are rare.

At the very least, I recommend knowledge of everything that enters a patient's body. Although I stand firm as regards the right of a patient to autonomy, I believe that the right of these purveyors of unproven potions to hawk their wares must remain under constant scrutiny. If a patient insists on certain types of CAM, I sometimes simply refuse therapy and state that it must be one or the other and that the patient must chose. Although the patient may abandon conventional therapy, the physician should give assurances that he or she will *not* abandon the patient. The best way to fight quackery is with facts and calm, critical thinking. It is sometimes an uphill battle that makes us appear as physicians protecting their own turf. So be it.

There is little complimentary to say about complementary and alternative medicine in patients with diagnosed malignancy. Level heads with decades of experience cannot say, "I know this cannot harm you." Proponents also cannot say, "I know this is safe to take and effective against your cancer." They cannot say they know the exact ingredients in their concoction. Supporters of CAM may not even know the purity, other ingredients, and effects from processing (since none of this is required), and they do not know how it interacts with all other chemotherapy drugs as tested under the rigors of clinical trials. Wake up, hear the call of your anxiety, and stop the craziness. CAM adherents cannot tell you any of those things, because they do not know them.

Sellers of CAM routinely do not do any testing except making sure your credit cards and checks are good. Harsh? Not harsh enough. With rare exception, you will not see them go through complete scrutiny of the FDA. At best, they will get FDA statements of purity of ingredients, but that is all. But just because something is 100% ineffective at treatment does not mean it is 100% inert. The fact is, it may be something that hurts you, and unless the FDA has thoroughly investigated it and stated it is safe and effective, beware.

Be aware that once a drug is proven safe and effective by the FDA for one indication, it is not illegal to use it as doctors see fit to use it for other off-label uses based on well-scrutinized peer-reviewed literature. This has led to the well-reasoned application of drugs off-label. This is not wrong, and you will find these are all building blocks, for the most part, of intelligent studies showing their benefit.

When some substance looks promising from the plant and animal kingdom, it is tested, not held back by some evil conspiracy. Think about how self-defeating that is. If it is sufficiently nontoxic and has some mechanisms of action that make sense and some minimal response rate, it will find its way into early-level trials (described later). A number of our frontline drugs that exist today came from the plant and animal kingdom. However, this is after extensive years of testing. Ignore the shaman and the gurus hawking claims they may really believe, as they have no high-quality data or relevant training. If what they had worked, it would not be complementary medicine; it would be frontline medicine.

There is also no rational reason to support any of the nonsense that "the man" or "Big Pharma" or whatever is holding CAM back. Ridiculous! Capitalism is doing just what one wants it to do: reward the real deal that will go the distance and not kill people or usurp their hope and resources. The system is not perfect, but it is, without any equivocation, the best in the world for declaring a new drug as safe and effective. Moreover, our system does the right thing by limiting patents, expediting highly promising drugs, and creating special tracks for enormously promising drugs. "The Man" or "Big Pharma" would be idiots and bankrupt if they were to proceed in any other way.

Furthermore, those of you who know how to read an annual report or balance sheet should ponder this: it takes almost seven years and over $600 million for a new drug to go on the market as safe and effective. Consider how much is spent on non-winners. Profit *margins*—not profits, but the real numbers, such as how much is finally left after everything is paid for—range from negative 7–10% in bad years and 5–20% in good years, with the overall average around 6–9%. Nobody is routinely getting ripped off.

The cost in lives, pain and suffering, manpower, and health-care-cost dollars wasted and clogging up the system because of CAM barkers and naive folks exercising their admittedly free choice is outrageous. Many have stated that one out of every six dollars is wasted in oncology by the pursuit of, application of, and costs from using complementary or alternative medicine.

Media Matters

Beware mass media; they are often hit-and-run news-du-jour artists without the time, temperament, or talent to clearly put any news or breakthroughs in perspective, let alone in individualized terms. Sometimes they get a lot right, especially when the content of their stories it based in fact and not predominantly emotional. Some incredible network and cable television shows highlight the exceptions of bad physicians and run the stories without comments about the overwhelmingly good data out there when it comes to the constancy and quality of oncology care.

Yes, the media have a crucial and welcome role to help watch, encourage, support, and, in a sense, police the field for the betterment of all. But remember, their job is not meet you in the ER, take your calls at three a.m., work with other consultants, calculate your chemotherapy, talk with the family, and be the responsible individual from rumor to tumor to treat and beyond.

Antidotes for Anecdotes

One of the biggest poisons in our field is the anecdote. It is the irresponsible presentation without hard, verified, in-context data of some patient response or treatment with an against-all-odds outcome or surprise ending (such things happen rarely) that the storytellers or listeners then wrongheadedly think presents new rules and lessons to all broadly, or especially to them.

Anecdotal medicine frequently causes suffering, and in oncology, where margins are slimmer, it can cause death.

For example, many seem to think that if you flip a penny ten times and get three heads and then seven tails in a row that tails is favored. But this is not true—not even if you get the same ratio doing it again.

Prognosis and the Future

It may or may not be premature to discuss prognosis early on. This is a case-by-case situation. It can be very confusing at first to present to individuals how groups have handled highly similar situations. Using comparative hypothetical or historical groups to predict an individual's prognosis can be relevant and helpful, but it is not a crystal ball into the individual patient's future. No one is to be hopeless. I have seen enough surprise turns to the positive to jewel a crown with joy rather than be jaded by some anchor around my heart. Odds are things patients beat from time to time.

Oncologists and patients would be wise to outline and explain the potentially long list of experts needed in future care early in the journey. The list may be long, confusing, and frightening. It may include ostomy nurses and physicians needed to perform further biopsies, diagnostic tests, or radiation treatments. Oncologists must prepare their patients for the entourage in their service rather than position patients for a frightening flood of new doctors and procedures.

Take the Time and Avoid Timelines

Most importantly, rendering the diagnosis takes time. The vagaries of managed care and reimbursement issues have private oncologists seeing enormous numbers of patients per day. This can be insane and inhumane. It is easy and understandable to state that there simply is not enough time. Somehow, some way, there must be. In the end, spending time will eventually save time. After all, it may be all the doctor has to give at some point.

Oncologists must not give Hollywood-style timelines. The best approach is to refer to the literature and the ranges that a patient most likely fits while stressing once again that patients are individuals, not statistics. Patients and providers should avoid attempting to quote dates or make dramatic pronouncements. That is pandering to fear and fatalism.

Odds should be explained both as relative odds and absolute odds. As an example of this explanation, I will relate what I do to illuminate these crucial concepts to the patient. I take out a dime, a penny, a one-dollar bill, and a ten-dollar bill in front of the patient. The difference between the penny and the dime in *relative* value is that the penny is one-tenth of the dime. The same is true for one dollar and ten dollars; one dollar is one-tenth of ten dollars. However, the difference between the *absolute* amount of ten cents and one cent is nine cents. The difference in *absolute* terms between the ten dollars and one dollar is nine dollars. Nine dollars is *absolutely* much larger than nine cents, yet nine cents is 90%, relatively speaking, of ten cents, just as nine dollars is 90%, relatively speaking, of ten dollars. However, the *absolute* difference between nine cents and nine dollars is *absolutely* quite large.

Why care? A 10% improvement in survival or response or duration of response can vary greatly, depending on what odds you started with. This concept is crucial when discussing adjuvant therapy. This is treatment given when statistics say there are high odds of recurrence of unseen lurking disease after apparent removal of the primary cancer and no visible evidence of cancer cells remaining anywhere. If adjuvant therapy is given, it is because it has a certain relative and absolute risk of preventing recurrence at some future point in time.

Oncologists offer many breast cancer patients adjuvant therapy—treatment after the primary surgery to kill hidden distant disease. The concepts of absolute and relative risk play a large role in this decision. It is crucial to know what the real difference, the *absolute* difference, is between those treated adjuvantly and those not. A 10% improvement in the odds of recurrence, when the odds of recurrence are only 10%, is just an improvement from 10% to 11%. However, a 10% improvement of odds of recurrence when the odds of recurrence were 80% is the difference between eight and eighty-eight. That is 8%. That is eight more people potentially alive out of one hundred.

Understanding basic statistical language does not end there, and the education to build understanding begins at the time of giving the diagnosis. Patients must be able to understand what the percent improvement stated really refers to. Is it an improvement in the odds of response to therapy or of the risk of recurrence? Does it translate into a 10% improvement in the time to recurrence? Is it referring to a 10% improvement in *the* odds of survival? Does it translate into how long one lives before eventually dying from the disease? On the other hand, and as is commonly the case, does the 10% apply to some, but not all, of these very different notions? These are all very large, practical quality-of-life issues, and they are very different concepts.

Remember, Statistics Can Be Your Friends

Statistics provide the numbers needed to tell you if a study had any ability or power to convey any useful information to you.

Statistics also give us wondrous definitions, such as the level of power (predicting the truth) of published studies. They tell you if you can definitely say yes or no is true with some degree of certainty and if the type of study and the evidence for it are rock solid.

They tell you whether or not you can know that the odds of an outcome experienced by others might be similar for you.

They are so important that they are discussed in multiple areas of the book.

Second Opinions

I address second opinions in the legal section in detail, but a few points are germane when initially discussing the diagnosis. They should be encouraged for all patients and families who broach the subject. A word to the wise: second opinions may be given for therapy that is either far more or far less aggressive than what was originally offered. Rarely, some who render second opinions may libel or slander the primary physician to the family and not condone what the primary doctor has done so far. Therefore, prudence, candor, and preplanning are wise when assisting the patient in obtaining second opinions or commenting on them. The only significant problems I have ever encountered in this regard occurred when complementary or alternative medicine practitioners got into the mix. This dilemma is addressed more fully in a later chapter.

The Contract

Although stated later in the legal section, it bears mentioning here that patients expect a contract, and the list of what is required is long. They expect doctors to listen, to teach, to be available, to address pain (almost all pain can be effectively treated), to help with sleep and bowel habits, and to prevent nausea and vomiting. Patients need to hear that we now have medications that may increase appetite and stamina. Providers must tell the truth and be clear on the schedule of progress reports. An often overlooked area is the golden rule that doctors must never "keep secrets" from the patient no matter what the significant other or family says. Patients must always be clear on what their policy is regarding messages and answering machines and receivers of physician calls other than the patient.

Remember Autonomy: It Begins and Ends There

Will the real patient stand up? It is you, but you are not your disease. *You* must have a relationship built on knowledge with your disease to lower your burden. There is immense power in the gift of autonomy as described earlier in the book. Go back and read the first few chapters again. Remember, this is your journey, and you call the steps.

A Final Few Words

One of the deadliest weapons—both against the cancer and, unwittingly, against the patient and family—is not chemotherapy; *it is the physician's mouth*. Clinicians must not only think about what they are about to say, but they must also say only what they are thinking—no more and no less. For example, more than once, I have heard stories of the devastating blow caused by an answering machine message thoughtlessly left for all to hear and often misunderstand.

In sum, this chapter is simply saying that the tongue, as well as the cancer, can be the "enemy of the neck," or the liberator of the patient's autonomous license to engage fully and vigorously in his or her treatments.

TREATMENTS

Example of Finding Just One Cancer Cell

What follows in this section is a much more advanced presentation of the major methods we use to treat patients, such as radiation, chemotherapy, and surgery, as well as some of the newer therapies. There is sufficient depth here for one who wishes to get a broad overview (about late high school level) of one way to embrace the basic science principles. There is also sufficient depth layered in that is more like a Discovery Chanel or *Nova* overview of how all the material connects. Again, I encourage you to look it over and certainly use it as a reference to better understand your options and, more so, the world of those professionals who are treating you.

You will be both amazed and awestruck at how we are wondrously assembled and how incredibly ingenious cancer cells disassemble the norm to their survival advantage. The sheer genius of the design and the methodical cleverness of the treatments being developed by talented men and woman worldwide as they unravel the nature of cancer may deeply move you. Thus, there is something here for the student of science as well as a wow factor for all as we look at these therapies and their rationales.

They are also included because it is patients such as yourself, who are supporting this work not only through taxes but also by enrolling in clinical trials (to be discussed later), that have brought us this far. Thank you, and I hope this walk through these wonders helps calm your anxiety and embolden your power to fight right along with your health-care team and, when appropriate, to cheer on this new age of enlightened endeavors that make the weapons in the oncologist's armamentarium grow.

Let us first look at the rationale and principles of treatment starting from the not-so-hypothetical situation of tests that find only one or only a few cancer cells in the blood. Large tumors above the level of detection (0.5 cm) are self-apparent; something must be done. However, there is a lot to be learned by looking at where technology is taking us in terms of early detection. There is a lot to be learned in terms of when to treat and why. So with that in mind, let us spend a little time examining lessons learned from the perspective of finding one or barely any malignant cells. What do we do, and what do we think? How did these cancer cells escape our own immune system—or did they?

Research at the cellular level looks for why one cell and its progeny survive, escape surveillance and destruction by our immune system, and grow beyond the limits of the normal counterpart cell that they mimic to some degree. Why do they spread, frequently homing in on specific normal tissues, displacing and destroying them? How do they do it? We do not have all the whys, but the quality of questions is growing with each high-quality answer.

No one wants to treat everyone who is found to have random malignant cells found accidentally or by intentional search just because they are there. No one wishes to ignore these cells all the time either. The same thinking applies when you think you have a complete remission. How do you know what is enough therapy? How do you know you have a durable remission or cure? Often we do not know, but our tests are growing in leaps and bounds in terms of cell-specific or cancer-specific signs, symptoms, and clues that cue us in that there is disease remaining. Our trials tell us what therapies work best alone or together and when it is time to either stop or offer highly experimental treatment since all conventional therapy has failed.

At the beginning of the present millennium, the National Cancer Institute established a goal of eliminating the suffering and death due to cancer by 2015. This was noble but unrealistic. Much research is aimed at finding both the primary tumor as well as any metastases (sites of tumor spread) as early as possible. Exactly when, where, how and why a distant metastasis of a primary tumor occurs is not clear in many cancers. In addition, it most certainly varies within patients with the same type of cancer as well as among different types of cancer. For solid tumors, a lot of data have been collected using both cellular-based techniques and imaging of tumor lesions of over 0.5 cm (our present most common detection threshold). These data provide us with general ideas of the personalities of both treated and untreated cancers in terms of the where and when of spreading.

Some cancers spread by direct invasion and may invade and spill over into lymphatic and vascular channels. Some not only seek out and enter the blood but also actually travel to predestined organs, manipulating our own machinery and building cell-sized canals to travel within. They also feed themselves by moving close to these new vessels.

A great deal of research has gone into detection beyond the level of the physical exam and human eye. We will delve a bit more deeply into this notion of applying critical thinking to observations made over the decades derived by pondering the exciting notion of trying to find just one cancer cell among billions.

Even if there is just one tumor cell found, is it clonagenic? That is, can it and will it anchor in some organ, find just the right conditions for growth, and produce offspring? Will it survive long enough to produce offspring before its own internal clock signals that it is time to die? Will all the essential nutrient requirements be present? Can it evade assault by antibody-producing cells and non-antibody-producing cells of the immune system before whatever clock it internally follows or whatever assault it is battered by (immune system, oxygen content, acid/base environment, and such) does it in? Is finding it once in the circulating blood an indication that many malignant cells are circulating undetected?

Is finding it once a sufficient marker of high probability that among the other tumor cells that are facing the same challenges, at least one will succeed? Is there high certainty that blood involvement on this test, seen once, is a marker for high likelihood of bone marrow involvement or brain involvement, as is the case with other cancers? Do cells in the blood constitute real and sufficient markers for patients to do poorly in some predictable way, as is known for some solid (excluding primary hematologic) malignancies? When would we want to listen to the presence of one such cell in the blood?

Put another way, is the finding of one test, or whatever number you have showing cells of the tumor in the blood, of clinical relevance? If so, what is it relevant to—total tumor burden, response rate, disease progression, overall survival, etc.? Or, as the title of the book implies, is this (the positive circulating blood results) a rumor that does not imply serious consequences and underlying meanings as listed above, or is it in fact the bellwether test that is saying, "Where you see few, trust there are many?"

In general, finding circulating leukemic cells in patients with acute leukemia must be taken in the context of where in the therapy you are. In chronic leukemia, the same concept is true, as by definition even stable disease and low-level disease will show the malignant cells. However, when so-called solid tumors cells are showing up in increasingly sophisticated assays of the blood, all the above big clinical questions arise.

Yes, the test is very important *if* a positive circulating malignant cell test means that where there are few there are many (such as a positive bone marrow with malignant cells in it). The standard reasoning (if the realistic intent is cure and not palliation) is to initially treat the patient full-dose on-time with chemotherapy. Patients may not handle this well, and if you undertreat, the malignant cells will overgrow and resist the less-than-optimal dosing because of the probable marrow involvement. If you do not cleanse the marrow, the marrow may never recover, and you may end up with the horrific possibility of a bone marrow packed with increasingly resistant cancer cells. You will also have dependency on blood products. All of this will have transpired because we believed finding one positive circulating cell in solid tumors meant the bone marrow was involved, which warrants, if treating for cure, full-dose on-time therapy.

As our technology grows, we need to understand what the implications of our technologies' sensitivities are. It is not yet standard care in clinical staging of solid tumors to assess patients' blood or bone marrow to see if there are any circulating cells from the original cancer present and actively circulating. Similarly, if the test is done, I am not clear as to what to do with a negative result.

If the test is negative and the patient has widespread disease, I feel you have added nothing. If it is negative with otherwise limited early-stage disease, I would be hesitant to treat an otherwise low-stage patient with therapy meant for high-stage without either new data showing the original staging was wrong or published research telling us how specific and sensitive the test is for predicting it behaving like advanced disease. The point is to be careful of what tests you do if careful review of published experience shows you that it is not clear what one is to do with the answer.

Might it make a difference if we could find cells circulating in the blood that presumably might be markers for cells trying to set up shop in distant lands? Intuitively, yes, but again, unless you have the data or are collecting it in an organized manner with patient consent to use it to get information that helps tailor your treatment, I would stay away from asking a question whose answer you do not know how to address. I do support aggressively finding out through trials.

This is why a number of companies have embarked to see if they can find circulating solid tumor cells in the blood. In the case of colon, prostate, breast, and lung tumors (and in the literature many other tumors), the answer is yes. However, it is not clear if such detection is meaningful in the setting of a complete remission elsewhere or in the setting of a partial response. What do you with that?

In the case of leukemia, a large portion of what you do is aimed at eradication of all leukemic clones (cancer cells capable of dividing) using all the tests there are to find them. These include looking for cell-specific staining techniques to find very specific molecules in or around or through the cell surface, making them unique to their benign counterparts. It continues to be our hope that earlier detection, even detection of the single circulating malignant cell in the bloodstream, might confer a different prognosis that might then argue for various therapies and combinations of treatments. In leukemia the argument holds true, as by definition the tumor is of the bone marrow and diagnosis depends primarily upon specific bone marrow findings.

However, for the so-called solid tumors, we just do not know what finding circulating cells really means. One promising technique employs monoclonal antibodies (discussed later in more detail)—manmade antibodies engineered to be specific for something on, in, or associated intimately with the cancer cell. You can put a marker or fluorescent tag or isotope on the antibody and look for the radiation these tags emit. Then one can count the cells in a fluorescent-activated cell sorter channel through which the blood flows, learning how many cells show the presence of the marker. Of course, this requires both high specificity and sensitivity of the marker for the tumor-cell-associated antigen and strong binding affinity so that the monoclonal antibody does not easily fall off. Another recent style of detection is to have the antibodies contain iron, which then allows for an iron-bound antibody complex if the antigen is present. Then, when the cells are run through a sorter under a magnetic field, only the cells with the marker will stay on the magnet.

All of this is to tell you that one should understand the natural history of the disease to which you are going to apply a test. Based on other results, is it in the realm of possibility that cancer cells could be in the blood? What is the pretest probability of this ? If it is profoundly low, you could be asking for confusion and get a result you have no use for except perhaps as research data. You would also want to know from prior controlled applications of the test in multiple scenarios and locations how sensitive (low false positive) and how specific (low false negative rate) the test was when tested against known positive and negative controls—in other words, how often its yes and its no (tumor cells in blood) are correct.

There may be a role for assays looking for single circulating cells in both seeming complete responders and major responders initially in collecting the data on all manners of patients to learn what the test can do, and in some cases directing further therapy as early as possible. The more we use tools to collect that information, the more they can teach us.

It is not yet clear in which cancers (other than most leukemias) this single-cell detection really identifies cells destined to survive in a new area and multiply. You cannot biopsy everywhere, as you will usually be taking a sample.

Before you choose to take a test, be sure you know how specific and sensitive it is before using it, and know whether there are any likely scenarios in which the test results will clearly change prognosis.

Beyond Single-Cell Detection

Our present conventional level of detection of internal gross tumor is about 0.5 cm whether we use a CXR scan or computerized axial tomography (CAT), the latter of which use specialized X-rays with computer assistance to create images at varying depths, akin to slices of a loaf of bread, to 0.5 cm detail. Magnetic resonance imaging (MRI) translates the movement of water under a massive magnetic force into images of incredible detail, again about 0.5 cm resolution. These are frequently used to supplement simple X-rays, ultrasound, and various so-called nuclear medicine scans, such as bone scans and PET scans. Ultrasound is good at looking at the flow of fluids as well as densities and cavities, and bone scan measures new bone being laid down in response to processes which have eaten away or destroyed prior bone, such as fracture and repair, arthritis, and, in some classic patterns by tumor of the bone or tumor that has spread to bone. PET scans elegantly track the metabolism of isotopes of simple sugars in the brain and can be useful in the evaluation of both primary brain cancers and tumors that have spread to the brain, which take up the simple sugar you give it, thinking it nourishment of a sort.

After initial responses to treatment, one will have a very difficult time knowing if therapy had a positive sustainable benefit if one cannot easily see the tumor(s) using the above tests. One also will not know how viable any residual disease is, whether one sees it or not. A spot on film might now be residual scar.

Ascertaining function of the cancer cells as mimicking normal counterparts will not be easy, as only a few malignancies readily do that, such as some thyroid cancers. Our tools of detection are imperfect, with limits stated above. There can be problems with the sensitivity of our studies when size is small, which means that there is a high false negative rate, wherein the test says the cancer cells are not there but, in fact, they are and are out of our range of detection. Assays can also have a problem of not being sufficiently specific and have a high rate of false positives, wherein the test incorrectly claims benign tissue to be cancerous.

Thus, an enormous of amount of research is looking into minimal residual disease and tests done of various biopsy-type specimens or body regions that try to inform the clinician as to whether cells are present with the ability to divide and have "children." This is not an exact science. There are many other factors occurring at the same time we are making these measurements: the clinical condition of the patient, prior therapies, the condition of the bone marrow, organs' abilities to tolerate further therapy, the order of therapy, and so on. Thus, the research that seeks to detect disease at its lowest level of tumor burden tries to understand how that translates into the risk of a local, regional, or systemically advanced disease.

With acute leukemia, the message is already clear: kill every cell visible using all means of detection, as just one cell could be clonal and lead to relapse. In solid tumors, this is not clear. No one wants to treat everyone who is found to have random malignant cells found after intentional search or just because they are there and no one wishes to ignore them out of hand. We must understand these delicate relationships before we miss an opportunity to improve therapy or choose wisely to stop when there is no proven disadvantage.

Breast cancer is a great example of how numerous factors mix in increasingly accurate mathematical prediction models to sort patients into risk groups and to define what groups will do best with which therapies. The hunt is on to add to the already considerable lists of factors we search for in all breast cancer patients and their cells. All of that informs us as to the risks and benefits of future therapy. This is poignantly true, though we do not see residual disease that in many is clearly there but not yet reliably detectable in most patients by any one particular assay.

Resolving the issue of benign versus malignant is, in the case of breast cancer, the realm of the pathologist looking at tissue. There is usually no need for anything further to ascertain if breast biopsy cells are malignant. However, their personality and their likely future behavior can be ascertained with incredible detail and power by studying those specimens hormonally, genetically, biochemically, antigenically, and immunologically. Some of these tests show either positive or negative results; others give actual numbers of cells. We look for the interior or surface of cell chemical binding sites, which, when present, predict behavior. One may be able to use various immunologic trackers (antibodies that bind to a very specific portion of molecules known as antigens, which are substances capable of eliciting an immune response, such as, but not only, antibody production). With these techniques, one can find individual cells among millions. Similarly, secondary chemical reactions can be triggered by the presence and interaction of a target seen only on malignant cells. Likewise, the measurement and location of radiation given off when radioimmunocongjugates (created by adding minuscule amounts of radioactive isotopes to the binding antibody) can prove the detection of a target protein seen in either only malignant cells or the more angry and apt-to-spread cells.

Sometimes we find receptors for common substances present or absent in the cancer cells, such as the receptor (think biochemical mailbox) for estrogen and progesterone. In the case of breast cancer, their presence is better than their absence, and their presence opens up a whole class of drugs that can powerfully suppress the spread and growth of the clones (daughter cells) of cells that have the markers. Early work suggests putting various toxins or powerful radioisotopes that can tag some breast cancer cells on the antibody and deliver a toxic payload lethal to nearby cancer cells as well as those directly taking up or linking with this " magic bullet" antibody or antibody/missile combination. Furthermore, you may see the breast cancer cells by looking for the radiation emitted by the injected isotope on targeted cancer cells.

I was fortunate to be on the first team to image breast cancer with a monoclonal antibody labeled with a radioactive isotope. This showed not only where the bulk of tumor was but also allowed us to find previously undetected areas of spread by looking for radiation emissions. In addition, our team had humanized the antibody. Previously, a major obstacle was that the antibodies were largely from mouse origin, and the human patient could react against them, confounding their utility.

Thyroid cancer shows similar possibilities for diagnosis that also looks for protein production of the cells as well as uptake of building blocks for the protein. The cancer is an easy target for diagnostic uptake of radioisotopes At higher doses, therapeutic radiotherapy can target the tumor, which absorbs it and thus receives a lethal dose.

Thus, we are trying to exploit the fingerprint of the cell surface, cell transmembrane, cell body, cell nucleus, nucleus-associated proteins, or genes and their products—anything the cancer cell possesses uniquely, slightly aberrantly, or in excess amount as compared to its benign counterpart. This type of targeted therapy is a type of rational drug design; we sleuthed for vulnerabilities using the intricacies of the cancer cell as opposed to its benign counterpart and built near-targeted bullets for only our intended prey.

Diagnostically, the more we understand any of the unique physical, genetic, molecular, or immunologic and antigenic fingerprints of cancer cells, the more we can develop tests that exploit those differences. We can then "find," perhaps with tagged chemical or radioactive dyes, depots of malignant cells at much higher resolution than with other techniques.

Therapeutically, finding the cells when they are less in number not only means less tumor burden, but probably better penetration into tumor depots and higher ratios of killed cells to viable cells. The tempo of such targeted therapy and rational drug design submissions to the FDA continues to pick up as the possibilities rumor of some wonder drug from the animal or plant kingdom. Similarly, the pace of thoughtful laboratory rational drug design based on finding more Achilles' heels that tumor cells have as opposed to their normal counterparts, which leads to rationally built drugs, is accelerating. The numbers are staggering. About five thousand or so ideas thought worthy of beginning the testing that starts with nonhuman toxicity studies turns into just a handful thought suitable for phased human toxicity studies and trials per year. It costs around $500 million up to $1 billion dollars to develop a major new drug and typically takes three to five years. Patents are not lifelong, and generic drugs do follow after reasonable times.

The FDA (and by extension the USA) does more drug development and testing with amazing track records of accuracy than any other nation or consortium. Drug companies and big pharmacies are neither robber barons nor angels. Their profit margin, what they actually return after all costs, is not spectacular, and they can go years working on reserves before the next great drug comes along. There has been no better system shown for providing mankind with safe and effective oncology medicines.

Some cancer treatments require the death or disabling of all cancer cells in the patient capable of dividing and growing and or spreading. Some treatment may not remove all viable cancer cells but remove the ability of those cells to repeat the havoc that preceded treatment. As a result, patients are living longer and often with a better quality of life. Some types of cancer are becoming more of a chronic disease that must be managed and controlled over the course of many years and maintained until new discoveries in treatment are made.

For the last several decades, the common cancer treatment methods have been surgery, radiation, and chemotherapy. While these treatments are focused on destroying the tumor cells, they can damage normal cells in the process or may have significant treatment-related toxicity.

The newest category of cancer treatments are targeted therapies that act in specialized ways to destroy or act against tumor cells, often not affecting normal cells. These are innovative therapies, many of which were scoffed at less than a couple decades ago but are now commercially available with bold new trials launching nearly weekly internationally. These therapies are based on discerning something unique about the cancer cell or some sort of potential Achilles' heel that can be exploited while not harming normal tissue. As a result, patients may experience less severe side effects than with other treatments. The newer treatments can also be combined with older therapies to enhance antitumor effectiveness.

The bottom line is that although all therapy is not individualized and may never completely be, the distance from laboratory bench to patient bedside is shrinking. Soon therapies will exploit singular or multiple areas of tumor vulnerability at the molecular and even genetic level, all as a result of fundamental research your tax dollars (in large part) support. Soon therapies will be more patient-specific.

Because of improved early detection and better cancer treatments, there are approximately 9.6 million cancer survivors alive today in the United States. This compares with only 3 million people with a history of cancer who were alive in 1971.

Another potent message is the marriage of technologies. As discussed a number of times already, we are often marrying the anitigenicity, chemical reactivity, or genetic fingerprinting of tumor cells with CAT scans and

MRI. This is done to detect and then "see" both the primary tumor and, with hope, early depots of spread—and in the case of marrow, presence even on the single-cell level. The notion of intellectual partnership in medicine is crucial. In oncology, our tools function best when in synergy (where, for example, one plus one equals three). Critical thinking and well-constructed trials based on good science cast a long shadow.

Staging

As was noted earlier, before treatment and after initial diagnosis, staging is done. Considering signs, symptoms, cues, and clues so far, and knowing the typical history of each disease, your oncologist will look where needed to assess the exact extent of the disease in exquisite detail. Some patients require bone marrow biopsies, some need scans of the brain, and so on. The goal, using internationally accepted conventions and definitions, is to stage the patient's cancer in a manner in which anyone hearing the stage has an understanding of the most clinically relevant way of knowing where your tumor is and is apparently not. Thus we can compare patients with the same stage, intelligently develop treatment regimens, and follow outcomes not just for you but also for all patients with similar stages. Before we look into how we treat it, we must understand the how and why of knowing where it is, as local versus systemic therapy, or some combination therein, depends on that as well.

Staging gives us information about the extent, spread, and severity of a patient's disease. This allows a more accurate and comprehensive treatment plan and can even infer a pretreatment prognosis by comparing to others similarly staged. The systems for staging have evolved, and the more we learn what really matters for each disease, the more we add criteria. Staging is a living science with a goal of having more patients live because of its work.

Typically, the so-called T, N, and M staging rules are used (the letters standing for tumor size, lymph node involvement, and metastasis, respectively). This system assigns patients to various levels or sublevels of stages 0–4. Physical exam, physical condition, certain laboratory tests, imaging scans, and microscopic pathology reports refine the system.

A clinically useful tumor classification would be able to compare similar cancers and similar patients. Such a schema must be tumor specific and reflect the natural history of the tumor as much as possible. A unified approach to the degree of spread and severity of the tumor is crucial, as prognosis, therapy, and the ability of scientists worldwide to talk to each other hinge on it. Thus, the staging classifications of the American Joint Committee on Cancer rely on the premise that thoroughly staged and described tumors will largely act similarly and have similar outcomes.

The TNM system attempts to organize our understanding of tumors. The system is dynamic and living and evolves with our knowledge of increasingly relevant prognostic factors. If the world categorizes tumors in detail in exactly the same way, there is no Tower of Babel effect whereby no single scientific language exists and is universally accepted. The problems that can occur when different languages are used disappear, and physicians then pave the road for rapid accumulation of information about highly similar tumors in highly similar situations. That information leads to clinical trials. Clinical trials lead to the future of better and evolving cancer care. Thus, precise tumor staging is crucial.

The most common mistake regarding staging that I see is that patients do not understand the implications of their stage and thus labor under erroneous conclusions. A frequent misconception is demonstrated when most patients describe their cancer. There is a tendency to name the cancer according to where it has spread rather than where it came from. This is not correct.

Let us look at a mythical explanation using the United States as our body. We name terrorists for the land they came from. They have a native culture, character, and craft of terrorism they conduct. Whether they are in California or Maine, we name them from their place of origin. Where they have spread to is crucial, but that only tells us how advanced their spread is. A real-world example of this in cancer medicine is demonstrated when patients with breast cancer that has spread to bone state they have bone cancer. This is incorrect. They have *breast* cancer that has spread to *bone*. This is not mere semantics. There are enormous differences in treatment and prognosis between breast cancer that has spread to bone and bone cancer.

The TNM classification system is also identical to the Union Against Cancer schema (UICC).They both have clinical and pathologic staging. Simply put, pathologic staging is determined when a tumor is physically seen and biopsied. The site of origin determines the *T* stage and refers largely to the size of the primary tumor at that site. The *N* refers to proven evidence of lymph node spread, and the *M* refers to proven evidence of distant spread, or metastasis. Clinical staging employs multiple different nonsurgical techniques, such as X-rays or CAT scans, MRI, ultrasounds, or PET scans, which may image or demonstrate findings that are extremely suggestive of spread.

Thus, clinical staging relies on what we can see, and pathologic staging relies on what we can feel or have touched as a result of tissue biopsy. In some cases, biopsy may be required to confirm suspicions of the presumed clinical stage, as the impact of incorrect assumptions of the degree of advance frequently have enormous consequences. Of course, we cannot biopsy all tumors that we see; they must be safely accessible. In addition, in many cases, such as breast cancer, biopsy of nearby draining regional nodes is routine. Immense knowledge is gained by systematically finding and assessing for cancer in what we call the sentinel lymph nodes, which regionally drain the primary cancer.

"Stage grouping" refers to combining the clinical or pathologic stage information (i.e. the T, N, and M information) and grouping it into larger numeric stages—usually 1–4, with occasional subsets. Stage 1 is the most limited and Stage 4 usually refers to being widespread. Different combinations of TNM can be in the same stage group, such as a large tumor with no involved lymph nodes or a small tumor with a few involved nodes. All stage grouping is specific for each tumor. These numeric groups are not used for convenience; rather, they reflect the spread of the disease and have enormous influence on prognosis and therapy.

The clinical stage guides therapy. The pathological stage ascertained after complete surgical removal of all visible disease can determine the need for further therapy, even when no remaining tumor seems to exist. Both breast and colon cancer are excellent examples of the stage seen as a result of surgery predicting the risk of future relapse from microscopic tumor cells that may still be present. As mentioned in the "Diagnosis" chapter, adjuvant therapy refers to when we see no remaining tumor cells but history tells us, based on the tumor type and stage, that there is a meaningful risk that viable cancer cells remain undetected. The utility of such therapy is very specific for the type of tumor. Adjuvant therapy is wise if evidence suggests that it can help improve the odds of preventing recurrence, delaying recurrence, or increasing the odds of survival. It is not wise for every tumor or every stage of any tumor. It is a very specific choice based on very specific clinical evidence; the benefit is very tumor- and stage-specific.

Therapeutic procedures, such as partial or total surgical removal, may alter a tumor's stage and the life history of the cancer. Thus, we have the rTNM restaging scheme, which yields different results than the original stage. Obviously, we use the rTNM for reestimation of prognosis and guidance for further therapy after total or partial surgical removal. Whenever patients are compared or treated in clinical studies, physicians always use the original pretherapy stage of the tumor so that everyone is on equal footing and starting at the same place. Not all patients with any given tumor type or stage will or can have surgical removal. Comparison that is more accurate can occur among patients owing to this rationale.

There are exceptions to the TNM staging criteria, and they usually include the so-called liquid tumors, such as leukemia, lymphomas, etc. They do not lend themselves easily to the TNM system because of the way patients with them typically present at diagnosis and their natural history. Thus, there are elegant, detailed criteria for staging. In the case of most leukemia, physicians use lists of definitive factors to give a prognostic score. Thus, we can group these diseases into various stages that predict response to therapy and odds and duration of survival. These factors are constantly evolving as molecular and genetic tests and knowledge that goes far beyond simple laboratory tests develop.

The beauty of such staging schemes that are internationally accepted is that they allow us to compare therapies stage-for-stage and design clinical trials intelligently with high likelihood of answering an important question. The staging schemes help us decide what adequate therapy is and assists in further refining treatment approaches.

In most cases, staging relies on the *anatomic* extent of the malignancy. We know where the tumor has physically spread. However, sometimes the degree of aberrancy—the bizarreness and abnormality in the appearance of the tumor under the microscope (histological grade)—and patient age can affect staging. Thus, two very similar tumors may have slightly different stages because the cancer cells are more primitive or angry in one case or the patients are different ages. The reasoning for the different stage is the same reasoning used for staging. In the example above, we know that more angry cells or an older age impact the prognosis of otherwise similar patients; thus, we name the stage differently.

Although cancer cells mimic their normal cell counterpart as discussed in "The Enemy," they often have very specific identifying fingerprints or products. Increasingly, molecular markers, which are the presence of highly specific molecules that identify or mark the disease; specific genetic fingerprints; abnormal proteins on the cancer cell surface; and other cancer-specific characteristics and tumor products aid in staging and directing therapy. In some cases, the degree of bizarreness of the cancer cells may be the most important staging criterion of all.

The challenge for any staging system is that it must keep up with the diagnostic advances in oncology as we find newer valid and crucial prognostic variables. Thus, original and future stages of the seemingly same tumor may not be similar. There is no widely accepted detailed staging system yet for tumors of the central nervous system, owing to inherent difficulties in defining landmarks, discovering the significance of those landmarks, and the frequent lack of biopsy material.

In conclusion, it is imperative to have an extremely accurate staging of any tumor, whether it is by anatomic site only or by biochemical, genetic and molecular, or immunologic measurements. Patients must be certain that their tumors are precisely staged and that they know what stage their tumors are. As mentioned, we understand treatments and prognosis largely in terms of the stage of the disease at the time of the diagnosis. *Individual* treatment decisions require thorough staging.

Patients must remember that they are individuals and not a group. Although the study of groups of similar patients have taught us enormously what the odds are for response, duration of response, and freedom from relapse and survival, *patients experience their diseases as individuals.* Individuals may beat or, less happily, lose against the odds.

Chemotherapy

The National Cancer Institute (NCI) has played an active role in the development of drugs for cancer treatment for over fifty years. This is reflected in the fact that approximately one-half of the chemotherapeutic drugs currently used by oncologists for cancer treatment were discovered and/or developed at NCI.

NCI's Developmental Therapeutics Program (DTP) has over four hundred thousand drugs in its repository that have gone through some kind of screening process. About eighty thousand compounds have been screened since 1990 using the current screening system. Compounds can enter at any stage of the development process, with either very little or extensive prior testing. NCI supports about 1,500 clinical trials through a variety of programs. NCI researchers at the National Institutes of Health in Bethesda, Maryland, conduct some, while others take place at cancer centers, hospitals, and community practices around the country.

It is far beyond the scope of this book to discuss in any depth all the nuances of the more than fifty common chemotherapy drugs available. Previously, in the overview section, we enumerated the major classes of drugs. Here we will delve a little more deeply into how the drugs we have work, as well as the most importance drug advances.

The first and most important concept is that, typically, specific drugs work for specific tumors. However, this is this is changing as new combinations are tried. Secondly, drugs try to hit the Achilles' heel(s) of the tumor. Yes, the majority of cancer cells have an Achilles' heel—a weak spot that drugs theoretically attempt to exploit. Although these drugs may damage normal cells in the process, such as those of the gastrointestinal tract and bone marrow, the bulk of the damage is intended to affect the tumor because of its Achilles' heel(s).

One particular area of concern is off-label use. Pharmaceutical companies initially apply to the FDA for approval of a new agent for a particular tumor in a particular setting. This requires an average of six years of development and more than $500 million. FDA approval means a drug is known to be safe and effective. It then receives approval for its use for a specifically tested indication. Once approved, hundreds of researchers and many patients with *other* tumors or different stages of the original tumor type compared to the original trials, participate in carefully designed phase 1–4 clinical trials of the drug, either alone or in combination with other drugs or radiation.

Remember, I am using a broad definition of "drug" to include novel immunologic agents, typical chemotherapy compounds, vaccines, and many other varieties of substances administered in many different ways. In this way, researchers can develop numerous extremely important uses for the original drug that go beyond the original FDA-approved use. After FDA approval, it is usually only a matter of time before we know, because of more trials, if the drug has additional uses. Typically, many do. Thus, patients need not be wary if the drug(s) they are treated with is off-label.

Normal cells have a life cycle. The creation of new cells from a parent cell is a reasonably well understood process with numerous genetic and biochemical markers that tell us where the cells are in that process. The phases of the process have different names. One technique of developing a new drug is targeting a potential vulnerability because of the phase a tumor cell may be in.

Cells that are resting are usually in a very chemotherapy-resistant phase. In the next phase, or interphase, cells become very active in making the building blocks that they need to live, maintain the household, and prepare to divide and have children.

The genetic material of all cells is contained in tightly coiled twisted ladders knows as chromosomes. Those ladders are made of DNA, and the nucleus inside the cell is the headquarters or home for the chromosomes. This genetic material contains all the directions and all the blueprints for everything that cell is and can do. In the DNA synthesis phase, the amount of DNA doubles in preparation of the cell dividing. In the Gap 2 phases, a fine meshwork of scaffolding appears inside the cells; the structure looks like an old-fashioned bingo spindle. This mitotic spindle is necessary for the duplicated DNA in our chromosomes to move across the nucleus before the cell divides into two cells. In the final phase, the M phase (for "mitotic") all the newly created and aggregated DNA material goes into the two daughter cells in identical amounts.

Chemotherapy drugs may be specific for a phase they affect the most. These drugs attempt to exploit the fact that most, but not all, cancers cells are more active than healthy cells and more prolific at having offspring. Some chemotherapy agents, however, are phase nonspecific and kill nondividing cells. Examples are the antitumor antibiotics, excepting bleomycin. Some drugs are simply specific for the whole cycle and do not need a particular phase. Rather, these drugs require only that the tumor cell be going through the cycle of life, not just a particular phase. Thus, these drugs can inflict injury at any point along the cell cycle. Examples are the so-called alkylating agents. Generally, these types of drugs have a linear dose-response behavior, in that the more that is given, the more tumor cells should theoretically be killed. Of course, two things limit this. One is the tolerance of normal cells (thus the patient's body), and the other is the multiple clever ways tumor cells can either acquire or already have inborn resistance to the agent.

As mentioned above, there are phase-specific drugs that are only effective if they are present during a particular phase of a tumor cell's life cycle. This type of drug usually has a limit in cell-killing ability. After a certain dose level, no further killing happens. However, if the drug is still present the next time that specific phase occurs in a tumor cell's life cycle, more tumor cells theoretically may die.

Tumor cell growth is very important to understand. First, it is highly variable, with the time required to double the number of cancer cells ranging from less than twenty-four hours to more than three hundred days. Furthermore, cells in the center of a tumor mass may not even be alive if they have outstripped their blood supply and delivery of nutrients and oxygen. Thus, tumor growth depends on the number of cells dividing over time. Usually, the larger the tumor, the smaller the percentage of dividing cells and the longer it takes cells to divide. There are elegant models; one of the most common is the Gompertzian model that I am discussing. Some general rules apply. Growth rate is most rapid and often exponential during the early days of a tumor. Thus, instead of 2 cells going to 4, then 8, then 16; two cells may go to 4, then 16, then 256. Therefore, the growth fraction, or the number of cells dividing, is high. The portion of tumor cells that are growing decreases as the tumor gets larger, and it often plateaus because of nutrient supply. This may help one to get a handle on these numbers. It takes one billion cells for just one gram (there are about twenty-eight grams to an ounce) of tumor tissue. One gram is about the lowest level at which we can detect cancer. That is equal to about a 1 cm mass in a breast or 1 cm nodules on a chest X-ray. One thousand and one million times that amount is about two to twenty pounds of cancer and usually results in severe organ damage, major medical problems, and death.

Sadly, tumor cells have multiple mechanisms of innate or acquired resistance to chemotherapy. Tumor cells within a given cancer may have some diversity in this regard. Some tumor cells are naturally (innately) drug resistant and eventually become the predominant cell. This is particularly true if chemotherapy eliminates all the sensitive cells. A theory called the Goldie–Coldman hypothesis asserts that the probability of a tumor having resistant cells is proportional to tumor size. Thus, tumors can become more resistant to chemotherapy as they grow. However, chemotherapy makes some tumor cells quickly produce enzymes or use other techniques to neutralize the drug. This is acquired resistance. Some tumor cells make substances in high concentration that not only lead to destruction of the chemotherapy drug but also quickly repair any DNA or other damage the chemotherapy drug may have caused.

DNA on chromosomes is tightly coiled. There are specific enzymes that let it uncoil so it can duplicate DNA for its children. Some chemotherapy drugs either try to inhibit the enzyme that allows the uncoiling or try to keep the DNA for the children cells stuck on the spindle on which this occurs. Once again, tumor cells can acquire resistance to this. Sometimes the mere exposure of a drug to a tumor cell prompts the tumor cell to make a transport protein to carry the drug actively out of the cell before it can do damage. Sometimes this tumor cell reaction not only leads to resistance to one chemotherapy drug but also induces the tumor cell to make a multidrug resistance gene. A gene is a portion of a chromosome that carries the code for one specific message—typically it is a message for a protein that has a very specific job. Human cells have tens of thousands of genes. The multidrug resistance gene helps the tumor cells create a very effective pump that pumps chemotherapy drugs out of the tumor cell before they can cause harm. There is more than one multidrug resistance gene, and unfortunately, there has been only minimal success in blocking these genes' actions. Many of the above reasons are why we use non-cross-resistant chemotherapy to try to hit the tumor from multiple angles. The concept is similar to using a cocktail of drugs against the cancer cells that are sufficiently different so that we hit the tumor cells in multiple ways.

Regarding how much chemotherapy is enough, more often than not, more is not better. Very high does, which only work for a few tumors, require the support of bone marrow transplants to rescue the patient from the damage the high dosages of drugs inflict on normal cells.

Thus, if caught early enough, a dozen or so of human tumors are clearly curable with chemotherapy alone. There are about seven or so that are very responsive, but cure is not typical with drugs alone. There are many, depending on their stage, that are highly treatable for long durations. Then there are the groups of only occasional responders, such as advanced melanoma, the common type of kidney cancer, many forms of brain cancer, and advanced cancer of the bladder and pancreas.

We previously discussed adjuvant chemotherapy. This is treatment given after the primary removal of the tumor when there is no evidence of remaining tumor but there is a well-known risk of recurrence. The intent is to prevent recurrence. Adjuvant therapy of breast cancer is the model for this concept, which changes the odds of survival for countless patients. Neoadjuvant chemotherapy is treatment given before primary surgical removal of a tumor to ease the removal, make surgery less invasive, and offer the benefit, in some cancers, of determining whether the drugs chosen are effective or not. Salvage chemotherapy is treatment given after failure of initial therapies. It is not synonymous with unsuccessful treatment, as many patients undergoing this type of therapy see prolonged survival free of progression or recurrence while enjoying a good quality of life.

Most chemotherapy drugs can also be categorized based on how they work rather than just when they work. Thus, there are alkylating agents that target tumor DNA and try to bind to it, thus disrupting a tumor cell's ability to have offspring. Some are antimetabolites. These drugs mimic small molecules the cancer cell needs to keep living. These function like a computer virus by not allowing the cell to proceed in cycles, as they are dysfunctional copies. There are antitumor antibiotics, which generally are drugs derived from microorganisms and are usually not cell-cycle specific. These are often useful in slow-growing tumors. There are plant alkaloids that function by not letting the spindle we talked about earlier form, thus preventing the tumor cells from dividing. These drugs may also make the spindle's structure unstable.

Finally, as will be touched on somewhat in the section "The Future," other agents exist that do not neatly fit any of these classes. These novel drugs may destroy essential enzymes or function as a hormone or hormone receptor manipulator necessary for tumor growth. If a receptor or keyhole needs to work for a tumor cell to grow, blocking the keyhole can be very effective. Some chemotherapy agents can be very disabling by affecting the ability of the tumor cell to eliminate harmful by-products it produces as it grows.

Some drugs interfere with molecules necessary for the tumor to grow. Some such drugs are estrogens, antiestrogens, and antiandrogens. An exciting, relatively new, and promising type of treatment is immunologic therapy and biologics. We will discuss this in more detail in "The Future." The earliest effective treatment of this type is interferon treatment. There have also been attempts to "beef up" immune cells of the patient outside the body of the patient and reinject them in hopes they will find the target tumor cell and help the immune system. Finally, there are agents that try to force tumor cells that are "stuck" in a primitive always-on-and-dividing phase to go through orderly, controlled cell growth and life. These drugs are trying to make the rogue cancer cells grow up, mature, straighten out, and become normal. These are known as differentiation agents and have met with some success in some forms of leukemia.

A very exciting breakthrough of only the last decade is not true chemotherapy to fight cancer but rather a method of employing genetically engineered drugs to fight the effects of the cancer on you and your bone marrow. All of our blood cells are made in the marrow. There is a complex army of specialized white blood cells to fight infection and red cells to carry oxygen. There are now genetically engineered drugs routinely available that are largely identical to the normal molecules in your body that stimulate production of red and white blood cells. Anemia and dangerously low white blood cell levels can occur either from the therapy or the presence of the tumor, or both. Enormous fatigue and poor quality of life are associated with anemia, and infections that can be life threatening are more common with low numbers of infection-fighting white blood cells. Both can now be very effectively treated. There is also a genetically engineered product to help your body make platelets (which help blood clot), though it is not as effective as the other two.

Thus, these hematopoietic (blood) growth factors have had an enormous impact on the ability to both fight, defray, and hasten recovery from chemotherapy-induced low blood counts and the secondary risks of infection and fatigue. These little miracle molecules are precise genetic replicas of your body's own growth factors that can now be mass-produced by recombinant genetic engineering. Furthermore, longer-acting versions are now available through manipulating the molecules, thereby decreasing the frequency with which injections must be received. Thus, we are more effectively fighting fatigue, avoiding transfusions, and decreasing the risk and expense of infection. Furthermore, oncologists are more frequently able to deliver full doses of chemotherapy on time in cases where cure and benefit depend on that.

The first widely used genetically engineered product was the red blood cell growth factor called erythropoietin. This can improve the anemia and fatigue of many cancer patients if needed. This is an injection, similar to an insulin injection, self-administered by the patient. Injections are needed as infrequently as every one to three weeks in some cases. The other billion-dollar-selling wonder drugs are G–CSF and GM-CSF, which, like the red cell drug, are administered subcutaneously. They support white blood cell counts. Both are available in daily and every-two-to-three-week forms. Such drugs have changed the practice of oncology. These two drugs alone have markedly improved the quality of life for millions of cancer patients.

In summary, not all tumors are the same in terms of chemotherapy sensitivity. We design drugs to exploit unique cancer cell weaknesses and take advantage of their usual higher rate of growth. There are numerous ways to attack the malignant cells. These cancer cells are clever, adaptive enemies that may be quick to find a way around our armamentarium. Wonderful new therapies exist to support patients undergoing some of the toxicities of therapy. As will be discussed in "The Future," exciting and novel treatment approaches have arrived. Thus, the sooner we get to the cancer, the better; the more we can do to prevent it, the better; and the more patients we can get on well-designed clinical trials, the faster we will conquer this frequently devastating disease.

Radiation Therapy

Radiation therapy uses high-energy radiation to kill cancer cells by damaging their DNA. Radiation therapy can damage normal cells as well as cancer cells. Therefore, treatment must be carefully planned to minimize side effects. The radiation used for cancer treatment may come from a machine outside the body, or it may come from radioactive material placed in the body near tumor cells or injected into the bloodstream A patient may receive radiation therapy before, during, or after surgery, depending on the type of cancer being treated. Some patients receive radiation therapy alone, and some receive radiation therapy in combination with chemotherapy.

The care of the oncology patient must be multidisciplinary. Pathologists, radiologists, clinical laboratory physicians, and immunobiologists are crucial members that render the correct diagnosis. In many cases, a team comprising the medical oncologist, surgeon or surgical oncologist, and radiation therapist assess what treatment techniques are needed. Finally, there are chemotherapy nurses, technicians, and social workers rounding out an integrated team.

Radiation oncology is a clinical discipline devoted to the use of ionizing radiation for patients with cancer as well as some other diseases. We give radiation alone or in combination with other treatments. The goal is to deliver the maximum lethal dose to the tumor and minimize any toxicity to surrounding normal tissues in hopes of eradicating the tumor while maintaining a high quality of life. Radiation therapy may also have a role in treating or preventing symptoms. Radiation can be used to reduce pain, restore the opening of blocked airways, prevent bone fractures owing to tumor having spread to the bones, and aid in other organ function, while again trying to minimize suffering. Just as with the medical oncologist, the radiation oncologist must assess all the factors relevant to the patient's situation and determine whether more radiation is safe and beneficial.

Many types of radiation are used. The most common kind is external beam radiation using photons or electrons. The photons used are X-rays or gamma rays and may be considered as bundles of energy that deposit a damaging dose to the tissue as they pass through it. These beams are carefully shaped by shielding the normal surrounding tissue. Depending on the voltage used, which can vary millionfold, these X-rays may travel from barely a millimeter to a depth of 3–4 cm with techniques used to spare the overlying skin. Radioactive isotopes, the most common of which is cobalt-60, emit gamma rays. Most facilities no longer use gamma rays because of the need to replace the isotope and frequently recalculate dosages as a result of the natural radioactive decay of the isotope. The gamma knife is an exception that radiates brain tumors with precise accuracy and employs up to 201 cobalt-60 sources.

Other sources of external beam radiation are protons and neutrons. Protons are positively charged particles that have the advantage of depositing dose at a constant rate over the majority of the beam, with most of it at the end of the beam. Protons, unlike photons, fall off quickly in their ability to do damage beyond the target. Although this vastly limits damage to normal tissue, the enormous expense in generating these rays has limited their use to only a handful of centers in the Unites States. Neutrons are uncharged heavy particles that are produced a number of ways. Neutrons collide with protons in the tumor cell nucleus and can be very effective. Experience with these units is limited because of enormous cost, but clinical trials comparing all these types of radiation are underway.

Brachytherapy is a physically different way of delivering ionizing radiation. In this technique, the physician places or implants sealed or unsealed radioactive sources very close to the target. Since the dose of radiation falls off very rapidly as distance increases, this is one technique that works better in most cases to deliver higher doses of radiation to the target than external beam radiation. The dose is generally delivered over days and is seen in use in some cervical, prostate, and breast cancers. Various radioactive substances are used as the radiation-emitting source.

Radiation therapy may be intended to be curative or rather be used simply for symptom control. Cooperation of all members of the team is essential to achieve these goals. Furthermore, tumors have highly variable sensitivity to radiation doses. Importantly, normal tissues have maximum doses that can be tolerated after which severe damage can occur. Thus, as is true for chemotherapy, the probable benefit of radiation must be weighed on a careful case-by-case basis against the probability of damage to normal tissue in the way of or near the beam. This is not a simple business, and extremely close coordination with the physicist, dosimetrist (physicist who calculates the right dose), and treatment planning staff is standard.

So why does radiation work? First, one can kill just about anything with enough radiation; the issue is that one cannot always safely give enough radiation to kill the intended target. High doses may be irritating or lethal depending on the tissue irradiated. Thus, so-called dose response curves exist for all tumors. These tell us the correct dose to get the desired effects of killing tumor cells. These curves also exist for each type of normal tissue (e.g., bone, brain, nerve, bone marrow, intestine, mouth, etc.). Furthermore, the sheer bulk, or lack thereof, of the tumor will also play a pivotal role in the maximal tolerated dose.

You may hear the term "boost volume," which is used to describe the residual tumor volume receiving the highest doses of irradiation. This is often necessary in larger tumors, where a higher dose is delivered to a location where viable tumor cells may well be and would, if left unchecked, multiply and grow. In addition, since radiation works better with plenty of oxygen and many of these cells are at the oxygen-poor core of the tumor, the boost is helpful.

Molecular oxygen must be present at the time of irradiation for maximal killing of tumor cells. The probable mechanism is that the radiation creates free radicals, which are very damaging to tumor DNA. Nearly all cell death from radiation results from disruption of cancer cell division and the new tumor cell formation process. Thus, tumor cell death in nondividing irradiated cancer cells is uncommon. It is also true that apoptosis, which is the name for the phenomenon of all cells being preprogrammed to eventually die from old age, appears to occur at an accelerated rate once cells are irradiated. That is, irradiation "ages" the cancer cells. Cancer cells attempt repair of nonlethal and potentially lethal cellular damage from radiation. This occurs within about five to six hours and is probably never complete. Although human cells have a narrow range of tolerance, compared to tumor cells they have a more efficient repair and recovery processes. We try to exploit this phenomenon by the daily or twice daily treatment, or fractionation scheme, of most radiation.

As one would imagine, there is clearly an array of adverse effects from radiation, depending on dose and intervals as well as type and duration. Three-dimensional planning is the biggest advance as regards not only focusing the beam precisely but also avoiding damage to normal tissue. In this technique, similar to a hologram, the radiation team can predict how much beam is going where. Nonetheless, there are both early and late radiation-induced reactions. The early reactions occur during or immediately following treatment and are usually self-limiting, although they may last for a few weeks. These may be local or systemic and include loss of appetite, nausea, fatigue, inflammation of the esophagus, diarrhea (if the GI tract is in the beam), skin reactions (redness and peeling), inflammation of the lining of the mouth, loss of hair, and low blood counts. The basic mechanism is damage to rapidly dividing cells. These symptoms can be modestly treated and usually resolve well.

Late radiation-induced reactions can be clinically important and may be apparent months to years later. They are often progressive and not self-limiting. Such reactions are typically local and include inflammation of nerves, death of bone, tightening of bowels, scarring of the lungs, loss of skin, kidney damage, and heart damage. These are usually very infrequent, owing to the careful planning discussed earlier. Since these late effects are usually irreversible, careful planning toward prevention is pivotal.

As one would expect, the side effects of radiation therapy influence other treatment methods, and vice versa. Certain chemotherapy agents can greatly accentuate skin inflammation during radiation, and thus we avoid simultaneous administration. Some may even create a radiation recall effect long after the chemotherapy is over. This is when, after the administration of particular types of chemotherapy, a previously irradiated area may inflame even though the radiation was delivered quite some time previously. Prior abdominal surgery may accentuate both acute and late radiation-induced bowel damage if bowels are placed in the path of radiation. Radiation can damage small blood vessels and thus may impair healing after surgery. Finally, a more recently recognized complication of radiation is the risk of bone marrow and blood disorders, as well as acute leukemia, years after the therapy.

The key is teamwork and careful planning. As with any therapy, one must always weigh the benefits against the harms while remembering the immense harm of not treating the tumor at all or treating it inadequately. The techniques of radiation are becoming more refined. The field of radiation sensitizers that may increase the vulnerability of tumor cells relative to normal cells is growing. Radiation will continue to have a prominent role not only for symptom control but also as an integral portion of a comprehensive approach to the treatment of many human malignancies as seen in cancers of the lung, colon/rectum, and breast, as well as Hodgkin's disease.

Principles of Surgical Oncology

Much of early cancer therapy focused largely on surgical excision as the primary treatment for solid tumors. A common thinking was that cancer spread in an orderly manner regionally, then into adjacent lymph nodes, and then on to distant sites. Thus, it was thought that removal of all cancerous tissue, if possible, would be associated with cure. It eventually became apparent that surgical removal of all cancerous tissue possible did not necessarily coincide with cure, and this led to the development of screening strategies and a search for adjuvant therapies. Thus, the role of the surgical oncologist has evolved into a broad spectrum of surgical procedures for cure, diagnosis, local control, and symptom control.

Once a tumor or mass has been identified, it is usually the role of the surgeon to obtain adequate tissue for definitive diagnosis. The type of surgeon who will take on this role is determined by the amount of tissue needed and the location of that tissue. The key is to use the most effective but least invasive technique to obtain tissue, fresh or fixed in preservative, with all the margins well aligned and labeled, with as little damage to surrounding tissue as possible. This may involve a fine-needle aspiration to study clusters of cells, a larger core biopsy, or a punch biopsy, done through the skin.

Open biopsy can be incisional or excisional. Incisional biopsies are done by making an incision in anesthetized skin and obtaining a wedge of tissue. This incision is planned carefully so as not to interfere with further surgery or leave a track for seeding of tumor cells. Excisional biopsies remove the entire mass and are best suited for small tumors. Depending on the size, these are either office-based or operating room procedures.

Another important role of the surgeon is staging, which determines the extent of disease and whether a tumor is truly removable. When distant disease is suspected, a number of scans may be ordered. There are bone scans, which measure and take pictures of the activity of bone cells responding to some form of injury. PET scans look at the metabolism of radioactive glucose by tumors as opposed to benign tissue. CAT scans are computer assisted X-rays that can image a part of the body and reconstruct it all into a picture, and MRIs measure the different reactions of various tissues to a magnetic field and reconstruct those differences into very detailed realistic maps and pictures. In many cancers, especially breast, lung, melanoma, some abdominal cancers, and some chest cancers, the surgeon may be more accurate at staging than less-invasive means.

Some of the procedures a surgeon uses are mediastinoscopies, in which a fiber-optic scope is placed behind the sternum to assess if a lung mass is malignant and too advanced for surgery that is more radical. Laporotomy, an exploration of the abdomen, is sometimes used for cancers of the uterus and ovary, as well as testicular cancers. Laparoscopy, where a fiber optic scope is inserted into the abdomen under a general anesthetic, has found a very large number of uses. Biopsies can be obtained, and organs directly visualized. In some cancers, the surgeon intentionally removes or samples lymph nodes in the abdomen for curative, diagnostic, and staging intent. Studies are continuing in some newer applications, such as cancers of the pancreas and stomach, to see if this has a role.

A more recent area of interest is the sentinel node biopsy, in which a radio-opaque dye is injected at the primary tumor site and, using both visualization and a gamma camera (similar to a Geiger counter), the presumed sentinel draining node is identified. More studies have suggested this as having a standard role in breast cancer, melanoma, and other cancers, and the results are often used to determine if further therapy is needed, as well as to determine the probable extent of the disease.

The surgical oncologist is pivotal in the primary resection of the tumor. This requires expert understanding of not only anatomy but also architectural planes of spread and knowledge of proven, effective extent of surgery needed. Occasionally, there are some cases in which the surgeon may remove one or a few sites of spread disease. In a few cases the natural history of a tumor has shown that removal of isolated recurrence will improve chances of survival even though seemingly isolated recurrences almost always mean that the horse is out of the barn, as the tumor is already blood-borne and has spread.

Surgery may be done on the colon or cervix based on premalignant changes as a preventive measure in hopes of avoiding full-blown cancer. Surgery may follow after initial chemotherapy is given to shrink the primary tumor, making surgery easier and perhaps of greater benefit. Such chemotherapy was labeled earlier as neoadjuvant. It is often given with the intent of saving or preserving an organ, such as a larynx, or to allow a lumpectomy instead of an entire breast removal.

Some surgical procedures may be for symptom control, such as placing a tube in the chest in an attempt to drain a malignant collection of fluid and then introduce a scarring agent to prevent further collection of fluid. Stents may be placed in an obstructed biliary tree or bowel if the obstructed area cannot safely be removed. In some cases surgery is done to bypass an obstruction even though the cancer is advanced. This is often associated with significant relief of pain and suffering. Tubes can also be placed in an obstructed esophagus to improve distressing symptoms.

Surgeons may play the pivotal role in both functional and reconstructive cosmetic surgery. This has gained great success in various techniques of breast reconstruction, use of skin flaps over wide surgical areas, restoration of the movement of muscles, covering of susceptible organs or structures, and improvement of general cosmetic affect.

Surgeons and invasive radiologists help us through the placement of both percutaneous (through the skin) and subcutaneous ports or catheters for the administration of blood products and various drugs, as well as for obtaining blood without constant use of arm veins. This can be extremely convenient and is generally very well accepted by patients. The ports can be under the skin and visible with no impairment of lifestyle; they simply require flushing at monthly intervals. The percutaneous catheters are usually shorter lived and require a bit more maintenance. In some cases, in specific centers, catheters are placed directly into the artery feeding the liver to aid in direct delivery of chemotherapy in relatively higher concentrations to either prevent tumor spread to the liver in high-risk people or treat spread that has already occurred.

Finally, surgeons can be of immense help to improve nutrition by placing tubes for nourishment directly into the stomach (gastrostomy tubes) or small intestine (jejunostomy tubes). The gastrostomy tube is also used at times to prevent obstruction by allowing an escape valve of sorts.

The role of the surgeon has thus evolved from primarily attempting total removal of all manners of tumors to being part of highly skilled teams whose skills address diagnosis, prevention, staging, cure, and symptomatic treatment of all manners of tumors. In particular, a fully trained surgical oncologist is invaluable to the comprehensive management of many of our most common malignancies.

Therapeutic Monoclonal Antibodies

One of the newer types of novel therapies available today is therapeutic monoclonal antibody therapy. Understanding what therapeutic antibodies are requires understanding the body's immune system. Antibodies are proteins found in the body that are made in response to foreign substances that have the ability to elicit an immune response. Such substances are thus antigenic, and the molecular portion of them that elicits the immune response upon being recognized as foreign is the antigen. Put differently, antigens are any substance that produces a sensitivity response by the body when it comes into contact with antigenic tissue. Think of antigens as anything foreign that produces a "fight" response by the body's immune system. However, some substances that have antigens as part of their structure do not elicit a response.

The body produces antibodies specific to specific antigens. The antibody attaches to the antigen, and a reaction is triggered that usually, but not always, results in the destruction of the antigen. This process is a crucial part of a complex immune system structured not too dissimilarly to a comprehensive national defense system with initial attack troops, as well as various types of antibody-producing cells, cells that eat foreign substances, and intelligence and memory cells that coordinate and remember the attack.

In the 1950s scientists began to explore methods of using the body's immune system to help fight cancer by looking for ways to make specific antibodies that would grab onto and destroy cancer cells. It took twenty years of research to develop laboratory methods that would produce a single antibody that recognized a single antigen. That singularity is actually molecularly based and leads us to call such antibodies monoclonal. This method, called the hybridoma technique, opened the door for scientists to make unlimited amounts of pure monoclonal antibodies. By the 1980s, scientists were sure that a "magic bullet" to cure cancer would soon be discovered. That was not the case, but many monoclonal antibodies are used today in some cancers with good responses.

Early monoclonal antibodies were produced using mouse cell factories, and understandably, a major problem was that human bodies recognized the mouse protein and severely reacted. It took two decades and a team at UCSD, of which I was a part, to image the first cancer with human antibodies. Now humanization techniques are widespread, with only some mouse protein involved. Allergic reaction remains possible but is not widespread.

Cancer cells are foreign, and the hope, in principle, was that antibodies could be made to the theoretical tumor-associated *specific* antigens presumed to exist. Although this is not so easily accomplished, considerable progress has been made, and therapeutic antibodies are now part of routine oncology practice.

Several therapeutic antibodies are now in use, and many more are being studied in clinical trials. They are designed to react with cancer cells in a way that triggers the body to fight a cancer more effectively or deliver a lethal payload or be directly toxic. They represent a growing family of "targeted therapies."

Here is how it works: Monoclonal antibody therapy aims to target tumor cells that have a certain protein antigen on the surface of the cell. When a monoclonal antibody binds with the protein antigen on a cancer cell, it helps the body's general immune response. The antibody acts like a key that fits only one lock on the cell surface (the antigen). Once the key is inserted into the lock, one of several actions may occur. The signals to the core of the cell (nucleus) can be blocked so normal cell functions, such as growth and repair, do not occur. The key can attract other cells of the immune system or other blood proteins to destroy the cell. Or the signal for cell death can be started. Any of these actions can result in stopping cell function or in cell death, which is the goal for targeting cancer cells.

Therapeutic monoclonal antibodies alone can interfere with cell functions, or they can work in partnership with agents that are attached to them to target and kill tumor cells. Thank of it as delivering a lethal, highly specific payload. Examples of agents that attach to the monoclonal antibody are radiation agents, chemotherapy drugs, or other biologic agents. Once the monoclonal antibody carries the other agent along to the target, the agent can direct its killing effect on the tumor cells to destroy the cancer.

Chemotherapy acts very differently when it is working with a monoclonal antibody than when it acts alone. Chemotherapy can be nonselective, which means that it can affect all cells dividing at certain phases. Thus normal cells can also be affected, and there may be systemic, body-wide effects.

Monoclonal antibody therapy is more tumor specific than chemotherapy, but it is not perfect. As stated, the monoclonal antibody targets a specific antigen on the surface of the tumor cell. Normal, healthy cells are not usually affected. Therefore, when the chemotherapy payload is delivered only to the surface of the tumor cell, the side effects can be much milder than if the chemotherapy were circulated throughout the entire body.

At the present time, the most common therapeutic monoclonal antibodies being used in cancer treatment include (1) anti-CD20/B-cell, (2) anti-EGFR, and (3) antiangiogenesis. Each is described in greater detail below.

Anti-CD20/B-cell monoclonal antibodies: Scientists have discovered that people with non-Hodgkin's lymphoma (NHL) have a specific antigen on the cell surface called CD20. In normal cells, the CD20 antigen helps in the growth and maturation of one type of lymphocyte called B-lymphocytes, which help in the immune system. CD20 antigens also play a role in helping tumor cell growth. A number of newly developed treatments target the CD20 antigen to stop the growth of the cancer.

A specific anti-CD20/B-cell monoclonal antibody, Rituxan (rituximab) was developed to attach to the CD20 antigen on normal and malignant B-cells in order to recruit the body's natural defenses to attack and kill the marked B-cells. The CD20 antigen is not present during the early development of B-cells; therefore, with Rituxan, B-cells can regenerate after treatment and return to their normal functions. Rituxan has been approved by the FDA for the treatment of relapsed or refractory non-Hodgkin's lymphoma and indolent B-cell NHL. It is also used for other diseases, such as chronic lymphocytic leukemia (CLL) or Waldenstrom's macroglobulinemia.

Current research is focused on evaluating Rituxan in combination with chemotherapy in indolent NHL and other cancers. It is generally administered as an IV infusion once a week for four or eight doses. There are side effects, such as infusion reactions and infection.

Another type of monoclonal antibody is used in conjunction with a radioactive isotope (radioisotope) in a type of treatment that is called radioimmunotherapy (RIT). Zevalin (ibritumomab tiuxetan) is an FDA-approved radioimmunotherapy treatment that also targets the CD20 antigen found on B-cell non-Hodgkin's lymphoma (NHL) patients. The monoclonal antibody has a radioisotope attached to it that delivers radiation therapy to the lymphoma cells. With this dual-action therapy, cancer cells are destroyed by both high-energy radiation and the cell-killing action of the monoclonal antibody. When used in non-Hodgkin's lymphoma, radio-labeled monoclonal antibodies target specific cells and destroy cancer cells while minimizing damage to normal cells. Side effects include risk of infection, fatigue due to anemia, and bleeding.

A more recently approved targeted radioimmunotherapy treatment is Bexxar, which is made of two parts—a monoclonal antibody named tositumomab and a monoclonal antibody with radiation attached named iodine-131 tositumomab. This two-part treatment is used in patients with CD20 positive non-Hodgkin's lymphoma whose disease is no longer responding to Rituxan and has relapsed after chemotherapy. The unlabeled tositumomab portion of the agent (with no radiation attached) binds to the tumor cells. It also attracts other cells of the immune system, such as T-lymphocytes, which then attack the tumor cell. The tositumomab portion labeled with I-131 (the attached radiation) also locks on to other lymphoma cells and delivers a low, continuous dose of radiation directly to the cancer cells. This therapy is somewhat complex to administer, and patients are given medications in advance to limit side effects and prevent damage to the thyroid gland by the radiation. Other side effects are similar to those already mentioned.

Anti-EGFR monoclonal antibodies: Another type of monoclonal antibody currently in use is called anti-EGFR. There is a family of receptors found on the surface of normal and cancer cells called human epidermal growth factor receptors (EGFR). Something called an "epidermal growth factor" binds to these receptor proteins, causing the cells to divide. In healthy cells, an amount of this protein on the cell surface reacts with the growth factors that come along, and cell division remains within normal limits. The problem comes when there are abnormally high levels of this receptor protein on the cell surface (such as in many types of cancer cells); scientists believe these elevated levels may be partly responsible for the fact that cancer cells divide and multiply uncontrollably. Specific tests can measure whether the amount of the EGFR protein on the cancer cells is abnormally high or not. This can affect the kind of treatment that is recommended for the person with cancer. There are at least four members of this genetic "family," and they are called HER1, HER2, HER3, and HER4.

One important member of this family, HER2, is used to identify whether there is risk for excessive growth in certain cells. If the HER2 growth signal is unusually strong ("HER2 positive"), the nucleus tells the cell to divide and grow rapidly, which contributes to the development of a more aggressive cancer. Studies in cancer patients have shown that about 25–30% of all women with breast cancer have too many HER2 receptors. This seems to be an important reason that tumor cells grow and divide so rapidly. Knowledge of a woman's HER2 status can affect her course of treatment for breast cancer.

Herceptin (trastuzumab) is the first monoclonal antibody created from human cells and approved by the FDA for the treatment of HER2-positive metastatic breast cancer. Herceptin works by targeting tumor cells that have too many HER2 receptors (also known as HER2 overexpression). When the cell signal is stopped, the cancer cells' ability to continue to grow and divide is also stopped. This process is unique because only cells with HER2 overexpression are targeted by Herceptin. Standard chemotherapy kills cells that are dividing, which means both breast cancer cells and normal cells are destroyed. This causes many of the side effects associated with chemotherapy, such as hair loss, nausea and vomiting, and risk of infection and bleeding. Since Herceptin interferes with the cell signaling in only the breast cancer cells, there are fewer side effects. However, some problems with cardiac toxicity may prevent some patients from receiving this antibody.

Herceptin is approved for women with breast cancer

- for first-line (first treatment after diagnosis) use in combination with a chemotherapy drug called Taxol (paclitaxel), and
- as a single agent (used alone) in second- and third-line treatment after the breast cancer has recurred.

Thousands of women have had a good response to this drug; their cancer has reduced in size or disappeared. It is not yet known how long the drug should be given, so research is ongoing. Herceptin has become a landmark biologic therapy for women with HER2-overexpressive metastatic cancer.

Erbitux (cetuximab) is another new anti-EGFR monoclonal antibody treatment, but it targets a different member of the EGFR family: the HER1 receptor, which is also just called EGFR. This monoclonal antibody has been found in clinical trials to bind with the HER1 or EGFR receptor to stop cell growth signals in people with colon cancer. It has been discovered that many people with colon cancer have EGFR overexpression (too many EGFR [HER1] receptors are found on the cell surface). When Erbitux binds with the receptor, the EGFR can no longer cause the tumor cells to grow and divide. Erbitux is approved by the FDA for patients with metastatic colon cancer, and it can be used alone or with another drug. It is administered intravenously.

Both of the anti-EGFR monoclonal antibodies listed here, Herceptin and Erbitux, can be given safely. However, infusion reactions can occur (fever, chills, nausea), especially during the first treatment. There are also side effects, such as an acne-like rash, weakness, and diarrhea. Many of these side effects can be lessened with medications.

Other Biological Therapies

Biological therapy is a type of treatment that works with your immune system. It can help fight cancer or help control side effects from other cancer treatments, such as chemotherapy. Biological therapy and chemotherapy are both treatments that fight cancer. Biological therapy helps your immune system fight cancer. Chemotherapy attacks the cancer cells directly. There is some overlap to this, but that is generally a good way to view the differences, as not all the ways in which biological therapies help are understood.

Generally these therapies tend to stop or slow the growth of cancer cells, make it easier for your immune system to destroy or get rid of cancer cells, and keep cancer from spreading to other parts of your body. They interact with your spleen, lymph nodes, tonsils, bone marrow, and white blood cells, which comprise the immune system. The white blood cells in particular have many subtypes with very specific ranges of functions; some attack right away, some assist, some make antibodies, and some create memories and oversee it all.

There are many forms of biological therapy. One is cancer vaccines. While other vaccines (like ones for measles or mumps) are given before you get sick, most cancer vaccines are given after you have cancer. (The vaccine to prevent cervical cancer is one notable exception.) Cancer vaccines may help your body fight the cancer and keep it from coming back. Doctors are learning more all the time about cancer vaccines. They are now doing research about how cancer vaccines can help people diagnosed with melanoma, lymphoma, and kidney, breast, ovarian, prostate, colon, and rectal cancers. To date, none have shown exceptional promise (except the vaccine to prevent cervical cancer), but the work continues.

Other types of biological therapy are as follows:

- BCG, or bacillus Calmette-Guérin, treats bladder tumors or bladder cancer.
- IL-2 or Interleukin-2 treats certain types of cancer, such as melanoma and renal cell cancer.
- Interferon alpha treats certain types of cancer, such as melanoma, renal cell cancer, and some unusual tumors of the immune system.

A subset of biological therapy is immunomodulatory agents, which are drugs that can modify or regulate the functioning of the immune system. One notable example is thalidomide. These appear to have multiple actions, including both anticancer and anti-inflammatory activities. They affect the immune system in several ways. They induce immune responses, enhance activity of immune cells, and inhibit inflammation. These agents appear to alter the levels of various growth factors and affect cells of the immune system. They may also directly enhance our bodies' natural killer cells while suppressing factors made by cancer cells that might inhibit them. They may also inhibit the growth of new blood vessels (angiogenesis) through inhibition of vascular endothelial growth factor (more on this in a moment). They can induce cell death in some notoriously resistant cancers, such as multiple myeloma, and somehow partner with other cells of only modest effect on myeloma and increase their power.

Angiogenesis Inhibitors

Angiogenesis is the formation of new blood vessels. Tumors need blood vessels to grow and spread. Angiogenesis inhibitors are designed to prevent the formation of new blood vessels, thereby stopping or slowing the growth or spread of tumors. FDA has approved several angiogenesis inhibitors for the treatment of cancer. Angiogenesis inhibitors may have side effects that are different from those of other cancer treatments. In addition, they may only stop or slow the growth of a cancer, not completely eradicate it.

The process of angiogenesis is controlled by chemical signals in the body. These signals can stimulate both the repair of damaged blood vessels and the formation of new blood vessels. Other chemical signals, called angiogenesis inhibitors, interfere with blood vessel formation. Normally, the stimulating and inhibiting effects of these chemical signals are balanced so that blood vessels form only when and where they are needed.

Angiogenesis plays a critical role in the growth and spread of cancer. A blood supply is necessary for tumors to grow beyond a few millimeters in size. Tumors can cause this blood supply to form by giving off chemical signals that stimulate angiogenesis. Tumors can also stimulate nearby normal cells to produce angiogenesis-signaling molecules. The resulting new blood vessels "feed" growing tumors with oxygen and nutrients, allowing the cancer cells to invade nearby tissues, move throughout the body, and form new colonies of cancer cells called metastases.

Because tumors cannot grow beyond a certain size or spread without a blood supply, scientists are trying to find ways to block tumor angiogenesis. They are studying natural and synthetic angiogenesis inhibitors, also called antiangiogenic agents, with the idea that these molecules will prevent or slow the growth of cancer.

Angiogenesis requires the binding of signaling molecules, such as vascular endothelial growth factor (VEGF), to receptors on the surface of normal endothelial (blood vessel wall) cells. When VEGF and other endothelial growth factors bind to their receptors on endothelial cells, signals within these cells are initiated that promote the growth and survival of new blood vessels.

The FDA has approved bevacizumab to be used alone for very malignant brain tumors and to be used in combination with other drugs to treat metastatic colorectal cancer, some non-small-cell lung cancers, and widespread renal cell cancer. Bevacizumab was the first angiogenesis inhibitor that was shown to slow tumor growth and, more important, to extend the lives of patients with some cancers. The FDA has approved other drugs that have antiangiogenic activity.

Angiogenesis inhibitors are unique cancer-fighting agents because they tend to inhibit the growth of blood vessels rather than tumor cells. In some cancers, angiogenesis inhibitors are most effective when combined with additional therapies, especially chemotherapy. It has been hypothesized that these drugs help normalize the blood vessels that supply the tumor, facilitating the delivery of other anticancer agents. This possibility is still being investigated. Angiogenesis inhibitor therapy does not necessarily kill tumors but instead may prevent tumors from growing. Therefore, this type of therapy may need to be administered over a long period.

These drugs are not free of side effects, and not surprisingly, studies have revealed the potential for complications that reflect the importance of angiogenesis in many normal body processes, such as wound healing, heart and kidney function, fetal development, and reproduction. Side effects of treatment with angiogenesis inhibitors can include problems with bleeding, clots in the arteries (with resultant stroke or heart attack), hypertension, and protein in the urine It is likely that some of the possible complications of angiogenesis inhibitor therapy remain unknown. As more patients are treated with these agents, doctors will learn more about possible side effects and their frequencies.

Bone Marrow and Stem Cell Transplantation

Blood-forming stem cells are immature cells that can mature into blood cells. These stem cells are found in the bone marrow, bloodstream, or umbilical cord blood. Bone marrow transplantation and peripheral-blood stem cell transplantation are procedures that restore stem cells that were destroyed by high doses of chemotherapy and/or radiation therapy. In general, patients are less likely to develop a complication known as graft-versus-host disease (GVHD; "graft" referring to the donor's cells and "host" referring to the patient's cells) if the stem cells of the donor and patient are closely genetically matched.

After being treated with high-dose anticancer drugs and/or radiation, the patient receives the harvested stem cells, which travel to the bone marrow and begin to produce new blood cells.

A "mini-transplant" uses lower, less toxic doses of chemotherapy and/or radiation to prepare the patient for transplant. A "tandem transplant" involves two sequential courses of high-dose chemotherapy and stem cell transplant.

Understanding the nature of a stem cell is crucial to grasping why science and medicine have looked, with some considerable successes, into giving very high, potentially lethal, levels of chemotherapy to patients with various malignancies (most of them of the bone marrow itself) and then rescuing patients with stem cells from bone marrow, circulating blood sources, or umbilical cord blood.

The bone marrow is the soft, spongelike material found inside bones. It contains immature cells known as hematopoietic, or blood-forming, stem cells. Hematopoietic stem cells are different from embryonic stem cells. Embryonic stem cells can develop into every type of cell in the body. Hematopoietic stem cells divide to form more blood-forming stem cells, or they mature into one of three types of blood cells: white blood cells, which fight infection; red blood cells, which carry oxygen; and platelets, which help the blood to clot. Most hematopoietic stem cells are found in the bone marrow, but some cells, called peripheral-blood stem cells (PBSCs), are found in the bloodstream. Blood in the umbilical cord also contains hematopoietic stem cells. Bone marrow transplantation (BMT) and peripheral-blood stem cell transplantation (PBSCT) are procedures that restore stem cells that have been destroyed by high doses of chemotherapy and/or radiation therapy. The hope is that the high doses, which otherwise might be lethal, will be lethal for the primary cancer being treated and the marrow cells will then rescue the patient and repopulate the marrow and blood.

There are three types of transplants:

- auotologous transplants, in which patients receive their own stem cells
- syngeneic transplants, in which patients receive stem cells from their identical twin
- allogeneic transplants, in which patients receive stem cells from their brother, sister, or parent, or from an unrelated donor who is a close match to the patient in the antigenic fingerprint of the blood

Furthermore, in some types of leukemia, the graft-versus-tumor (GVT) effect that occurs after allogeneic BMT and PBSCT is crucial to the effectiveness of the treatment. GVT occurs when white blood cells from the donor (the graft) identify the cancer cells (the tumor) that remain in the patient's body after the chemotherapy or radiation therapy as foreign and attack them.

BMT and PBSCT are most commonly used in the treatment of leukemia and lymphoma. They are most effective when the leukemia or lymphoma is in remission (when the signs and symptoms of cancer have disappeared). BMT and PBSCT are also used to treat other cancers, such as neuroblastoma (cancer that arises in immature nerve cells and affects mostly infants and children) and multiple myeloma. Researchers are evaluating BMT and PBSCT in clinical research studies for the treatment of various types of cancer.

Matching of the graft from the donor to the recipient on a genetic basis is necessary, as the recipient's immune system still will have enough retained ability to recognize the donor as foreign and can begin to attack it. Thus, transplants between identical twins have some advantages, and matching of genetic similarity to special classes of antigens is necessary before attempting transplant. People have different sets of proteins, called human leukocyte-associated (HLA) antigens, on the surfaces of their cells. The higher the number of matching HLA antigens, the greater the chance that the patient's body will accept the donor's stem cells. In general, patients are less likely to develop GVHD if the stem cells of the donor and patient are closely matched. Close relatives, especially brothers and sisters, are more likely than unrelated people to be HLA-matched. However, only 25 to 35% of patients have an HLA-matched sibling. Large volunteer donor registries can assist in finding an appropriate unrelated donor.

The stem cells used in BMT come from the liquid center of the bone, called the marrow. In general, the procedure for obtaining bone marrow, which is called harvesting, is similar for all three types of BMTs—autologous, syngeneic, and allogeneic. Harvesting the marrow takes about an hour.

The harvested bone marrow is then processed to remove blood and bone fragments. Harvested bone marrow can be combined with a preservative and frozen to keep the stem cells alive until they are needed. Stem cells can be cryopreserved for many years.

The stem cells used in PBSCT come from the bloodstream. Aphaeresis (selectively removing and harvesting them) typically takes four to six hours. The stem cells are then frozen until they are given to the recipient. Stem cells also may be retrieved from umbilical cord blood.

The stem cells used for autologous transplantation must be relatively free of cancer cells. The harvested cells can sometimes be treated before transplantation in a process known as "purging" to get rid of cancer cells. This process can remove some cancer cells from the harvested cells and minimize the chance that cancer will come back.

After entering the bloodstream, the stem cells travel to the bone marrow, where they begin to produce new white blood cells, red blood cells, and platelets in a process known as "engraftment." Engraftment usually occurs within about two to four weeks after transplantation. Complete recovery of immune function takes much longer, however—up to several months for autologous transplant recipients and one to two years for patients receiving allogeneic or syngeneic transplants. Doctors evaluate the results of various blood tests to confirm that new blood cells are being produced and that the cancer has not returned.

The major risk of both treatments is an increased susceptibility to infection and bleeding as a result of the high-dose cancer treatment. Doctors may give the patient antibiotics and blood products. Patients who undergo BMT and PBSCT may experience short-term side effects, such as nausea, vomiting, fatigue, loss of appetite, mouth sores, hair loss, and skin reactions. Potential long-term risks include complications of the pretransplant chemotherapy and radiation therapy, such as infertility, cataracts of the eye, secondary (new) cancers, and damage to the liver, kidneys, lungs, and heart.

With allogeneic transplants, GVHD sometimes develops when white blood cells from the donor (the graft) identify cells in the body of the patient (the host) as foreign and attack them. The most commonly damaged organs are the skin, liver, and intestines. This complication can develop within a few weeks of the transplant or much later. To prevent this complication, the patient may receive medications that suppress the immune system. GVHD can be difficult to treat, but some studies suggest that patients with leukemia who develop GVHD are less likely to have the cancer come back.

A "mini-transplant" is a type of allogeneic transplant. This approach is being studied in clinical trials for the treatment of several types of cancer, including leukemia, lymphoma, multiple myeloma, and other cancers of the blood. A mini-transplant uses lower, less toxic doses of chemotherapy and/or radiation to prepare the patient for an allogeneic transplant. The use of lower doses of anticancer drugs and radiation eliminates some, but not all, of the patient's bone marrow. It also reduces the number of cancer cells and suppresses the patient's immune system to prevent rejection of the transplant.

Unlike traditional BMT or PBSCT, cells from both the donor and the patient may exist in the patient's body for some time after a mini-transplant. Once the cells from the donor begin to engraft, they may cause the GVT effect and work to destroy the cancer cells that were not eliminated by the anticancer drugs and/or radiation. To boost the GVT effect, the patient may be given an injection of the donor's white blood cells. This procedure is called a donor lymphocyte infusion.

A "tandem transplant" is a type of autologous transplant. This method is being studied in clinical trials for the treatment of several types of cancer, including multiple myeloma and germ cell cancer. During a tandem transplant, a patient receives two sequential courses of high-dose chemotherapy with stem cell transplant. Typically, the two courses are given several weeks to several months apart.

Targeted Cancer Therapies

Targeted cancer therapies are drugs or other substances that block the growth and spread of cancer by interfering with specific molecules involved in tumor growth and progression. We have already addressed monoclonal antibodies as well as thalidomide and antiangiogenesis. There are some more remarkable examples of the notion of having a specific molecular target with targeted drugs. Targeted cancer therapies that have been approved for use in specific cancers include drugs that (1) interfere with cell growth signaling or tumor blood vessel development, (2) promote the specific death of cancer cells, (3) stimulate the immune system to destroy specific cancer cells, and (4) deliver toxic drugs to cancer cells. By focusing on molecular and cellular changes that are specific to cancer, targeted cancer therapies may be more effective than other types of treatment, including chemotherapy and radiotherapy, and less harmful to normal cells.

Many targeted cancer therapies have been approved by the FDA for the treatment of specific types of cancer. Others are being studied in clinical trials, and many more are in preclinical testing (research studies with animals).Targeted cancer therapies are being studied for use alone, in combination with other targeted therapies, and in combination with other cancer treatments, such as chemotherapy.

The general idea is that targeted cancer therapies interfere with cancer cell division (proliferation) and cancer spread in different ways. Many of these therapies focus on proteins that are involved in cell-signaling pathways. Signaling pathways form a complex communication system that governs basic cellular functions and activities, such as cell division, cell movement, cell responses to specific external stimuli, and even cell death. By blocking signals that tell cancer cells to grow and divide uncontrollably, targeted cancer therapies can help stop cancer progression and may induce cancer cell death through a process known as apoptosis. Other targeted therapies can cause cancer cell death directly, by specifically inducing apoptosis, or indirectly, by stimulating the immune system to recognize and destroy cancer cells or by delivering toxic substances directly to the cancer cells.

The development of targeted therapies, therefore, requires the identification of good targets—targets that are known to play a key role in cancer cell growth and survival. It is for this reason that targeted therapies are often referred to as the product of "rational drug design."

For example, earlier in the text we briefly addressed the Philadelphia chromosomes present in a chronic type of leukemia. Most cases of chronic myeloid leukemia (CML) are caused by the formation of a gene called *BCR-ABL*. This gene is formed when pieces of chromosome 9 and chromosome 22 break off and trade places. One of the changed chromosomes resulting from this switch contains part of the *ABL* gene from chromosome 9 fused to part of the *BCR* gene from chromosome 22. The protein normally produced by the *ABL* gene (Abl) is a signaling molecule that plays an important role in controlling the multiplication of tumor cells. Therefore, *BCR-ABL* represents a good molecule to target.

Once a target has been identified, a therapy must be developed. Most targeted therapies are either small-molecule drugs or monoclonal antibodies. Small-molecule drugs are typically able to diffuse into cells and can act on targets that are found inside the cell. Most monoclonal antibodies cannot penetrate the cell's exterior walls and are directed against targets that are outside cells or on the cell surface.

Candidates for small-molecule drugs are usually identified in studies known as drug screens, which are lab tests that look at the effects of thousands of test compounds on a specific target, such as BCR-ABL. The best candidates are then chemically modified to produce numerous closely related versions. These are tested to identify the most effective and specific drugs.

The first molecular target for targeted cancer therapy was the cellular receptor for the female sex hormone estrogen, which many breast cancers require for growth. When estrogen binds to the estrogen receptor (ER) inside cells, the resulting hormone-receptor complex activates the expression of specific genes, including genes involved in cell growth and proliferation. Research has shown that interfering with estrogen's ability to stimulate the growth of breast cancer cells that have these receptors (ER-positive breast cancer cells) is an effective treatment approach. Several drugs that interfere with estrogen binding to the ER have been approved by the FDA for the treatment of ER-positive breast cancer.

Some molecules cause cancer cells to die by interfering with the action of a large cellular structure called the proteasome, which degrades proteins. Proteasomes control the degradation of many proteins that regulate cell proliferation. By blocking this process, they cause cancer cells to die. Normal cells are affected too, but to a lesser extent. Ontak is approved for the treatment of some patients with cutaneous T-cell lymphoma (CTCL). It consists of Interleukin-2 (IL-2) protein sequences fused to diphtheria toxin. The drug binds to cell-surface IL-2 receptors, which are found on certain immune cells and some cancer cells, directing the killing action of the diphtheria toxin to these cells.

Gene Therapy for Cancer

Gene therapy is an experimental treatment that involves introducing genetic material into a person to fight or prevent disease. Researchers are studying gene therapy for cancer through a number of different approaches.

A gene can be delivered to a cell using a carrier known as a vector. The most common types of vectors used in gene therapy are viruses. The viruses used in gene therapy are altered to make them safe; however, some risks still exist with gene therapy.

Genes are the biological units of heredity. Genes determine obvious traits, such as hair and eye color, as well as more subtle characteristics. Complex characteristics, such as physical strength or musical aptitude, may be shaped by the interaction of a number of different genes along with environmental influences. They are located on chromosomes inside cells and are made of DNA, which was discussed previously. We have between thirty thousand and forty thousand genes carrying instructions for proteins or enzymes in our bodies.

Only certain genes in a cell are active at any given moment. As cells mature, many genes become permanently inactive. The pattern of active and inactive genes in a cell and the resulting protein composition determine what kind of cell it is and what it can and cannot do. For example, "liverness" is turned on in liver cells, while everything but that is turned off.

Gene therapy is an experimental treatment that involves introducing genetic material (DNA or RNA) into a person's cells to fight disease. Gene therapy is being studied in clinical trials (research studies using people) for many different types of cancer It is not currently available outside a clinical trial. Some approaches target healthy cells to enhance their ability to fight cancer. Other approaches target cancer cells, to destroy them or prevent their growth. In one approach, researchers replace missing or altered genes with healthy genes. Because some missing or altered genes may cause cancer, substituting "working" copies of these genes may be used to treat cancer.

Researchers are also studying ways to improve a patient's immune response to cancer. In this approach, gene therapy is used to stimulate the body's natural ability to attack cancer cells. In addition, scientists are investigating the insertion of genes into cancer cells to make them more sensitive to chemotherapy, radiation therapy, or other treatments. In other studies, researchers remove healthy blood-forming stem cells from the body, insert a gene that makes these cells more resistant to the side effects of high doses of anticancer drugs, and then inject the cells back into the patient. In another approach, researchers introduce "suicide genes" into a patient's cancer cells. A pro-drug (an inactive form of a toxic drug) is then given to the patient. The pro-drug is activated in cancer cells containing these suicide genes, which leads to the destruction of those cancer cells. Other research is focused on the use of gene therapy to prevent cancer cells from developing new blood vessels.

Most genetic material cannot be directly inserted into a person's cell. It must be delivered to the cell using a carrier, or vector. The vectors most commonly used in gene therapy are viruses. Viruses have a unique ability to recognize certain cells and insert genetic material into them. The insertion of these viruses is sometimes done by inoculation and sometimes by removing cells and exposing them to the desired virus and then reinfusing these new cells.

Scientists alter the viruses used in gene therapy to make them safe for humans and to increase their ability to deliver specific genes to a patient's cells. Depending on the type of virus and the goals of the research study, scientists may inactivate certain genes in the viruses to prevent them from reproducing or causing disease. Researchers may also alter the virus so that it better recognizes and enters the target cell.

Viruses can usually infect more than one type of cell. Thus, when viral vectors are used to carry genes into the body, they might infect healthy cells as well as cancer cells, causing mutation, and there is a remote chance of their being introduced into reproductive cells. Other concerns include the possibility that transferred genes could be "overexpressed," producing so much of the missing protein as to be harmful. Alternatively, the viral vector could cause inflammation or an immune reaction, and theoretically the virus could be transmitted from the patient to other individuals or into the environment. Scientists use animal testing and other precautions to identify and avoid these risks before any clinical trials are conducted in humans, as well as a number of ethical and scientific reviews.

Scientists working on the Human Genome Project (HGP), which has completed mapping and sequencing all of the genes in humans, recognized that the information gained from this work would have profound implications for individuals, families, and society. The Ethical, Legal, and Social Implications (ELSI) Research Program was established in 1990 as part of the HGP to address these issues. The ELSI Research Program fosters basic and applied research on the ethical, legal, and social implications of genetic and genomic research for individuals, families, and communities. The ELSI Research Program sponsors and manages studies and supports workshops, research consortia, and policy conferences on these topics.

Hyperthermia

Hyperthermia is a type of cancer treatment in which body tissue is exposed to high temperatures (up to 113°F) to damage and kill cancer cells. Hyperthermia is almost always used with other forms of cancer therapy, such as radiation therapy and chemotherapy. Several methods of hyperthermia are currently under study, including local, regional, and whole-body hyperthermia. Many clinical trials (research studies) are being conducted to evaluate the effectiveness of hyperthermia.

Research has shown that high temperatures can damage and kill cancer cells, usually with minimal injury to normal tissues By killing cancer cells and damaging proteins and structures within cancer cells, hyperthermia may shrink tumors. Hyperthermia is almost always used with other forms of cancer therapy, such as radiation therapy and chemotherapy. Hyperthermia may make some cancer cells more sensitive to radiation or harm other cancer cells that radiation cannot damage. When hyperthermia and radiation therapy are combined, they are often given within an hour of each other. Hyperthermia can also enhance the effects of certain anticancer drugs.

Several methods of hyperthermia are currently under study, including local, regional, and whole-body hyperthermia. In local hyperthermia, heat is applied to a small area, such as a tumor, using various techniques that deliver energy to heat the tumor. Different types of energy may be used to apply heat, including microwave, radiofrequency, and ultrasound. Depending on the tumor location, there are several approaches to local hyperthermia. External approaches are used to treat tumors that are in or just below the skin. External applicators are positioned around or near the appropriate region, and energy is focused on the tumor to raise its temperature.

Intraluminal or endocavitary methods may be used to treat tumors within or near body cavities, such as the esophagus or rectum. Probes are placed inside the cavity and inserted into the tumor to deliver energy and heat the area directly. Interstitial techniques are used to treat tumors deep within the body, such as brain tumors. This technique allows the tumor to be heated to higher temperatures than external techniques. Under anesthesia, probes or needles are inserted into the tumor. Imaging techniques, such as ultrasound, may be used to make sure the probe is properly positioned within the tumor. The heat source is then inserted into the probe.

Radio-frequency ablation (RFA) is a type of interstitial hyperthermia that uses radio waves to heat and kill cancer cells. In regional hyperthermia, various approaches may be used to heat large areas of tissue, such as a body cavity, organ, or limb. Deep-tissue approaches may be used to treat cancers within the body, such as cervical or bladder cancer. External applicators are positioned around the body cavity or organ to be treated, and microwave or radio-frequency energy is focused on the area to raise its temperature.

Regional perfusion techniques can be used to treat cancers in the arms and legs, such as melanoma, or cancer in some organs, such as the liver or lungs. In this procedure, some of the patient's blood is removed, heated, and then pumped (perfused) back into the limb or organ. Anticancer drugs are commonly administered during this treatment.

Continuous hyperthermic peritoneal perfusion is a technique used to treat cancers within the peritoneum (the space within the abdomen that contains the intestines, stomach, and liver), including primary peritoneal mesothelioma and stomach cancer. During surgery, heated anticancer drugs flow from a warming device through the peritoneal cavity. The peritoneal cavity temperature reaches 106–108°F.

Whole-body hyperthermia is used to treat metastatic cancer that has spread throughout the body. This can be accomplished by several techniques that raise the body temperature to 107–108°F, including the use of thermal chambers (similar to large incubators) or hot-water blankets.

Most normal tissues are not damaged during hyperthermia if the temperature remains under 111°F. However, because of regional differences in tissue characteristics, higher temperatures may occur in various spots. This can result in burns, blisters, discomfort, or pain. Perfusion techniques can cause tissue swelling, blood clots, bleeding, and other damage to the normal tissues in the perfused area; however, most of these side effects are temporary. Whole-body hyperthermia can cause more serious side effects, including cardiac and vascular disorders, but these effects are uncommon. Diarrhea, nausea, and vomiting are commonly observed after whole-body hyperthermia.

A number of challenges must be overcome before hyperthermia can be considered a standard treatment for cancer.

Laser

Laser light can be used to remove cancer or precancerous growths or to relieve symptoms of cancer. It is used most often to treat cancers on the surface of the body or on the linings of internal organs. Laser therapy is often given through a thin tube called an endoscope, which can be inserted in openings in the body to treat cancer or precancerous growths inside the trachea (windpipe), esophagus, stomach, or colon. Laser therapy causes less bleeding and damage to normal tissue than standard surgical tools do, and there is a lower risk of infection. However, the effects of laser surgery may not be permanent, so the surgery may have to be repeated.

The term "laser" stands for light amplification by stimulated emission of radiation. Ordinary light, such as that from a light bulb, has many wavelengths and spreads in all directions. Laser light, on the other hand, has a specific wavelength. It is focused in a narrow beam and creates a very high-intensity light. This powerful beam of light may be used to cut through steel or to shape diamonds. Because lasers can focus very accurately on tiny areas, they can also be used for very precise surgical work or for cutting through tissue (in place of a scalpel).

Lasers are most commonly used to treat superficial cancers (cancers on the surface of the body or the linings of internal organs), such as basal-cell skin cancer and the very early stages of some cancers, such as cervical, penile, vaginal, vulvar, and non-small-cell lung cancer. Lasers can be used to shrink or destroy a tumor that is blocking a patient's trachea (windpipe) or esophagus. They may also be used to remove colon polyps or tumors that are blocking the colon or stomach.

Laser therapy can be used alone, but most often it is combined with other treatments, such as surgery, chemotherapy, or radiation therapy. In addition, lasers can seal nerve endings to reduce pain after surgery and seal lymph vessels to reduce swelling and limit the spread of tumor cells.

Laser therapy is often given through a flexible endoscope (a thin, lighted tube used to look at tissues inside the body). The endoscope is fitted with optical fibers (thin fibers that transmit light). It is inserted through an opening in the body, such as the mouth, nose, anus, or vagina. Laser light is then precisely aimed to cut or destroy a tumor.

Lasers are more precise than standard surgical tools (scalpels), so they do less damage to normal tissues. As a result, patients usually experience less pain, bleeding, swelling, and scarring with laser therapy than with traditional surgery. With laser therapy, operations are usually shorter. In fact, laser therapy can often be done on an outpatient basis. It takes less time for patients to heal after laser surgery than traditional surgery, and they are less likely to get infections.

Laser therapy also has several limitations. Surgeons must have specialized training before they can perform laser therapy, and strict safety precautions must be followed. Laser therapy is expensive and requires bulky equipment. In addition, the effects of laser therapy may not last long, so doctors may have to repeat the treatment for a patient to get the full benefit.

Photodynamic Therapy

Photodynamic therapy (PDT) combines a drug called a photosensitizer or photosensitizing agent with a specific type of light to kill cancer cells When photosensitizers are exposed to a specific wavelength of light, they produce a form of oxygen that kills nearby cells. Each photosensitizer is activated by light of a specific wavelength. This wavelength determines how far the light can travel into the body. Thus doctors use specific photosensitizers and wavelengths of light to treat different areas of the body with PDT.

In the first step of PDT for cancer treatment, a photosensitizing agent is injected into the bloodstream. The agent is absorbed by cells all over the body but stays in cancer cells longer than it does in normal cells. Approximately twenty-four to seventy-two hours after injection, when most of the agent has left normal cells but remains in cancer cells, the tumor is exposed to light. The photosensitizer in the tumor absorbs the light and produces an active form of oxygen that destroys nearby cancer cells.

In addition to directly killing cancer cells, PDT appears to shrink or destroy tumors in two other ways. The photosensitizer can damage blood vessels in the tumor, thereby preventing the cancer from receiving necessary nutrients. PDT also may activate the immune system to attack the tumor cells.

The light used for PDT can come from a laser or other sources. Laser light can be directed through fiber-optic cables (thin fibers that transmit light) to deliver light to areas inside the body. For example, a fiber optic cable can be inserted through an endoscope (a thin, lighted flexible tube used to look at tissues inside the body) into the lungs or esophagus to treat cancer in these organs. Other light sources, include light-emitting diodes (LEDs), may be used for surface tumors, such as skin cancer.

PDT is usually performed as an outpatient procedure. PDT may also be repeated and may be used with other therapies, such as surgery, radiation, and chemotherapy.

Extracorporeal photopheresis (ECP) is a type of PDT in which a machine is used to collect the patient's blood cells, treat them outside the body with a photosensitizing agent, expose them to light, and then return them to the patient. The FDA has approved ECP to help lessen the severity of skin symptoms of cutaneous T-cell lymphoma that has not responded to other therapies. Studies are underway to determine if ECP may have some application for other blood cancers, and also to help reduce rejection after transplants.

PDT has its limitations. The light needed to activate most photosensitizers cannot pass through more than about one-third of an inch of tissue (one centimeter). For this reason, PDT is usually used to treat tumors on or just under the skin or on the linings of internal organs or cavities. PDT is thus less effective than other methods in treating large tumors, because the light cannot pass far into these tumors. PDT is a local treatment and generally cannot be used to treat cancer that has spread (metastasized). The skin and eyes of a patient who has undergone PDT will be sensitive to light for approximately six weeks after treatment. Thus, patients are advised to avoid direct sunlight and bright indoor light for at least six weeks.

CLINICAL TRIALS IN ONCOLOGY

A clinical oncology trial is a defined treatment regimen of highly similar patients that is performed for testing a drug, device, surgical procedure, or other intervention to determine effectiveness and safety in preventing, alleviating, or curing cancer. This mandates that there be obvious room for improvement regarding the benefits of conventional therapies.

Current definitions of good clinical practice in clinical trials can be found in the World Medical Association's *Declaration of Helsinki*, the *Belmont Report*, or *Good Practice: Consolidated Guidelines*. These documents underscore and emphasize all of the areas of medical law and ethics covered in this book. The single most important principle of clinical trials is that the rights of the patient must come first and their ability to give informed consent via extensive and thorough informed consent documents written at the eighth-grade level is mandatory. Institutional review boards must ensure this and monitor studies frequently as they progress. Using ethical vocabulary, the principle of autonomy is assured through the informed consent process. Consents of patients to participate in clinical trials must not be coerced, and all alternatives to participation must be presented in detail and in a manner that the patient can clearly understand. The patient has the right to have all questions answered and may remove himself or herself from the study at any time. There must be no fear that medical care will be suboptimal or withheld if the patient does not participate. Consent must be obtained again if the trial is amended or as new data become available. The principles of beneficence (acting for the welfare of the patient) and justice must apply where known. Anticipated risks must be clearly weighed, and the goods must outweigh the harms. All participants must have a fair share in any benefit. The trial must have clinical scientific merit that can be supported by the best available data at the time as reasonable, rational, prudent, doable, and timely. A mechanism for scrupulously monitoring safety and unexpected developments must be established.

There are various types of trials conceptually. There are prevention trials, which are concerned with the health and prevention of cancer in those without cancer but at risk. There are diagnostic trials, which focus on means of identifying a tumor earlier or more accurately. Therapeutic trials are concerned with improvement of symptoms, improving rates of response to therapy, duration of response, duration of freedom from relapse, or odds of survival.

Rather than treat patients prospectively with experimental therapy versus standard or conventional therapy and following them for long periods, trials may be retrospective. This refers to the comparison of treatment groups to markedly similar patients from the past. Although there are inherent shortcomings and pitfalls with retrospective trials, they may be the only type of trial feasible in some circumstances, such as very rare disorders. Prospective trials try to demonstrate whether there is equivalence or superiority of one treatment over another in highly similar patients that differ only in the therapy they received. A longitudinal trial collects and measures all manner of information about the patients being treated perpetually and longitudinally over time. A cross-sectional trial measures predefined parameters from the same participants at one point in time. Participants in parallel trials and crossover trials are followed longitudinally during treatment, and then, after a predefined period, allowing for a "washout" of effect of the first treatment, they may cross over to the other parallel arm of treatment in the trial. Scientists are able to calculate in advance for each trial how many patients are needed in each treatment group to assure that meaningful statements can be made with statistical certainty at a high level that the results observed were not by chance and are thus reproducible for future patients treated similarly.

The National Cancer Institute Cooperative Group program is paid for by tax dollars and has approximately eight thousand investigators at 1,500 institutions enrolling over twenty thousand patients per year. That is not a lot when one considers that it represents at best 5–7% of all eligible patients for clinical trials and is how clinical oncology treatments are developed. At least one dozen multi-institutional groups receive funding this way. We are finally seeing international studies involving thousands of patients from dozens of countries with remarkable progress.

A patient should be informed as to what exactly the end points being measured are. There are common clinical end points. A complete response is disappearance of all disease for at least four weeks. A partial response is a 50% reduction in the bidimensional or, if feasible, three-dimensional sum of the products of all the diameters of all the areas of tumors and no new areas. As an example, if there is one area of 3×5 cm, another of 2×6 cm and a third of 1×3cm, then one first calculates the dimensional products (15cm, 12 cm, and 3 cm) and then adds them together (30 cm). This is done at two points at times, and the results are compared to see mathematically just how much, overall, the total amount of measurable tumor decreased or increased in size. If different areas of tumor increase as well as decrease at the same time, it is a mixed response. Stable disease is when neither of the above applies. Progressive disease is when there is at least a 25% increase in the bidimensional or three-dimensional sum of the products of the diameters of all measurable disease. Overall response is the sum of partial and complete responses. In extremely aggressive tumors, we sometimes add to this calculation the areas of tumor that have not changed in size, as this represents a clinically meaningful success.

Event-free survival is the duration of time before something of clinical consequence occurs, such as establishment of disease-free status, death, or development of a certain advance in stage. It is common when portraying these landmarks to refer to the median, not the average number of events. The median is the point at which 50% are above and 50% are below the measured parameter, such as the point where one-half of the patients survived at a certain period or one-half responded to some degree. This is much more useful in reproducibly predicting the performance of future patients than the mathematical average. A few very high or low numbers can affect averages greatly. This could result in an artificially higher and lower result than would most likely occur over time if the same question was studied repeatedly.

It is critical that investigators do all they can to avoid introducing bias. Common examples of bias are enrolling too many patients from one institution, as that may overrepresent a certain demographic or healthy group; or the investigator, nurse, or patient knowing their treatment or selecting the treatment in advance. Thus we have single blinding or double blinding, where no one but a data coordinator, who knows the patient by number only, has the code of encryption that assigned a treatment. Thus, randomization, which is not as simple a process as tossing a coin or picking treatments according to even or odd social security numbers, is employed. Using a sophisticated statistical set of tools, a random (mathematically speaking) assignment of patients to treatment regimens is performed. Another enormously important point is stratification, whereby all reasonable or probable variables that could alter a patient's chance are equally balanced between treatment groups. Otherwise, for example, one could be comparing young, strong folks with older, frail individuals with the same stage of the same tumor.

There must be very strict inclusion and exclusion criteria. Simply put, one must know that the population studied is relevant to the question and that its results will be referable to the general population of similar cancer patients—the whole point of the study. Once again, there is no room for cutting corners or skimping on details of prescreening patients.

A controlled study means there are at least two distinct treatment approaches in the study to which patients are randomly assigned. These are called arms. One arm receives the known conventional therapy and is referred to as being in the control arm. Another population, as identical as possible, receives an experimental treatment. It is best to have active contemporaneous controls rather than "historical" patients from prior studies that seem to be similar, as this increases the chance that whatever outcome is seen is going to be valid and, most importantly, reproducible for future patients. Nonetheless, there are always confounding variables, often called covariates; thus stratification, as discussed earlier, is needed. This refers to various clinical parameters, demographics, prior therapies, and all manner of variables that may be out of balance in one group versus the other and could potentially influence the results and thus confound them. Thus, immense expertise is essential, and well-constructed monitoring is the rule. On a happy note, the field of oncology is as close to a paradigm or gold standard for how to perform clinical trials in medicine as there is. The specialty was born from them, is sustained by them, and advances because of them.

There are four phases of trials. Phase 1 trials are not intended to be specific for the treatment of an individual tumor type. These trials occur only after very extensive laboratory and animal testing suggests that they may be of some benefit and toxicity is largely predictable, acceptable, and manageable. The intent of these trials is to investigate if there is any possibility of benefit from a new treatment. They are targeted at patients for whom there is no known conventional therapy that holds any greater meaningful promise. The goal of these trials is not to establish or define odds of response; rather, these trials are designed as the first step of clinical research. Thus, they are designed to establish the maximum tolerated dose of the treatment regimen in humans. Statistically and practically, this means they require no more than thirty to forty patients, in most cases, to answer that first crucial question. Some patients may respond, and if so, that drug is destined for further study in more advanced trials.

Phase 2 trials are done based on responses seen in phase 1 trials. These trials are for those patients for whom there are no phase 3 or conventional therapies available. The intent is to obtain an estimate of the response of a specific tumor type. Thus, the tumor areas in these patients must be measurable, not just evaluable. An example of disease that is only evaluable would be a positive bone scan or fluid around the lungs. It is clear that the tumor is there, but it cannot be reliably measured. Phase 2 trials are usually limited to twenty-five to fifty patients. Researchers also determine what minimum rate of successful response must be seen for the trial to continue forward. This varies with each tumor, as there some tumors for which a very high response rate is expected. A large response rate from a phase 2 trial, which must be at least equivalent to presently available conventional therapy and not highly toxic or practically burdensome, is necessary for the treatment to proceed to the next phase of trials. However, in notoriously resistant cancers, a relatively low rate of response of, say, 20% may still mean a breakthrough or some promise.

A phase 3 trial enrolls a predefined minimum of patients with the same tumor type who are as similar to each other as practical. Phase 3 trials compare a conventional therapy to a promising new therapy that is believed to have benefits at least equal to those of the conventional therapy. The hope is that the new treatment will be superior, whether that means it is less toxic, less costly, easier to administer, faster to respond, longer lasting, more likely to cure, or more likely to prevent relapse. The more patients who are similar in the treatment groups from different institutions, the more reliable the results will be in terms of reproducibility for future patients. It is not surprising that single-institution studies usually have better results than when other physicians in different locations try to reproduce the results. This is predictable and is known as institutional bias. The most meaningful results are those that can be replicated largely irrespective of the locale. Some studies have thousands of patients in multiple countries and may even take years to accrue enough patients. Some never meet enrollment goals.

A phase 4 trial is large-scale and occurs after the drug has received approval from the FDA as safe and effective. Such trials are known as post-marketing studies. They are essential in detecting rare but potentially serious side effects, as well as previously unobserved beneficial effects from the new therapy. Such studies are invaluable because the sum total of all the phase 1–3 prior study patients leading to approval are only stepping stones to fine-tuning the new therapy and appreciating all of its applications.

There is enormous misinformation regarding the speediness, skill, and quality of effort expended in the discovery and development of new therapies. There are literally tens of thousands of enormously committed and gifted researchers involved in drug development internationally.

Although it is a bit of political hot potato with strong opinions held in every corner, it is essential to dispel some myths regarding the pharmaceutical industry that are simply not deserved. Yearly, over fifteen thousand potions are considered for phase 1 trials. Less than 5% ever make it to FDA approval in a highly regarded, exemplary process that takes five to seven years, although fast tracks exist for particularly promising wonder drugs. The cost to bring a drug to the FDA is over five hundred million dollars.

Responsibility for the sustenance and development of clinical trials is shared. The government has a role in funding, education, and public awareness. Treating physicians must be advocates as well, assuring availability of trials for their patients. Patients must volunteer to enroll in trials and possibly help themselves. Once made aware that trials exist and are the lifeblood of progress in oncology, it is incumbent upon patients to investigate the possibility of participation. It should now be clear that those who participate are *not* guinea pigs. They are, in fact, heroic and responsible citizens of the world, making a great contribution, whose safety is *never* in question. To all the patients present and future, I say the world needs you and I need you. It will be my lymph node or nasty nodule someday. We are connected to another through these trials, and we must share, physicians and patients alike, in the collective embarrassment that only 5–7% of patients who are eligible enroll in clinical trials. Yet, even still, advances are overwhelming (read "The Future") with this mere pittance of participation. Imagine if we only doubled that. Unbelievable results would follow.

The world has agreed to classify and characterize the levels of evidence derived from trials, from those with strong support to those based only on expert opinion and no data. They range from I–V and are below:

- Level I: Evidence obtained from at least one properly designed and randomized controlled trial.
- Level II: Evidence obtained from well-designed controlled trials without randomization.
- Level III: Evidence obtained from well-designed cohort or case-control analytic studies, preferably from more than one center or research group.
- Level IV: Evidence obtained from multiple runs of the trial series with or without intervention. Dramatic results in uncontrolled trials might also be regarded as this type of evidence.
- Level V: Opinions of respected authorities, based on clinical experience, descriptive studies, or reports of expert committees.

Here are some practical suggestions for improving familiarity with the world of clinical trials. This material will complement the section pertaining to the Internet. The PDQ clinical trial database provides detailed information on trials currently going on in oncology regarding particular diseases. It can be found at cancernet.nci.nih.gov/pdq.htm. It can be searched by phase of study, disease site, drug name, geographic location, and institution. It also has separate user-friendly search forms for health professionals and patients. Cancerlit (cnedtb.nci.nih.gov/cancerlit.shtml) allows access to clinical trial abstracts that are presented at conferences but not yet available as manuscripts. Cancer Trials (cancertrials.nci.nih.gov) provides research news and background reading on clinical trials in oncology.

NCI CTC 2.0 (ctep.info.nih.gov/CT3/ctc.htm) is the commonly used rating system for grading of treatment-related toxicities. The FDA MedWatch program (www.fda.gov/medwatch) allows reporting for serious drug-related adverse events for off-label use. Lastly, detailed descriptions of predicted toxicities of experimental and conventional toxicities are always in the treatment protocol. This document is the detailed guidebook of exactly how treatment and monitoring is to proceed. *Everything* regarding the trial is present in it. Patients should become familiar with it but must keep in mind that it will list all toxicity that has ever been reported, not their probability of experiencing such toxicity. That probability is usually much less for an individual than he or she may think.

Some important sites for trial information are below:

- CALGB Cancer and Leukemia Group B
  www.calgb.uchicago.edu
- ECOG Eastern Cooperative Oncology Group
  ecog.dfci.Harvard.edu
- NCCTG North Central Cancer Treatment Group
  ncctg.mayo.edu
- NSABP National Surgical Adjuvant Breast and Bowel Project
  www.nsabp.pitt.edu
- POG Pediatric Oncology Group
  www.pog.ufl.edu

- RTOG Radiation Therapy Oncology Group
  www.rtog.org
- Southwest Oncology Group
  www.swog.saci.org
- European Org for Research Treatment of Cancer
  www.eortc.be
- National Cancer Institute of Canada Clinical Trial Group
  www.ctg.queensu.ca

The above sites contain ongoing protocols, inclusion and exclusion criteria, geographic sites of investigation, points of contact, and summaries of results from prior studies that the physician may base therapeutic recommendations on. Another excellent resource is "Should I enter a Clinical Trial? A Patient Reference Guide for Adults with a Serious or Life Threatening Illness" www.ecri.org/documents/bctoc2.html.

Statistics

Statistical analysis must be done on the results of all clinical trials. Those results, coupled with results reported from all the tumor registries, help us generate the data that tells us all those odds you are told, and they help us build better trials. Although the subject is rather dry and for only some readers, it bears mentioning that an understanding of statistical thinking is extremely helpful for the patient and irreplaceable for the treating team.

The Surveillance, Epidemiology, and End Results Program (SEER) is the focal point of the largest body of data regarding the rates of cancer over time in the United States. These rates are adjusted in a manner so that we can make intelligent observations relevant for specific age groups. If this were not done, cancer rates would increase over time simply because the US population is getting older, as the risk of cancer is higher in older age groups. It is thus critical to understand the language and vocabulary used when responsible scientists talk about risks. This is well explained on the NCI site at "An Overview of the SEER Cancer Statistics Review."

The National Cancer Institute (NCI) updates cancer statistics annually in a publication called the *SEER Cancer Statistics Review* (CSR).

This report summarizes the key measures of cancer's impact on the US population. NCI monitors these cancer statistics to assess progress and to identify population subgroups and geographic areas where cancer-control efforts need to be concentrated.

The CSR consists of a series of publications that have been produced annually by the SEER Program in NCI's Division of Cancer Control and Population Sciences. Data included in the books are compiled by the SEER Program, which has monitored occurrence of cancer and survival of patients since 1973 in 10% of the US population.

The tables, charts, and graphs of the SEER CSR present cancer incidence rates (the number of cases per one hundred thousand persons), cancer mortality rates (the number of deaths per one hundred thousand persons), and five-year relative survival (this five-year survival data estimates only the patients' risk of dying from cancer-related causes, not from other illnesses).

Data are given for all major cancer sites by age, sex, and race. Cancer incidence and survival data are collected by the SEER Program, while mortality data come from the National Center for Health Statistics (NCHS). The reports also provide data on trends in cancer incidence and mortality rates, American Cancer Society estimates of new cancer cases and cancer deaths, and measures of the years of life lost prematurely by those dying of cancer. These books contain estimates of the lifetime probabilities of developing cancer and probabilities of dying of cancer. These probabilities are presented by race, sex, and cancer site. In addition, probabilities of developing cancer up to a specific age are also included.

The SEER Program web page provides an online version of the CSR that may be viewed on computers equipped with Adobe Acrobat Reader software. To access this version of the report, go to the SEER web page (http://www-seer.ims.nci.nih.gov) and then click on "Publications," which will yield a list of options including the most recent CSR. Single print copies of the most recent edition of the SEER Cancer Statistics Review may be obtained by writing the Office of Cancer Communications, National Cancer Institute, 31 Center Drive MSC 2580, Building 31, Room 10A16, Bethesda, MD 20892-2580, or calling the NCI's Cancer Information Service at 1-800-4-CANCER (1-800-422-6237).

You will need some help with the terms and their definitions, so let's review some crucial concepts now.

Incidence—the number of newly diagnosed cases for a specific cancer or for all cancers combined during a specific time period. When expressed as a rate, it is the number of new cases per standard unit of population during the time period. Incidence rates can be calculated based on a number of factors, such as age, race, or sex.

Example: 9.0 cases of pancreatic cancer per 100,000 persons annually (all races, both sexes, for the period 1990–1994).

Mortality—the number of deaths for a specific cancer or for all cancers combined during a specific time period. When expressed as a rate, the number of deaths during a specific time period are per 100,000 persons. Mortality rates can be calculated based on a number of factors such as age, race, or sex. Example: 3.1 deaths from multiple myeloma per 100,000 persons annually (all races, both sexes, for the period 1990–1994).

Age-adjusted rate—an incidence or mortality rate that has been adjusted to reduce the effects of differences in the age distributions of the populations being compared. An age-adjusted rate is computed by weighting the age-specific rates in the population of interest by the proportions of persons in the corresponding age groups in a standard population, usually the 1970 US population. In addition, some rates are presented adjusted to the world standard population, permitting comparisons of rates in SEER Program areas with those from other countries that have also published rates adjusted to the world standard. Unless labeled "age-specific," all incidence and mortality rates in the CSR are age-adjusted rates.

Relative survival rate—an estimate of the percentage of patients that would be expected to survive the effects of their cancer. This rate is calculated by adjusting the observed survival rate so that the effects of causes of death other than those related to the cancer in question are removed. Observed survival is the actual percentage of patients still alive at some specified time after diagnosis of cancer. It considers deaths from all causes, cancer or otherwise.

Percent change—a measure of the change in incidence and mortality rates over a specified time interval. Percent changes are also provided for two five-year periods.

Estimated annual percent change (EAPC)—a measure of the estimated yearly percent change in incidence and mortality rates over a specified time interval.

Person years of life lost (PYLL)—the sum of years of life lost by all persons in a population who died of a particular cancer. Actuarial (life-expectancy) tables are used to project the years of life that would have remained for persons who died of cancer at a particular age. Example: In 1994, lung cancer had a PYLL of 2.23 million years for the United States (all races, both sexes).

Average years of life lost (AYLL)—the average years lost to a particular cancer among all persons who died of that cancer. It is calculated by dividing the PYLL for a particular cancer by the number of deaths from that cancer. Example: In 1994 melanoma had an AYLL of 19.4 years for the United States (all races, both sexes).

Significance—when comparing rates, statistical significance means differences between or among rates that are unlikely to have occurred merely by chance. For example, the probabilities that differences occurred by chance may be given as less than 1 in 10 (0.10) or less than 1 in 20 (0.05).

Standard error—a measure of the variability associated with a reported cancer statistic.

Time trend—the change in a cancer incidence or mortality rate (increasing, decreasing, or not changing) over time and the magnitude of that change.

The performance of screening tests is usually measured in terms of sensitivity, specificity, and positive and negative predictive values (PPV and NPV). Sensitivity is the chance that a person with cancer will have a positive test. Specificity is the chance a person without cancer will have a negative test. PPV is the chance that a person with a positive test has cancer. NPV is the chance that a person with a negative test does not have cancer. PPV and, to a lesser degree, NPV are affected by the prevalence of disease in the screened population. For a given sensitivity and specificity, the higher the prevalence, the higher the PPV.

Briefly, relative risk (RR) compares the risk of developing cancer among people who have a specific characteristic being studied (like smoking one pack a day) compared to those who do not. If the relative risk is greater than one, the exposure or characteristic is associated with a higher cancer risk; if the relative risk is one, the exposure and cancer are not associated with one another; if the relative risk is less than one, the exposure is associated with a lower cancer risk.

An odds ratio (OR) is often used as an estimate of the relative risk. It is similar to how most laymen use the expression "What are the odds of my getting cancer if I smoked one pack a day for twenty years?" It also indicates whether there is an association between an exposure or characteristic and cancer. It compares the odds of an exposure or characteristic among cancer cases with the odds among a comparison group without cancer. When you compare the odds ratio—the relative risk (that is, the chances of two groups of folks who largely differ only in the "risky" behavior being studied, such as smokers versus nonsmokers)—you develop what is called risk or rate difference (or excess risk). This compares the actual cancer risk or rate among at least two groups of people, based on an important characteristic or exposure. This can be used in public health to estimate the number of cancer cases that could be avoided if an exposure were reduced or eliminated in the population. If we then apply this knowledge of how a risky behavior (smoking) causes cancer in individuals, and different rates of cancer between groups who do and do not smoke, we can understand what are called population-attributable risk measures. It really is simple and commonsensical. Putting all of these observations together carefully can then help us understand and estimate the proportion of cancer cases in a population that could be avoided if an exposure (such as smoke) were reduced or eliminated. Basically, in this case, it would tell us how many cases of lung cancer a society could avoid.

A screening test utility is also affected by understanding how many folks are needed to undergo the test in order, statistically—odds-wise speaking—to save one life. This number estimates the number of people that must participate in a screening program for one death to be prevented over a defined time interval. Then, once a screening test finds something, another important measure of the power of that test whether it made a meaningful difference and just how big that difference was.

A statistic termed "average life-years saved" estimates the number of years that an intervention saves, on average, for an individual who receives the intervention. This reflects mortality reduction as well as life extension (or avoidance of premature deaths).

SYMPTOM CONTROL AND SIDE EFFECTS

Advances have been made in the development of newer cancer treatments with fewer side effects and in the utilization of effective medications to address some of the traditional side effects from chemotherapy and radiation. Many people assume that the severe nausea and vomiting caused by cancer treatments two or more decades ago still exist. In fact, the incidence of nausea and vomiting has been greatly decreased, even prevented altogether in some instances, by some revolutionary medications available today. In addition, the risks of infection and fatigue have also been reduced with other medications that reduce the extent of time that a patient has low blood counts as a result of treatment, as well as the severity of those counts.

Advances in these areas have changed the cancer experience for millions of people and have made it possible to maximize the potential anticancer impact of chemotherapy and radiation. However, side effect prevention and management remains a critical issue for people with cancer today. It is important that you learn to read your physical signs, keep track of symptoms and side effects, and communicate with your health-care team regularly. More often than not, the signs and symptoms you experience are temporary and related to treatment as well as changes that are occurring in your body as the treatment works to control or destroy the cancer. If you experience a side effect from therapy, it is important to become vigilant and maintain open communication with your health-care team and family so you can proactively manage the side effects throughout treatment.

To be active in your cancer care, become informed about side effects *before* you select your treatment program. Consider asking your doctor the following questions as you select the best treatment option for you:

- What side effects commonly occur with the treatment or drug regimen that is being recommended?
- What is the likelihood that I will have those side effects, and how mild or severe could they be?
- Do the benefits of the recommended treatment outweigh the potential side effects?
- Are these side effects compatible with my lifestyle and expectations during cancer treatment?
- How will the potential side effects either be prevented or be managed effectively so they do not interrupt my treatment schedule or decrease my quality of life?

In addition to some of the most common side effects associated with cancer treatment—namely nausea and vomiting, low blood counts, emotional distress, and diarrhea—there are a few newer side effects that have become common with the newest treatments, such as skin rashes and nail and nerve irritation.

The side effects of cancer treatment are due to the specific agent or agents you are receiving. They can be mild to severe. Most side effects can be minimized and generally do not require interruption of treatment. You may not experience these side effects or others. Each person reacts differently to cancer treatment. However, some side effects do interfere with quality of life. There is continued research to find ways to minimize the side effects of cancer treatment, and there are several good tips to manage or control side effects until more medical solutions are found.

There is a great variety and broad range of effects from therapy. No one patient usually suffers them all, and more than a few have a relatively easy go of it. In this section, I will alphabetically discuss some of the more common adverse events that transpire in some, but not all, patients. Rather than be scared by these things, I urge patients to be prepared, as they may occur at some point. I will not review all of the complications of cancer and all of the treatments for those complications in the manner of a physician's medical text, but I will rather cover the most common ones in sufficient depth. Pain control is addressed in a separate chapter owing to its importance and the anxiety and suffering associated with it.

Alopecia

Alopecia is the loss of all or part of the hair from any part of the body, including the scalp, eyebrows, eyelashes, face, and pubic area. This is a direct effect of some forms of chemotherapy and sometimes radiation. It occurs because of temporary destruction of rapidly growing cells, such as hair follicles. The most common drugs that cause this are bleomycin, carboplatin, Cytoxan, dactinomycin, doxorubicin, epirubicin, etoposide, 5-FU, idarubicin, ifosfamide, irinotecan, mitoxantrone, paclitaxel, and topotecan. The loss is temporary. It may begin two to three weeks after the start of treatment. Hair might thin or fall out at once. It grows back after treatment, sometimes thicker, darker, and curlier than before, usually around three to four months after therapy. Simple hair care with a mild shampoo is all that is needed. A soft brush should be used, and one should avoid any hair treatments, hair dryers, curling irons, mousse, and hair spray. Many consider cutting their hair before it falls out, as it looks fuller and thicker. Other patients buy wigs, hairpieces, or false eyelashes before their hair falls out, as it is easier to match at that time. These may be tax-deductible medical expenses. One can cover his or her scalp with these items, turbans, various hats, etc. The American Cancer Society can help with advice on this. It is important to use sunscreen, as the scalp will be sensitive to heat and cold.

Radiation therapy and many chemotherapy drugs can cause hair loss, or alopecia. Some chemotherapy drugs cause people to lose some of their hair, and some cause total hair loss, including body hair, eyebrows, and eyelashes. Some newer treatments do not cause any hair loss. Talk to your doctor about what you can expect regarding hair loss with your specific treatment regimen. You may read or hear others talk about placing ice on top of their head or tying a tourniquet (a tight rubber band) around their head to prevent hair loss. There is little truth to any of these tales.

Some helpful hints for dealing with hair loss include the following:

1. Use mild shampoos and soft hairbrushes.
2. Use low heat when drying your hair.
3. Buy scarves, wigs or hats, or a ***scalp prosthesis.***
4. If you're thinking about buying a wig, try to do so before you lose your hair so the hair stylist can more easily match your color and preference.
5. Do not dye your hair or get a permanent or body wave.
6. Use sunscreen and wear a hat or scarf to protect your scalp from the sun.
7. Call your local American Cancer Society to see if a Look Good, Feel Better program is being held in the area. This program is for both women and men undergoing cancer treatments.

Anorexia

Anorexia is the loss of desire for food or a decrease in the appetite. Sometimes it is severe enough to effect proper nourishment and cause a condition of wasting called cachexia. Many factors can cause this, including radiation to the belly, changes in sense of taste from the chemotherapy, the cancer itself, depression, fear and anxiety, fatigue, and tiredness. Numerous chemotherapy drugs can do this. The best defense is to eat small meals and snacks whenever you want. It is wise to eat at least five or more small meals a day and to try different foods.

Occasionally, one glass of wine can boost the appetite, but patients should always ask or be informed about potential interactions of alcohol with their medications. It is best to drink liquids before meals instead of with them. Some have found that cooking with lemon, basil, oregano, and rosemary helps. Marinated meals often work well, and when cooking, it can help to prepare meals in advance of feeling tired or ill. Inquiries should be made of the nurses or social workers for arranging to have Meals on Wheels bring food for those unable to cook for themselves. Food can be made bright and colorful. Consider setting a pleasant table. I often recommend doing things differently, such as eating in an unusual place or taking a walk before meals to increase hunger. Food will taste better if the mouth is clean, so maintenance of good dental hygiene is essential There are many supplemental shakes the oncologist probably has samples of that provide excellent calories. Many patients are candidates for Megace, which is a liquid that can stimulate appetite and weight gain in some cases. There are other medications that are of some use, such as steroids and cannabinoids.

Treatments and the stress of the cancer experience can affect your interest in eating or your actual taste buds. Adequate nutrition is an important part of the body's recovery from cancer, yet it is often a challenge for patients undergoing cancer treatment. Many cancer centers have a registered dietician available to assist with eating concerns.

Some helpful hints for loss of appetite include the following:

1. Eat small meals or snacks whenever you want, rather than eating three meals a day.
2. Vary your diet. Try new foods and recipes.
3. Use liquid nutritional products that are high in calories and protein.
4. Try to take in at least four ounces of protein each day.
5. Snack on nutrition bars or power bars.
6. Consider taking a walk before meals to make yourself feel hungrier.
7. Arrange to eat with family and friends, or watch TV while eating if you are alone.
8. Avoid food odors. Cold foods have fewer odors than piping-hot foods.

Bleeding and Thrombocytopenia

Thrombocytopenia is a decrease in the number of platelets in the blood. These are like little patches and plugs that help blood clot normally. Some types of chemotherapy cause this more than others do. Other than the so-called liquid malignancies, such as the leukemias, or in cases of a marrow severely packed with tumor or a depleted marrow, this is not common. A normal platelet count is 150,000 to 400,000. When the count falls below

50,000, the tendency to bleed begins to become clinically relevant. Most oncologists today tend not to deliver chemotherapy if the platelet count is under 100,000. A patient should look for bleeding he or she cannot control, an old injury that starts bleeding again, tarry black stools, blood in urine, blood coughed up from the lungs, blood in the stool, nosebleeds, bad headaches, pain in joints or muscles, pinpoint red spots on the skin, unexplained bruises, or heavier menses than usual.

It is wise to keep the skin moist and prevent it from cracking. I suggest using an electric razor. Feet should be protected, and care should be taken when using knives and such. Protective gloves should be worn if doing garden work or other odd jobs. One should use a soft toothbrush or oral swab to clean teeth. A common mistake is failing to blow one's nose gently or placing fingers or cotton swabs in the nose. Women should avoid douches and tampons and use feminine napkins. Stool softeners and generous oral intake of fluids will help avoid constipation. It is important to avoid aspirin as well as other anti-inflammatory medications, such as Celebrex, Vioxx, Motrin, Advil, or Nuprin, unless told otherwise. Intramuscular injections are to be avoided, as is the consumption of alcohol and the use of enemas or suppositories. Care should be taken during sexual intercourse. Obviously, one should avoid contact sports. If bleeding occurs, it is important to stay calm and apply pressure. If it does not stop, apply ice, and if it occurs in the mouth, one should swish with icy water or apply frozen tea bag compresses. More serious bleeding mandates a visit to the emergency department and a call to the doctor.

Constipation

Constipation means passing fewer bowel movements than normal for the individual. This is highly variable among people, so personal norms are the gauge. Three bowel movements a day or three a week can be normal. If one is constipated, the stool may be hard, dry, and difficult to pass. One may need to exert more effort to pass it, and that can increase the risk of both bleeding and infection. Many factors can cause constipation, from decreased fluid and fiber intake to bowel or stomach surgery, inadequate exercise, bed confinement, and abnormally high calcium levels, as well the psychological factors of stress, anxiety, or depression. Many common medications (too many to list here), such as antacids, narcotics, and some chemotherapy can cause this. Fluid intake, fruit intake, whole grains, raw and cooked vegetables, and especially peas, nuts, and popcorn can help prevent this. Cheeses and refined grain products should be avoided. Fluid intake should be eight to twelve cups of water a day. A fiber-containing laxative may help if recommended by the doctor. The same is true for stool softeners such as Colace. It is important to stick to routines and always go to the toilet when feeling the urge. Sometimes a hot drink beforehand is helpful. Exercising at least fifteen minutes a day is wise.

If constipated, continuing whatever regimen one is on and adding at least one glass of prune juice daily often helps. Some patients will need medications like Colace, Senokot or Dulcolax. This is for the physician to decide and not patients on their own. It is crucial to always check with the physician before ever using a suppository, as this may be very unwise because of a low white blood cell count from therapy, which increases the risk of seeding harmful bacteria into the body and starting what could be a life-threatening infection.

Certain drugs, including pain medications, can cause constipation. If you are receiving chemotherapy or radiation and have mild or infrequent constipation or other bowel problems, talk with your doctor and consider some of the following suggestions:

1. Drink plenty of fluids. Warm and hot fluids are especially good to help loosen the bowel.
2. Consider eating high-fiber foods, such as bran, whole-wheat breads and cereals, and fruits and vegetables.
3. Try to be as physically active as possible.
4. Consult your doctor before you use an enema, because if your platelets are low, an enema could cause bleeding. Also your white blood count could be low, and you could get an infection from an enema.
5. If you are on narcotic pain medication, talk to your doctor about taking a laxative and/or stool softener (do not use these products without checking with your doctor first). It is much easier to

think "prevention" than to have to deal with the consequences of constipation.

6. Call your doctor immediately if you have been constipated for more than three days or you have difficulty breathing. Constipation can cause fecal impaction (a buildup of hardened feces), which can be fatal and should be treated immediately.

Dental Problems

Both chemotherapy and radiation therapy of certain head and neck cancers can cause what is called xerostomia, which is drying out of the mouth, causing the loss of the protective effect of saliva. This may also cause mouth sores known as stomatitis or mucositis. Cleaning of the teeth daily after a full dental evaluation before receiving a radiation treatment can speed recovery from the effect of radiation on the teeth.

It is a wise idea to have a thorough dental exam and cleaning before starting therapy. That is the time to treat cavities and fit dentures well. Sometimes a fluoride gel is prescribed. Teeth should be brushed gently after each meal using a soft brush. Patients with painful gums can use cotton swabs, foam-tipped swabs, or gauze if their gums hurt, and they may try using a non-abrasive toothpaste or baking soda and water. The toothbrush needs to be rinsed well after use and allowed to dry thoroughly to avoid contamination. Dentures should be removed and cleaned after every meal and left out at night. Flossing is important and should be done unless the platelet count is low. Foods that stick to the teeth, such as caramels, chewy candy bars, and gummy bears, should be avoided.

Patients should look at their mouth every day with a flashlight and mirror and tell the doctor of any changes seen in the mouth or saliva, including red areas, blisters, white spots, coatings, ulcers, or bleeding. Mouthwashes with alcohol can make the mouth drier and are not to be used. The pharmacist can help with the right choices. Mild cases of mouth irritation can be treated with a saline solution made by dissolving a teaspoon of salt in hot water; swish with this solution, but do not swallow it. More severe cases of mucositis should be treated by a physician.

Depression

Depression is a mood of sadness, despair, and discouragement. It may just be "the blues" or something far more serious, requiring both medication and talk therapy. It is the inability to find pleasure in everyday life or the feeling that there is no reason to live. People with depression may or may not be as aware of their mood as keenly as friends and family are. There are agreed-upon clinical criteria used to make the diagnosis, but in general, patients and family should be concerned and seek professional help when at least six of the following are present for more than two weeks continuously: (1) feeling sad every day for two to three weeks in a row with weeping or crying more than usual; (2) having decreased interest in or pleasure from everyday activities; (3) having decreased interest in sex; (4) experiencing weight loss with no appetite or weight gain with an increased appetite; (5) being unable to sleep or sleeping more than usual; (6) feeling either agitated or sluggish persistently; (7) being tired or having decreased energy; (8) feeling worthless or guilty without rational cause; (9) having trouble thinking, concentrating, or making choices; (10) withdrawing from family and friends, and (11) thinking or talking about death or suicide.

Many cancer patients feel depressed transiently; it is not a chronic state for the majority. Things that may "tip you over" are a change of routine, inadequate exercise, confinement to a bed, a lost or decreased sense of well-being, grief or sadness because of changes in health, tiredness, fatigue or pain, uncertainty about prognosis, money, or finances, and, lastly, a long list of medications. The latter is a cause commonly forgotten and should always be considered. Simply being in the hospital away from family and friends or being in a strange or unfamiliar place is a very common cause of depression. A sense of loss of control or worry over tests is quite common and natural. Two frequently forgotten causes are lack of exercise and lack of adequate sunlight.

There should be no delay in relating any of these symptoms to the treating physician. Too many wait and suffer silently, feeling it is part of the package, to be expected, and something they should simply try to "gut out." Anyone can become depressed; it is not a sign of weakness. It can be treated successfully in the vast majority of people. Common sense tells us that all mood-altering substances, especially alcohol, should be avoided by people suffering from depression, except those prescribed by a doctor. Sufficient rest is essential, as well as exercise. There is no substitute for getting up and getting outside. As more than one therapist has said, a good adage is "Fake it until you make it." Always seek help. Medications to treat anxiety are extremely effective, very well tolerated, and made to be taken orally. Do not stop taking your medication unless your doctor says so. They may work in days, but it is not uncommon for them to take three to four weeks. It may also take two to four different medications before the best one for you is found.

Diarrhea

Diarrhea is a condition in which one has more bowel movements than normal, usually three or more loose stools in twenty-four hours. Both chemotherapy and radiation to the gut can cause this. Some types of bowel surgery are well known to be associated with this, as are certain medications. Other common causes are some antacids, antibiotics, chemotherapy, magnesium supplements, nonsteroidal anti-inflammatories, laxatives, bowel infections, stress, and anxiety. It is best to call the doctor when there is blood in the diarrhea, when the diarrhea lasts more than twenty-four hours, when there are more than five to six liquids stools per day, or when the diarrhea is accompanied by a fever, pain and cramping, rectal sores or cracks, or symptoms of dehydration, such as decreased urination, dizziness, lightheadedness, dry mouth, or increased thirst.

One possible solution is to eat small meals more frequently and lessen the intake of high-fiber foods, such as beans, dried fruits, nuts, popcorn, raw fruit, seeds, raw vegetables, and whole-grain breads. Rather, more low-fiber foods, such as ripe bananas, canned or cooked fruit, cottage cheese, rice, pureed vegetables, cream cheese, grape juice, white bread, and yogurt, should be chosen. Food or drinks that cause gas, such as beer, beans, cabbage, greasy or fried foods, spicy foods, and sweets, are to be avoided. It is wise to drink less alcohol and consume less caffeine and less chocolate. Many of us are lactose intolerant to a degree, so in general it is wise to be careful of milk and dairy products. Nicotine-containing products can be a significant problem as well.

If diarrhea develops, regular foods can be replaced with rice and warm milk (if one is not lactose intolerant), and fluid intake can be improved with simply water, flat ginger ale, apple juice, or Gatorade—but nothing containing caffeine. Room-temperature fluids are usually best. It is not uncommon for two to three quarts a day to be required. Low-fat cheese and yogurt can be helpful. Diarrhea causes the loss of potassium; thus, eating foods high in it, such as asparagus, bananas, oranges, saltwater fish, skinned apricots, skinned potatoes, and apricot and peach nectar, is wise.

The rectal area must be kept clean and dry. Washing with mild soap and water or taking sitz baths is often soothing. It is best to use alcohol-free baby wipes instead of toilet paper to clean oneself. Sometimes vitamin A&D ointment is soothing to irritated skin.

There are potent medications that are oral, subcutaneous, and intravenous if the diarrhea cannot be controlled otherwise. Most importantly, there must never be a delay in starting antidiarrheal medications, presuming that the problem will be self-limited.

Dysphagia

Dysphagia is trouble swallowing food, liquid, or saliva. A simple sore throat or an inflamed esophagus (esophagitis) may cause this. Many factors related to cancer can cause this. Radiation given to the direct area is one obvious cause; surgery in that area is another. In addition, a small number of chemotherapy agents are known to cause this in about 10–20% of the patients who receive them. It is usually transient, lasting one week. A few other less common medications uncommonly cause this.

It is time to call the doctor when there is a clear choking feeling, when food gets stuck, when pain is not tolerable, when there is hoarseness, cough, fever above 100.5 degrees, or when there are shaking chills or flulike symptoms.

Some steps at home that may work are pureeing foods or cooking foods until they are mushy and tender and cutting them into small bites. I tell patients to concentrate on foods that are naturally soft and to take plenty of supplemental nutritional drinks. Other good items are baby food, cooked cereal, bananas, applesauce, fruit nectars, soft-boiled eggs, cottage cheese, custard, and pudding or gelatin. Moistening foods as much as possible is wise, and if dryer foods cannot be avoided, it often helps to use butter, margarine, or melted cheese. Dry foods should be avoided, as should acidic foods, such as anything from the citrus family and tomatoes. Spicy and salty foods, chili, and nutmeg should also be avoided. Although it may not be as palatable, eating foods at colder temperatures is wise, as warm foods will cause irritation. Be sure to take sips of liquid with every bite. It is wise to drink through a straw to avoid too much bulk entering the esophagus at one time.

Edema

Edema is swelling caused by the abnormal buildup of fluid in the tissue spaces of the body outside of the blood and lymph vessels. It also is referred to as fluid retention. Fluid may collect in the legs, arms, feet, lungs, heart, or abdomen. Severe edema can cause the kidneys, heart, and lungs to be overworked and damaged. Symptoms of edema are puffiness of the affected area and, often, around the eyes.

Ascites is a related problem in which abnormal amounts of fluid accumulate in the abdominal cavity, which becomes tight and shiny as a result of stretching. There is an intense feeling of fullness sooner than usual after eating, and in many cases, distended skin veins over the abdomen may be seen more clearly.

People with cancer are at an increased risk for edema because the cancer itself may be lining a body cavity or organ and causing weeping. It may also be due to kidney failure and fluid retention, as nutrition may be so poor that there may not be enough protein in the blood to "hold" fluid inside the blood vessels, as normally occurs.

There are some medications, both chemotherapy and otherwise, that cause blood vessels to leak or cause shifts of salt and water into and out of the vessels. Some of these drugs cause this to happen only as the dose increases, whereas some cannot be as well predicted but are well known to cause it. Many of the drugs are those that are used to help cancer patients with other symptoms. Thus, the problem is not that common in non-advanced, non-high-dose settings. Nonetheless, edema caused by cancer may be permanent. Edema caused by malnutrition or most medications is usually reversible. However, if vital organs are damaged, it is often permanent.

It is time to inform the doctor when wheezing, difficulty eating, severe swelling; difficulty breathing, chest pain or tightness, rapid weight gain, or urinating smaller amounts than usual occurs. The most important things one can do is reduce the amount of salt in the diet at once and eat small, frequent meals if the abdomen is swollen. Increased protein intake may be helpful, as well as increased carbohydrate intake. The doctor can enlist the aid of a dietician to ensure the right combination of supplements. Fluid intake should not be changed unless recommended by the physician. That is a common mistake. Pillows or cushions should be used to raise the feet and legs above the heart when sitting or lying down. Severe edema warrants rest for several hours each day. The wearing of elastic graduated compression stockings for both the lower and upper extremities can be very effective, and many communities have edema clinics.

As stated above, foods high in salt must be avoided. The list is long, and reading labels is wise. Some high-salt items are convenience and snack foods, fast food, pizza, salted fish, ham, bacon, sausage, salted nuts, peanut butter, salted butter, processed grains and food mixes, olives, pickles, cheeses, and salad dressings. Another common mistake is cooking with monosodium glutamate (MSG), baking soda, baking powder, bouillon cubes, cooking sherry, wine, and meat tenderizers. It is wise to avoid strenuous exertion and sitting with feet on the floor for prolonged periods in cases of severe edema. The feet should be elevated whenever possible.

Fatigue

Fatigue is continuous and pervasive tiredness. It does not abate with sleep. There is a tendency to tire more easily with usual activities or simply not have the energy for everyday activities. Sometimes this can affect thinking, making choices, or just getting about.

The causes are highly varied. For some, just a change in daily routine or lack of exercise or bed confinement is sufficient. For many it is anemia, either from the cancer or from its treatment. Radiation therapy alone can also cause it. Of course, psychological stress factors of agitation, anxiety, and depression should be looked for, as well as chronic pain. There is a small handful of mostly hormonal or biologic drugs that can cause fatigue also; perhaps the most common and well know is interferon.

The doctor should always be alerted regarding fatigue, especially if there is lightheadedness, dizziness in general or when standing up, chills even in a warm room, difficulty breathing, or shortness of breath.

There are steps patients can take to combat fatigue, and they are intuitive and simple. One must believe his or her body and not push activities beyond what one feels capable of. Rest is pivotal. Sometimes an earlier bedtime is wise, as well as daytime naps. Short rest is often more effective than long rest periods. Light exercise is essential and should be engaged in daily if possible. Once again, the effect of inadequate nutrition and fluid intake is not to be underestimated. Unnecessary activities should be eliminated, and some chores delegated. It is a good technique to set slightly challenging goals that can be reached. Setting ones that are more difficult can lead to guilt and more fatigue. Mindset is also important. The focus should not be on fatigue. Rather, enjoy music, relaxing, and reading; see something stimulating on television or rent a movie. Some authorities suggest a fatigue journal, where one can see what makes him or her the most tired and help one start identifying what to cut back on.

Most importantly, there is excellent treatment for fatigue from anemia or chemotherapy in the form of a simple subcutaneous injection of erythropoietin, which may be administered every week, every two weeks, or every three weeks. More than 50% of patients with anemia or chemotherapy-induced fatigue will respond to erythropoietin. This chemical is the body's own red blood cell stimulant hormone; it is genetically engineered and is commercially available under a number of proprietary names.

Flulike Symptoms

Fever, muscle aches, chills, headaches, tiredness, and occasionally nausea and a poor appetite may start in a minority of patients a few days after chemotherapy, as a result of the drugs used. There are other causes, however, some of which are very serious. This may be the first sign of infection due to a low white blood cell count and lowered immune resistance. This generally can start about seven to fourteen days after chemotherapy treatments. In some cases, this low blood count is delayed further.

Biological antitumor medications like interferon, IL-2, BCG, Neupogen, Rituxan and Herceptin may cause fatigue. This is a sign of the immune system acknowledging the presence of the drug and is not usually indicative of a bad outcome; it is more the norm. Of course, the cancer itself can do this by making various chemicals that then circulate and elicit fatigue.

It can be hard to tell the difference between flulike symptoms and a real infection, so it is usually wise to call a physician when such symptoms appear. This is especially true if the drugs given are known to potentially transiently lower the white blood cell count. It is mandatory to seek help if there is a temperature above 100.5 degrees, shaking chills, profuse sweating with chills, runny nose, sore throat, productive cough, difficulty breathing, painful urination, pain or stiffness in the neck, unusual vaginal or penile discharge, pain or burning near the rectum, or persistence of general flu symptoms longer than anticipated.

As always, a mother's advice is right. Stay warm when necessary and cool when necessary by layering bedclothes. There is nothing like a good electric blanket or heating pad, and it is common sense to avoid any extremes of temperature. The timeworn remedy of a tepid bath can do wonders. Dehydration can occur with a fever through insensible loss, thus fluid intake should be approximately doubled. A good gauge is whether urination remains frequent and relatively light in color. It is very important not to take antipyretics—these are medications like aspirin, Tylenol, Motrin, etc.—unless told to by the physician, as they may falsely mask a dangerous fever or a real infection. Finally, many of the medications that can cause these symptoms can be taken at bedtime with less risk of them adversely affecting quality of life.

Heart and Cardiovascular Changes

Surgery, radiation, and some common chemotherapy drugs for cancer may cause problems with heart function. Symptoms may include chest tightness or pain, difficulty breathing, unusually slow or rapid heartbeat, or numbness in the left arm or shoulder. If you are deciding what type of chemotherapy might be best for you, ask your doctor about the potential adverse effects that certain chemotherapy drugs could have on your heart.

- Be sure your doctor knows about any past problems with your heart.
- An echocardiogram, stress electrocardiogram, or MUGA test may be done to determine your heart function before treatment is started.
- Contact your doctor immediately if you experience chest pain, changing heartbeat, or numbness in the left arm or shoulder.

Infertility and Sterility

The risk of reduced or lost ability to conceive or produce adequate viable sperm either long- or short-term is highly variable with age and chemotherapy regimen. In some cases it is unavoidable and sperm banking is recommended. In some cases with the same drugs, it simply depends on the individual. Radiation can also cause sterility if a sufficient dose is delivered to the gonads either intentionally or because of scatter despite shielding of the gonads. Some women will stop menses temporarily, some permanently; the same is true for sperm production and viability in men. It is also true that psychological factors can be at play, such as stress, anxiety, depression, fatigue, and drugs that have been prescribed. The doctor should be informed promptly if menstrual periods are missed, there is a change in menstrual bleeding, or bleeding after intercourse occurs.

The key is prevention and to inquire with the doctor about sperm banks and banks for frozen harvested eggs for use in the future. Communication among all, in advance, is the best course of action.

It is essential during chemotherapy that effective birth control is used flawlessly. Miscarriages, therapeutic abortion, and deformed children are all possible outcomes of being pregnant at the wrong time during chemotherapy, radiation treatment, or diagnostic imaging.

Insomnia

Insomnia is difficulty sleeping and has many forms. It may be the inability to get to sleep, the inability to stay asleep, early wakening, or poor sleep. This is a very common ailment among us all, not just cancer patients. There is a wide diversity of sleeping patterns, but concern should be aroused when there is persistent (more than one week) disturbance from whatever is the norm for an individual.

One of the more common causes of insomnia is effects from medications given as part of the therapy program. It may be possible to alter both doses and time of administration without changing effectiveness. Cancer patients have all the expected psychological stressors known to disturb sleep, whether it be at home or in the foreign environment of the hospital with all of its distractions. Such changes in daily routine can easily be the culprit, as well as getting less sunlight and exercise than usual.

Although it may seem counterintuitive, one of the worst things one can do is stay in bed when unable to sleep. It is wise to try some home remedies before resorting to the limited armamentarium for long-term insomnia. This is because medications may be highly effective for short-term treatment but rarely exceeding two to three weeks. If administered for longer periods, they generally wear off, cause a mild addiction, and worsen sleep with rebound insomnia. Benadryl is perhaps the only exception, but it may leave you groggy the next day.

Try some warm milk, herbal tea, relaxing music on a timer, or relaxation tapes. I hesitate to advise a single glass of beer or wine, as it works for some but it very frequently causes poor sleep and early awakening. Although you should exercise, you should not do so within the three hours before bedtime, as exercise will arouse many wakefulness chemicals.

Certainly, you should recognize the need to discuss psychological problems with the appropriate people, even if those people are just family members. Perseveration and dwelling will haunt you into the wee hours. Maintaining a routine is also essential. Get up and go to sleep at the same times, and plan meals well before bed. Absolutely avoid chocolate. Also avoid cola, caffeine, and nicotine for four to five hours before sleep. Plan to mellow out for the few hours before sleep. "Plan" is the key word; structure your day so it can happen. Some find that wearing earplugs helps, while others find it a nuisance. One overlooked area is the right temperature. It needs to be what you want, but you may find that keeping the sleeping area a few degrees cooler while snuggled in a comforter will do the trick. Plan your pain meds with your physician so you can pretty much count on not trying to sleep in pain or having them wear off while asleep. Your physician can make all kinds of manipulations that are very effective. Usually by following the above advice and telling your physician, the problem will be short-lived.

Lymphedema

Lymphedema is a specific form of edema owing to buildup of lymph fluid from blocked, removed, or destroyed lymph nodes. Our body has a vast network of microscopic canals that collect excess fluid and, especially, cellular debris, very much like a sewage system with collection stations for sterilization. When lymph nodes are surgically removed, blocked, or replaced and there are not enough others in the same location to take up the load, swelling of the affected extremity can occur, and downstream tissues may have a harder time fighting infection. Radiation can also destroy lymph channels and nodes. Certainly, the cancer itself, if strategically located, can alter or destroy local lymph drainage.

Lymphedema may not be transient. New lymph vessels may grow back immediately or years after therapy. The best preventive measures are daily exercises to stay limber as soon as possible after therapy. These include both aerobic exercises as well as weight-bearing exercises to build and tone musculature and help the venous return system of the affected limb. It is important to try to keep the skin clean and dry as well as moisturized to prevent cracks or deep peeling. This can be done by wearing gloves and using a mild antibacterial soap when cleaning an affected limb. Similarly, maintenance of nail hygiene is important to avoid becoming infected through scratches.

Lymphedema clinics perform therapy to assist drainage of affected limbs as well as fit compression stockings, often for the long term. Sizes may need to be changed regularly as progress is made. All activities that elevate the affected limb are useful and should be done three to four times. The physician should be contacted when there is weeping of the skin, new redness, signs of infection, open or nonhealing wounds, streaks going up the limb, a sudden increase in swelling or pain, or the onset of numbness.

There are definite things to avoid if possible. Blood should not be drawn from the affected limb, nor should blood pressure be taken on that side if possible. One should avoid using the limb to carry heavy objects—and even lighter ones if the limb will be mostly pointing downward. Sports or violent exercises posing the risk of trauma to the affected limb are to be avoided as well. Garments should fit loosely, as should jewelry. Hot areas will increase swelling. Obviously, intoxication can invite falls, causing trauma to the affected limb.

Menopausal Symptoms

Symptoms of menopause include hot flashes, vaginal dryness and tightness, swings of mood (sometimes to a large degree), painful intercourse, and irregular menses. These symptoms will occur in all women at some point in time, but the range of age is actually quite variable, ranging from the early forties to, rarely, as late as sixty years old. The duration of symptoms is usually two years or so, but there is considerable variation in both severity and duration. The average age for the onset of menopause is about fifty. Menopause is due to a woman's ovaries making less estrogen and progesterone, which control the normal menstrual cycle.

Cancer care may involve surgery, radiation, hormonal modalities, and chemotherapy, which can herald the onset of menopause. The physician should be informed if any of these symptoms appear, especially if periods are erratic, missed, or heavy. Other symptoms to look for are decreased sexual desire, hot flashes, and bleeding after sex.

There are some things one can do, and those do not include rushing out to the health-food store and getting the latest craze for menopause. This is a common mistake. Fluid intake will need to increase somewhat, and clothing should be loose and layered. Panty hose should have a ventilated cotton crotch, and nonbreathing, tight-fitting clothes should be avoided. Exercise is actually quite effective, especially long-term and weight bearing exercise, as loss of bone density will accelerate at this time. Some find that a hot flash journal helps them discover what foods and activities seem to bring on the flashes. Use of a water-based vaginal lubricant, such as K-Y Jelly, Astroglide, and Lubrin, may be of great assistance in intercourse. A vaginal moisturizer, such as Replens, may help. Occlusive and oil-based products are unwise, as they increase the risk of infection, as do scented products if they irritate.

There is a host of medications for menopausal symptoms and bone loss, and they are largely quite effective and generally worth the very small absolute risk they pose for breast or uterine cancer. Patients on antiestrogen therapy, however, have a more limited list of available medications. Nonetheless, great strides have been made in the treatment of hot flashes, and there is hope of success in at least 60% of women on antihormonal therapies with our new drugs.

Mucositis

Mucositis is inflammation of the mucous membranes of the mouth and throat, often marked by the presence of sores or ulcers in the mouth and throat. These can be very painful and seriously impair eating, speaking, and swallowing. These mucous lining cells are rapidly dividing cells, so they are particularly sensitive to many, but not all, forms of chemotherapy, as well as radiation. symptoms usually start three to five days after therapy. Their severity can vary widely, and they do resolve, usually by the second or early third week after chemotherapy. The appearance after radiation may be a little later, closer to ten days from treatment.

It is always wise to inform the doctor if mucositis symptoms develop, especially if they impair the ability to talk, eat, or swallow, if they last longer than expected, or if they are associated with a fever of 100.5 degrees or higher. Some things that can be done at home to alleviate these symptoms include drinking more fluid and avoiding all alcohol. As we discussed earlier, it may help to eat soft foods, such as pureed food, baby food, milkshakes, pudding, and custard, as well as to avoid all acidic food, such as foods in the citrus family and tomatoes. Spicy or salty foods are a bad idea as well. Cold foods may be tolerated better than hot foods. Patients should take an active role in maintaining oral hygiene and check themselves twice a day with a flashlight and a mirror, looking especially for blisters, red and white patches, and deepening or bleeding ulcers. Nasal breathing is more comfortable than mouth breathing, and lip balm may be soothing. All nicotine products will impair healing.

There are various medications that can relieve mucositis symptoms, ranging from home swish-and-swallow mixes of an anesthetic plus Maalox and Benadryl to oral, subcutaneous, and IV narcotics. Sometimes the physician will give preventative oral medicine for thrush in various forms and medications. Saltwater and chlorhexidine rinsing can help, and there are some agents a radiation therapist can use before radiation to decrease the risk of mucositis. If an anesthetic mix is to be used, it should be used just before meals; if the physician says it is all right, it may be swallowed. Extra caution is warranted when using these medications, as the numbness they cause may cause you to choke, bite yourself, or even burn yourself with a liquid you did not know was too hot.

Nausea and Vomiting

We all know what a horrendous feeling nausea is, and the great news is that we have outstanding therapies available to prevent it in more than 80% of patients. This field has advanced dramatically, and the group of agents that can be given with very few side effects is highly effective in preventing chemotherapy-induced nausea and vomiting. Furthermore, there are medications that prevent delayed nausea and vomiting in the vast majority of people. Thus, the horror stories so many believe are the rule are actually the exception. Radiation that involves the gut and sometimes the brain can cause some degree of nausea that may be more prolonged or low-grade. Patients are urged to request that their physician consider the whole cocktail of drugs available that can prevent nausea the first time, including a mild sedative. If this is successful, it is unusual for patients to have the problem further down the road. Certainly, one's anxiety and psychological state can alter the likelihood of nausea and vomiting occurring; thus, reading this book should help. Narcotics can occasionally cause nausea, but again, there are excellent medications that can be taken to prevent this in almost everyone.

The more difficult nausea or vomiting to treat is usually due to chemicals made by the cancer (rare) or direct obstruction of the gastrointestinal tract. In the latter case, surgical intervention ranging from actual open surgery and removal to bypassing the blockage to placement of a tube into the intestine through the skin in order to relieve pressure from the outside may need to be done.

It is time to call the doctor if nausea continues for more than a day, if eating is impossible, or if dehydration and weakness are occurring. Certainly, any blood in the vomitus requires immediate attention.

It is generally wise to not drink or eat anything for several hours before chemotherapy and to avoid any sights or smells that seem to cause nausea. Often, chilling liquids before a meal (for about an hour) can also help prevent nausea. Meals should be small, frequent, and eaten slowly while chewing food carefully and swallowing small portions. Some have found that, if they do not have mucositis cereal, toast and crackers in the morning are helpful. It is wise to avoid sweet, greasy, or fatty food when nauseated. Most nausea medications should be taken to prevent nausea. Similar to pain control, nausea control is usually much more effective if begun beforehand rather than treating the nausea once it has started. Clothing should be loose-fitting, and both alcohol and nicotine should be avoided. Sometimes it is possible to sleep through the nausea with the aid of medication. Although it is not commonly needed, those patients with intense anxiety or clear premonitions regarding the high likelihood of nausea may benefit from acupuncture, relaxation techniques, hypnosis, or biofeedback.

If vomiting does develop, the mouth should be thoroughly rinsed, and all other food should be avoided. Once the nausea has passed, small sips of fluid, such as water or Gatorade, may be of some aid. Occasionally tea, flat ginger ale, and apple juice will also help.

Neutropenia

Neutropenia is a decrease in a particular type of white blood cell in the circulating blood. The neutrophils are frontline fighters for most commonly developed bacterial infections. Neutrophils are a type of white blood cell, and as the neutrophil count lowers (the nurse can explain how to calculate this easily, and you *do* want to understand this), the risk of infection and the likelihood of a serious infection grow. These cells do not fight fungi or viruses. Other than in certain less common situations, that is not the initial concern. This is crucial because chemotherapy kills short-lived, rapidly dividing cells such as these. The period of the low count is called the nadir, and it usually occurs between seven and fourteen days after chemotherapy, but that can vary. It is essential for patients to know when their time of vulnerability is. Radiation, if it is applied to bone containing marrow, can have a similar and cumulative effect. In general, cancer, per se, can increase the risk of infections. Also, recent surgery that has broken through the protection of the skin and other tissue barriers can increase the risk of infection.

The doctor must be called if there is a fever of 100.5 degrees or greater, especially if it occurs during the vulnerable time when the neutrophil count may be the lowest. Signs of infection besides fever are a sore throat, pus drainage from any area of the body, unexplained redness of skin or a joint, eye and ear drainage, burning on urination, a painful rectal area, swelling around an IV, nonhealing sores that may also be draining, and unusual vaginal discharge.

The time-honored technique to prevent neutropenia, besides knowing and understanding the period of vulnerability, is vigorous hand washing before eating, after going to the bathroom, before touching the eyes or nose, and after blowing the nose. Feet should always be protected and kept well cushioned. Nail hygiene is essential. Hands should be protected from random forms of routine trauma as well. Daily bathing or showering is a must, and daily inspections of the skin for signs of infection are important. When there are low numbers of white blood cells, infections may not hurt as much or be as readily apparent; thus, a high level of suspicion is warranted. All wounds must be cleansed immediately with antibacterial soap and water. Dental hygiene is imperative with a soft, and preferably warmed, toothbrush after every meal and at bedtime. Gentle brushing is appropriate; vigorous brushing may seed harmful bacteria into the blood. It is wise to avoid constipation, as straining may cause fissures or cracks and allow the entry of bacteria locally and systemically. In addition, women should neither douche nor use tampons, as these, too, can cause bacterial contamination.

During the period of vulnerability, patients must stay away from sick people, fresh fruits, and plants and always wash their hands before and after preparing food. Medication that can lower a temperature should be used very carefully, as the last thing one wants to do is mask a fever during the time of a low white blood cell count. Once again, it is crucial to remember that if the white blood cell count is particularly low, one may not see pus or significant redness or feel significant tenderness. The key is to be suspicious during the vulnerability period. Some commonsense items to keep in mind are avoiding contact with stagnant water and refraining from cleaning pet litter and eating raw eggs. Patients should consult a physician before getting any vaccination.

Neurological Symptoms

As humans come hardwired, almost any part of the body can be affected if there is a neurological problem. Problems can range from numbness and tingling in fingers and toes to muscle weakness or seizures. There may be sleeplessness or too much sedation, loss of coordination and balance, hearing loss, constipation, and even jaw and neck pain. One of the most common problems is peripheral neuropathy caused by chemotherapy drugs and, rarely, some tumors. Symptoms from damage to peripheral nerves (nerves outside the central nervous system of the spinal cord, brain stem, and brain) can be numbness or tingling in hands, fingers, toes, and feet; difficulty with dexterity; burning; and weakness.

There are many causes for neurological symptoms that include the cancer, per se, particular chemotherapy agents, radiation to the head or spine, infection in or around the spine, simple stress and anxiety, and a host of medications, including antidepressants, narcotics, and multiple chemotherapy agents. Fortunately, in most of these cases, the symptoms are largely reversible. Some authors believe that adding glutamine and vitamin B_6 to chemotherapy in moderate doses as a preventative measure can help. The time to call the doctor is when symptoms are clearly not passing or are unusually severe, such as profound muscular weakness, severe headaches, seizures, unexplained sleepiness, any loss of consciousness, and the onset of paresthesias (numbness, tingling, or burning pains). Care must be taken when walking, especially on stairs. Handrails, shoes with good traction, and bath mats in the shower are wise. Alcohol will make neurological symptoms worse. There are medicines that can make anyone dizzy, such as antihistamines. These should be taken only as directed and with great care. It is wise to both protect and inspect the feet, as trauma may not be sensed as well as heat and cold. Caution should also be exercised when using sharp implements, such as when cooking, doing chores, or gardening.

Palmar-Plantar Erythrodesia

Palmar-plantar erythrodesia is more commonly referred to as hand-foot syndrome and has been occurring more frequently now that an oral formulation of 5-FU, called Xeloda, has found so many uses. It is a discomforting or painful feeling in the palms of the hands and soles of the feet, with occasional swelling, tingling, and burning. Frequently, the skin will turn dark red, worse than sunburn; blisters may develop, as well as peeling, and even ulcers may form in advanced cases. Sometimes skin just continues to peel off. Usually the hands are more affected than the feet, for reasons we do not fully understand.

The present thinking is that palmar-plantar erythrodesia occurs as chemotherapy builds up in the affected tissues, owing to there being fewer sweat glands and thicker skin in those areas. We are not clear on this, though. There are a number of other agents that can do this commonly, including *bleomycin, ara-c, Cytoxan, Adriamycin, methotrexate* and a few more. Generally, the higher the dose, the greater the risk there is of palmar-plantar erythrodesia developing. Fortunately, this condition is temporary, with symptoms occurring from a few days into chemotherapy to after a number of treatments. the condition usually resolves in a few weeks after stopping chemotherapy. The best self-care is to keep feet protected and skin clean and dry. The use of moisturizing lotion is fine. Patients suffering from palmar-plantar erythrodesia should pay close attention to nail hygiene, wear gloves in the kitchen and in the garden, and take care when using cutting implements. Hot showers may be unwise, as they can dry the skin out too much. Pillows may help to keep affected extremities elevated. All clothing should be loose-fitting and soft. Frequent mistakes patients make are to peel skin themselves, pick at sores, cause pressure with tight jewelry, or expose the affected extremity to too much heat or cold.

To date there are no magical medicines for palmar-plantar erythrodesia other than those that can control the pain associated with it.

Photosensitivity Reactions

During chemotherapy treatment, the skin may become more sensitive to sunlight than normal. Reactions include radiation enhancement, radiation recall, and sunburn, as well as discoloration and dark streaking due to some chemotherapy drugs.

The two radiation reactions can occur when chemotherapy is given even without sun exposure. The enhancement reaction occurs concomitantly with administration of the chemotherapy or within a week. The recall reaction may occur weeks or years after radiation treatment. When these reactions occur, the irradiated skin turns pinkish-red and begins to burn and itch, sometimes peeling. It may last a couple of hours or days.

Skin cells are rapidly growing, and radiation and chemotherapy can kill those cells, as well as damage their ability to heal, thus making some areas more susceptible to sunburn. There are a number of drugs, such as dacarbazine, 5-FU, methotrexate, mitomycin C and vinblastine, that can do this. Radiation therapy can cause this with the same drugs, plus bleomycin and Adriamycin. Radiation recall can also occur with epirubicin, VP-16, idarubicin, and interferon, Taxol or vinblastine.

Hair loss can increase the odds of sunburn; thus, it is wise for patients to stay loosely covered up. It is also wise to inquire with the local pharmacist as well as the treating physician regarding certain antibiotics and nausea medications that can worsen photosensitivity.

The time to call the physician is when there is redness or darkening of irradiated skin, blisters, wounds or sores, any fever over 100.5° after sunburn, or if symptoms of dehydration develop. Any fluid-filled blisters after sunburn should be looked at, and any sunburn that hurts too much to move requires attention.

The best self-care is to cover up, avoid exposure, and use a highly protective sunscreen of SPF 15 or higher. It should be worn every day during treatment whether the patient goes outside or not. The physician can indicate if a sunblock, such as zinc oxide, needs to be used. Application of the sunscreen should be generous, and it should be reapplied after swimming or sweating. A common mistake is not using lip balm. Clothing should include long sleeves and pants, sunglasses, and a hat. Sunscreen should be used on the scalp if hair loss has occurred and a hat is not worn. Deodorants, perfumes, or powders may be irritating, and the use of adhesive tapes on exposed skin should be avoided. If methotrexate is planned to be used, it is essential to avoid sun exposure before it is given, as many develop a severe sunburn afterward. The best home therapy is to use cool, wet compresses and perhaps a cool bath. Blisters *should not be opened*, as they can easily become infected. Direct sunlight, tanning salons, and sunlamps must be avoided.

If a photosensitivity reaction is sufficiently severe, there is medicine that can be either directly applied or injected. Pain relief is often best with aspirin or one of the local anesthetics applied to the skin. Antihistamines can reduce the itching, and steroid creams can relieve some of the itching and inflammation.

Sexual Dysfunction

Sexual dysfunction is *not* uncommon among cancer patients. It includes changes in desire, impotency, and longer time to orgasm. There may be *increased* sexual desire in some. Both men and women can be affected by sexual dysfunction. Surgery, radiation, and chemotherapy can hurt or damage the ovaries or testicles and affect how much estrogen, progesterone, and testosterone is produced. This directly affects sexual drive. Some women may stop having periods; some men may have little to no sperm production, and perhaps impotency.

The cancer itself is not the only cause for sexual dysfunction, as dramatic changes in physical appearance can occur with hair loss and have psychological implications. Stress and anxiety alone can affect performance, as can fatigue, tiredness, and nerve problems owing to surgery, especially in men. Some chemotherapy medications can do this, especially drugs that manipulate hormones, such as tamoxifen, and the aromatase inhibitors, such as Femara and Arimidex. Other culprits are busulfan, Cytoxan, and estramustine.

Physicians should be contacted whenever there are any sexual problems—not just impotency. One of the best therapies is communication between partners. Most of these changes are temporary, and therapies exist. Knowledge will help immensely, as the problem is often due to therapy and not something intrinsically or permanently wrong with the individual per se. It bears repeating that the brain is the largest sex organ; attitude is important, and relaxing is key. There are many ways to share love besides intercourse. Intimate touch includes so much more: cuddling, kissing, hugging, and all manners of touch. Some patients find that a diary of daytime sexual thoughts helps them gravitate toward things that make them or their partner feel more prone to sex and feel more sexual. *Never* underestimate the value of the imagination. Most women will not lose the ability to orgasm, although some positions may become more uncomfortable. The lubricants mentioned earlier may also be of use. Lubricated condoms and vaginal dilators are also available if needed. The American Cancer Society has specific literature on this issue.

Men need to know that the ability to have an orgasm is not actually controlled by the same mechanism that controls the ability to have an erection, and thus the ability to orgasm is often not lost. Medications are available for erection problems due to decreased blood flow or nerve dysfunction. Some are taken by mouth, such as Viagra, Levitra, and Cialis; some are injected into the penis, such as Caverject and PAP; and some are inserted into the urethra at the end of the penis, such as Muse. Most oral medications need thirty to sixty minutes to work and may last up to thirty-six hours. The injectable medications should be used within five to ten minutes and last up to one hour. Vacuum erection devices can help sustain an erection but may make some positions uncomfortable. There are also very effective semi-turgid and inflatable devices that can be implanted surgically.

Xerostomia

Xerostomia is principally a dry mouth. The condition usually occurs as a result of the patient not making enough saliva. This can lead to more severe problems, as saliva fights cavities. Xerostomia may develop from direct radiation to the mouth or salivary glands, or it may be caused by some forms of chemotherapy. Maintaining fluid intake and avoiding alcohol, which dries the mouth, are important. I recommend developing the habit of taking sips between every bite of food or eating ice chips or cubes, as well as eating sugarless hard candy and popsicles and chewing sugarless gum rather than their sugar-containing counterparts. As we have discussed before, one should be careful by eating softer, moister food, such as milkshakes, baby food, bananas, applesauce, and puddings. Dry, crisp, cereal-like food can be very problematic. Xerostomia increases the risk of cavities; thus, careful dental hygiene is essential. A home humidifier and practice at nose breathing can be very effective, as can artificial saliva. There are some medications of modest effectiveness one can get from one's physician to treat this condition.

THE PROBLEM OF PAIN

There is probably nothing more vexing to the clinician and frightening to the patient and family, while still being amenable to successful treatment, than the problem of pain. The problem has many aspects, principal of which is that, although our prioritization of the treatment of pain and the techniques available have improved, we are often too far behind in the prevention of pain as part of its treatment. Although the problem now has the international spotlight and pain assessment is considered "the fifth vital sign," we still have issues of physician inexperience regarding the numerous options available or presuppositions shared by physicians and patients alike regarding addiction and all the adverse things they think go with it. In brief, addiction is *very* uncommon in the appropriately treated cancer patient, and the treatment of pain can actually be one of the most rewarding aspects of cancer care, as over 90% of patients need not be in pain, including those with a terminal diagnosis.

One-third of all Americans will develop chronic pain at some point in their lives. It remains the number-one reason to seek medical care, and it is estimated that the total cost in lost wages and treatment may be as high as $100 billion per year. Cancer can cause pain from the direct invasion or stretching of organs, tissues, and bones. Radiation, chemotherapy, and surgery may also variably cause pain. There are approximately three-quarters of a million patients with cancer-associated pain in the United States yearly. The risk of cancer-associated pain varies enormously with tumor type and, unfortunately, often signals to the nonprofessional and patient alike that the patient is dying, which is *not* necessarily so. The most conservative estimates are that 45% of cancer patients who could be free of pain have their pain undertreated. More sadly, studies of populations of cancer patients suggest that minorities and the elderly—especially women—are the least well treated. Another problem with pain is that acute pain is often visible; you can almost see it as a third party. However, the much more unpleasant chronic pain may appear to be invisible, leading to occasional episodes of physicians doubting the level of pain the patient is experiencing.

The data of undertreatment is daunting regarding pain management, but it is getting better. Physicians typically inadequately assess pain at least half of the time. Furthermore, more than 20% of treating physicians appear to have an unrealistic fear of opiates or are simply not knowledgeable regarding their use. This ignorance is magnified when considering the more sophisticated, highly successful techniques of pain treatment available that employ multiple types of medications. Patients also share some of the responsibility for undertreatment in that there is a reluctance to report pain and a reluctance to take medicines as prescribed at least 50% of the time. Nonetheless, the caregiver is ultimately responsible in that it matters not what the patient's preconceived ideas are; rather, it matters what the physician does about them. Providers have to ask and believe their patients, give them permission to state their level of pain, and assure them they will not become addicts or lose competency when effectively treated.

Studies from over twenty-five major cancer centers have shown that the aggressive treatment of cancer pain invariably leads to better outcomes, even occasionally greater duration, as well as better odds of survival. It is not so much the improvement of the pain per se, but rather that aggressive treatment is often associated with more attention to detail by all, as well as less development of other problems that can occur simply because the pain is so debilitating when not controlled. Furthermore, as the pain cycle progresses unabated, there is increasing psychological distress and desperation that only fuels the cycle and increases the perception of pain as painful, ominous, and foreboding of imminent disaster or even death. It is well known but frequently not put into practice that aggressive treatment of pain *before* the cycle gets well underway *always* requires *less* total medication, thus decreasing the risk of adverse effects from pain treatment. It invariably takes significantly more medication to treat pain once it is of even modest duration or escapes control.

I ask patients to look at a simple pain scale that is no more than a line ten inches long, with zero being no pain and ten being the worst they have ever experienced. This is also the recommendation of the World Health Organization and is called the Visual Analogue Scale for Pain.

Physicians should also assess the *nature* of the pain, not just its level. Many types of pain respond to different modalities. Is it a body ache and internal, such as with twisting, traction, or distention? Is it referred to another area and thus poorly localized? Is the pain psychogenic and somatoform, which means real to the patient but beyond objective findings? Is it neuropathic, such as burning, tingling, altered sensations, or is it electrical, from damage to the central nervous system, peripheral nervous, system, or both?

The *initial* goal of a provider is to obtain at least a twelve-hour baseline of the patient's pain with a treatment goal of *at least* less than four on the scale for constant pain. Pain that escapes control episodically is called breakthrough pain. The goal should be to have this be no more than a three initially. The ultimate goal is zero around the clock, and this goal is obtainable.

The World Health Organization has published a staircase like stepwise approach to pain which starts with mild nonsteroidal anti-inflammatory drugs (such as *Motrin, Naprosyn, Mobic, Celebrex,* etc.). This may be with or without non-opiate drugs that act additively and have other more common uses, such as antidepressants, antiseizure medications, and even some types of steroids. Treatment of moderate pain involves the same medications with mild opiates added. Severe pain is treated with all of the former, substituting strong opiates and long-lasting sustained-release forms of opiates for short-acting opiates in the case of breakthrough pain.

Additive medications that can enhance pain treatment are called adjuvants. Common examples are Tylenol, low-dose antidepressants that can work in as little as one week, and anticonvulsants—especially the relatively nontoxic Neurontin and corticosteroids. There are also drugs known as neuroleptics, antihistamines, benzodiazepines (such as Valium and Ativan), antispasmodics, muscle relaxants, and systemic and local anesthetics. The provider must know the drugs well, however, so he or she can advise on effects and look out for adverse effects.

One of the most common mistakes is to the use of too much Tylenol while not considering kidney and liver toxicity. Another error is to dose too highly with anti-inflammatories, such as Motrin, and neglect stomach and kidney toxicity.

Local invasive procedures can sometimes be pretreated with EMLA (eutectic mixture of local anesthetics), which is a topical anesthetic. This is usually is a 1:1 mixture of procaine and lidocaine. It may be helpful in nerve pain from herpes, known as herpetic neuralgia, as can capsaicin, the ingredient that gives chili peppers their hotness. EMLA and capsaicin have both been useful in treatment of chest wall pain in mastectomy patients.

Another often overlooked drug is Decadron, a potent steroid used in high doses of 20 mg three times a day up to 100 mg per day for bowel obstruction pain or pressure from compression of the spinal cord or tumor in the brain.

Some patients with cancer that has spread to bone can benefit from the administration of radioactive substances like strontium-89 and samarium-159, which peak in four to eight weeks and last three to five months but can cause suppression of the bone marrow. These isotopes can do wonders for prostate cancer and other cancers that frequently spread to bone.

Major steps have been made in the method of delivery of opiates and other pain medications. There are now many forms of sustained-release, long-acting strong opiates as well as lozenges and transdermal patches (which are absorbed continuously through the skin over a few days). The FDA is presently reviewing inhaled opiates for extremely rapid relief. Even chemotherapy drugs are receiving FDA approval because one of their major benefits appears to be a decrease in the pain the cancer is causing. This has been seen with gemcitabine in pancreatic cancer and mitoxantrone in prostate cancer.

Ziconotide is a new synthetic drug similar to the venom of the sea snake. It is administered into the spinal canal with an implanted pump and is nonaddictive and more potent than morphine without the risk of addiction or withdrawal. However, it can lower blood pressure, cause dizziness, and cause alterations to one's mental state on occasion.

Little known to patients, except perhaps to prior heavy exercisers, is that exercise can be effective at reducing pain. God made us with both endogenous opiates and receptors for them in many locations. This is one of the reasons one may see tolerance to an opioid dose; very high doses may be tolerated well without risk of overdose once a patient has accommodated to them over a modest period. I have shocked more than a few score of trainees by administering almost a gram—one hundred times a beginning dose—of morphine, to a patient who had slowly become very tolerant. There is no ceiling dose for these drugs if they are handled correctly.

One drug that should not be used is Demerol. It can have long-acting metabolites and can cause seizures in higher doses. There are superior drugs. There are many long-acting opiates—some oral, some transdermal—and they all work. Common reasons for lack of success are too low a dose of the long-acting opiate and infrequent dosing of short-acting opiates for breakthrough pain. There should always be doses available for predictable pain before it happens—an enormous mistake invariably made. The total dose needed will be less if the pain is controlled. As said, there is no maximum opioid dose. The goal is to adjust for both side effects and pain relief while ensuring that pain relief is around the clock. As an example, if a patient is at a baseline of four or more on the pain scale, the twenty-four-hour dose should be increased by 25–50%, and supplemental doses for breakthrough pain of 10–15% of the total twenty-four-hour dose should be administered.

Some drugs are just not that effective but are popular for legal reasons. A classic example is Darvon, which is a poor analgesic. In addition, I never use codeine, as it often is nauseating and can cause horrendous constipation in the 5–15% of patients who have enzymes that metabolize it, thus leaving it with no analgesic effect. I find that Vicodin and its relatives are also somewhat weak opiates. A commonly underused drug is Dilaudid, which is effective both orally and by the continuous subcutaneous route. It is a marvelous analgesic. There are good points to methadone, but it is best left in the hands of the most experienced, as it can have a long duration of action and presence in the body with a tendency to accumulate. Fentanyl is available transmucosally, like a lollipop, with an onset of twenty to thirty minutes, but this has no correlation with the three-day-duration fentanyl patch dosing. Thus, although both together are good, one must carefully find the right dose of each. Furthermore, patients will need to be treated for pain control for the first twelve to twenty-four hours of the first patch, as it may not take full effect until after that period. The intraspinal route can also be used to deliver drugs, although this takes considerable expertise and is often reserved for specific indications, with a common one being treatment of severe pain in the near-terminal patient in whom an IV is unwanted or ineffective. Minute amounts of medication can cause profound analgesia. This is usually a last resort option.

There are alternative and, some would say, complementary forms of pain management for which there is some supporting data from clinical trials. None has been shown *conclusively* and *reproducibly* to be of benefit in the majority of patients with cancer pain. Most importantly, there appears to be no harm from these therapies other than if they are blindly chosen over the more conventional proven and reliable options discussed above. I do support their role as adjuncts that may be of help.

Acupuncture is an ancient therapy whereby tiny needles are inserted under the skin to "balance the energy flow." This has been shown to be useful for low back pain, musculoskeletal pain, arthritis, headaches, and for cancer pain in some patients. There are documented case reports of various types of surgery being performed with acupuncture as the only form of analgesia. Hydrotherapy refers to when water, under pressure or not, is applied to parts or all of the body to relieve pain. Some common examples are sauna, water massage, simple showers, tepid baths, and compresses. The philosophy behind this is that toxins are causing pain and this therapy effects their removal while stimulating circulation. There are clear studies that show that whirlpools may aid in the relief of severe mechanical low back pain, but the benefit of routine use for other forms of musculoskeletal pain or arthritis has been shown to be inconclusive and not reliable.

Massage is focused on the belief that pressure to painful soft tissues will decrease tensions and increase circulation. It is commonly used in musculoskeletal pain, fibromyalgia, low back pain, arthritis, and migraine. Prolotherapy injects irritants, such as simple sugars (typically dextrose), into ligaments and tendons. This approach supposedly stimulates inflammation that then facilitates healing. This is also known as nonsurgical ligament reconstruction. Tai Chi has grown considerably in popularity. The slow, patterned movements with controlled deep breathing, guided imagery, and mental focus are intended to facilitate stretching, increase strength, improve coordination and balance, and enhance the mind–body connection. Yoga consists of assuming and holding postures involving considerable stretching with the intent of achieving balance between the mind, body, and spirit. Many varieties are widely practiced. The principal ones are Lyengar, Anusara, and integral yoga. As with Tai Chi, there is no mistaking the benefit of meditation, stretching, and mentally reframing oneself in relation to the physical world.

As will always be the case in the healing arts, there are some techniques that are clearly fringe, unproven, potentially harmful, and without much credibility. This does not diminish their popularity, however, and it is wise to be aware of them. The Graston technique employs stainless steel instruments that are rubbed over painful areas to prompt the destruction and disruption of supposed scar tissue. Magnetic therapy has a very long history. Small magnets similar to those used in elementary school for science class are placed over strategic areas of skin or in the clothes near a painful area or "special" points. The claim is that they improve blood flow and cellular function. Meilus muscular therapy involves the use of a robotic arm that applies pressure to some muscles to prompt the release of lactic acid (a byproduct of routine cellular metabolism that increases when energy sources and oxygen supply are lower). Lactic acid is a known irritant linked to muscular fatigue. The concept is once again that toxins will be released, improving pain. Ozone (three oxygen atoms linked together) has been injected into joints based on the erroneous belief that this will somehow increase the breakdown of toxins and improve their removal. This is ineffective and raises safety concerns.

There are some rules of thumb one should never forget owing to their simplicity, the reward of following them, and the enormous discomfort that can occur when they are ignored. The most important is to start a cathartic as well as a stool softener when starting an opiate. Waiting for constipation will compound the problem of pain. Medications like Sennakot, Dulcolax, Metamucil, magnesium citrate, Reglan, and cisapride can do wonders when correctly prescribed. Stool softeners are only additive but often not sufficient. Another word to the wise is that when on narcotics, patients should be instructed to rise slowly, as transient low pressure and dizziness upon rising are not rare, as are initial dizziness, sedation, itching, dry mouth, decreased urination, confusion, nausea, vomiting, sweating, and, lastly, respiratory depression, which is rare if care is taken to not overdose.

Patients often say they are allergic to medications for pain. True allergies are rare. Less than 1% experience asthmalike attacks or hives. Most patients who say they are allergic are referring to nausea, vomiting, and constipation. If there is disturbing sedation, which often wears off, Ritalin (5–10 mg at the morning and 5 mg at noon) is very effective and will not interfere with the pain relief. Patients should be cautioned about the possibility that their natural reflexes may be slowed when they are out and about in their daily lives, which could affect driving and such. The vast majority of patients find that the right dosages of analgesics do not significantly impair them.

Rarely, the dose required for adequate pain control of a terminal patient might cause respiratory depression severe enough to precipitate death. Philosophers, ethicists, legal minds, and theologians have rigorously looked at this. If it occurs, it is considered death by double effect, in which the goal was treatment of pain in a terminal patient and *not* physician-assisted suicide or euthanasia.

If tolerance develops to the opioid, one simply increases the dose. Tolerance is *not* addiction. Physical dependency is also *not* addiction and occurs when abrupt cessation of the medication creates a well-defined withdrawal syndrome. One simply goes more slowly. Addiction is all of the former plus drug-seeking behavior and interference with activities of daily living in an adverse manner. Take this to heart; all of you frightened patients and less-than-well-informed physicians: addiction is usually a rare or unimportant concept in a cancer patient. The incidence rate of this is less than one in three thousand.

Terminal pain in the uncommunicative patient often signals itself by facial grimacing and signs of agitation. If present, physicians should judiciously give whatever dose is necessary for the patient not to suffer. It is ethical, legal, and our duty.

The diagnosis of cancer is *not* synonymous with death or a sentence for life with constant pain. Although pain is realistically and metaphorically part of living, it does *not* need to be constant, uncontrolled, or an unwelcome companion as we pass. It does *not* have to hurt to heal.

ALTERNATIVE AND UNPROVEN FORMS OF CANCER TREATMENT

Introduction

Motivated by the desire to improve their quality of life, get relief from symptoms and side effects, and feel more in control, many people with cancer are exploring therapies in addition to mainstream cancer care. The National Center for Complementary and Alternative Medicine (NCCAM), part of the National Institutes of Health, defines complementary and alternative medicines (also known as CAM) as a "group of diverse medical and health care systems, practices and products that are not presently considered to be part of conventional medicine." Some examples of CAM therapies include meditation, relaxation techniques, prayer, music and art therapy, acupuncture, biofeedback, and visualization.

CAM refers to more than specific treatments or practices. In essence, it is a broad social movement that continues to attract more and more people each year. In a recent government survey, 36% of US adults use some form of CAM. In a study done by Eisenberg et al in 1998, it was estimated that 629 million visits were made to providers of CAM services in 1997, costing between $12–20 billion in out-of-pocket expenses.

In contrast, strictly alternative medicines are usually independent treatments that are promoted as something to use instead of conventional therapies. An example of this is using a diet or herbs to treat cancer instead of treatment that has been proven and suggested by an oncologist.

Though they may seem to offer hope when conventional treatments fail, alternative medicines are often unproven and can be dangerous. This is particularly true when choosing to delay treatment of cancer in order to use unproven alternative methods, which can lessen the likelihood of remission and cure.

Some CAM therapies have been scientifically studied to find out if they are effective. For many other therapies, however, important questions remain about whether they are safe, how they work, and whether they actually treat the diseases for which they are being used. Currently, no scientific studies have shown that complementary or alternative therapy alone can cure disease. However, CAM might be effectively used to do the following:

- relieve symptoms and side effects of cancer and its treatment
- control pain and improve comfort
- relieve stress and anxiety
- enhance physical, emotional, and spiritual well-being
- improve quality of life

If you are thinking about using CAM, it is important to educate yourself. Always remember, when choosing complimentary alternative medicine,

1. tell your doctor about your CAM use,
2. carefully select the CAM practitioner to ensure high quality and professionalism,
3. do not assume just because a product is called "natural" that it is safe, and
4. use only information from trusted resources.

When patients wade into this mishmash and quagmire of largely a mixture of misrepresentation and the fears of man, I am tempted to advise them to just say no. However, when all conventional hope from conventional medicine (allopathic medicine) is lost, it is unwise to take such a position. It implies that the plant and animal kingdom has not brought us legions of drugs and leads, and that is clearly *not* true and never will be. Such an easy dismissal of the topic also denies patients' autonomy, and it is also intellectually irresponsible for an author to omit what is reality for many patients. Nonetheless, my sentiments are clear; these are risky waters, and patients, before choosing to wade in, must talk with their board-certified oncologist.

Few things can be as annoying in medicine than another huckster (especially when they are "doctors"—usually non-clinician PhDs or self-styled actors) carnie-barking some new snake oil that cures Uncles Lou's lumbago, little Johnnie's libido, and everything in between. The success of such endeavors is really a sad testimonial to how we mere mortals are obsessed with youth and immortality, but not health per se. We only obsess on health when we do not have it, and most still do too little to maintain and promote it. Frankly, the world of the wacko witch doctor is both a reflection of this obsession and a testimonial to capitalism. Those are the prime drivers of outrageous claims of cure, irrespective of passionate, tear-filled testimonials, plaintiff wails to the contrary, and altruistic proclamations of helping humanity.

We need to rekindle our brains and review the existence of the placebo effect. Remember the differences between an anecdote and a clinical trial, and have some confidence in the FDA. Hucksters thrive on the first two and escape the third and fourth by way of idiosyncrasies of federal law.

First, the majority of these whiz-bang potions escape the scrutiny of the FDA by being regarded as food supplements; they do not need to be, and have not been, proven as effective. Furthermore, all that is needed to practice any medicine in the United States is a valid license, a successfully completed postdoctoral internship in an accredited institution, and a passing score on the board examinations. One can then call himself or herself any type of physician he or she chooses, as well as invent an unrecognized specialty. Such individuals may not get hospital privileges without more extensive training and certification by a national board of examiners, but they may open an office or clinic and hang a shingle.

In addition, the FDA does not regulate these wonder potions. Since the FDA does not (cannot by law) regulate these wonder concoctions or treatments, there are almost no correctly done clinical trials supporting their use. Why would there be, as there is no regulation, financial incentive, or competition that would foster them. There is no $500–$600 million invested and no phase 1, 2, 3, and 4 research. There is no quality control and no pressure of scientific scrutiny or peer review. Patients will never know, and purveyors of the potions are not obligated to promise or guarantee that the jungle juice one is putting in some orifice is uncontaminated, let alone nontoxic or effective. Most studies that can be funded to examine this show that contamination and lack of purity is the rule. Patients may never know if the substance is pure, whether the amount taken is an effective concentration, what adverse effects in carefully controlled trials it can have, or whether it can have unwanted or even dangerous interactions with other drugs.

"Alternative medicine" is a somewhat argued term for a diverse assortment of philosophies, theories, and diagnostic, therapeutic, and preventive practices not generally regarded with any respect by the more Western allopathic medical community. People from other cultures use many of these remedies as their primary source of health care. However, in most developed countries these alternative methodologies are used along with conventional Western practices. Thus, the terms "complementary medicine" and "integrative medicine" are commonly used. It is also true that the word "complementary" can be used to refer to classically proven methods and modalities used in unconventional ways or to achieve unconventional endpoints thought to be of value.

In April 1995, the National Institutes of Health Office of Alternative Medicine established a panel on definition and description. It was charged "to establish a definition of the field of Complementary and Alternative Medicine (*CAM*) for the purposes of identification and research and to identify factors critical to thorough and unbiased description of (CAM) systems and practices that would be applicable to both quantitative and qualitative research." The panel defined CAM as follows: "CAM is a broad domain of healing resources that encompasses all health systems, modalities and practices and their accompanying theories and beliefs, other than those intrinsic to the politically dominant health system of a particular society or culture in a given historical period. CAM includes all such practices and ideas self defined by their users as preventing or treating illnesses or promoting health and well-being. Boundaries within CAM and between CAM and the dominant system are not always sharp or fixed."

It's important to be an informed consumer. Learn as much as you can about therapies you are thinking of trying. Understand the risks, potential benefits, and evidence of effectiveness for CAM therapies. Few scientific studies of their effectiveness have been conducted. The National Center for Complementary and Alternative Medicine (NCCAM) is a good source for learning about existing studies.

Information from websites should be viewed with a critical eye. The Internet is a wonderful resource that allows you to obtain volumes of information with the click of a mouse, but not all information on the Internet is accurate. For this reason, it is important to evaluate websites with a critical eye. Look for sites that have been established by government agencies, universities, or reputable medical or health-related associations. Be wary of sites that are paid for by a manufacturer of products, drugs, etc. Ask yourself, "What is the purpose of this site?" Educational sites are more credible than those designed to sell a product. Information on the website should include clear references from scientific journals. (Personal stories are not adequate to back up statements.) The information should also be current and recently updated. Be skeptical of sites that ask you for money or make claims that sound too good to be true.

Check with the federal government for information about therapies you are considering. If you are considering a therapy, check with the FDA's website, www.fda.gov, to see if they have information about it. The FDA's Center for Food Safety and Applied Nutrition website has information about dietary supplements at www.cfsan.fda.gov. You can also visit the FDA's website on recalls and safety alerts at www.fda.gov/opacom/7alerts.html. The Federal Trade Commission (FTC) offers information about consumer alerts for fraudulent therapies at www.ftc.gov. Also, visit the NCCAM website, www.nccam.nih.gov, to see if it has information on the therapy.

Always check credentials. Licensed and credentialed practitioners can provide higher-quality care than unlicensed ones. Credentials do not ensure that a practitioner is competent, but they show he or she has met certain standards to treat patients. The training, skill, and experience of the practitioner affect safety, so ask your physician or someone you believe is knowledgeable regarding CAM for recommendations. Hospitals and medical schools sometimes keep lists of area CAM practitioners, and some may have a CAM center or CAM practitioners on staff. You may want to contact a professional organization for the type of practitioner you are seeking. Finally, many states have regulatory agencies or licensing boards that may be able to tell you about practitioners in your area.

Quackwatch and other watchdog groups may be helpful. Quackwatch is one example of a nonprofit organization that aims to identify health-related frauds, myths, fads, and fallacies. This group primarily tries to expose quacks, or "pretenders to medical skill ... [those] who [talk] pretentiously without sound knowledge of the subject discussed." Quackwatch is useful for gaining background information on a questionable CAM topic or for finding information that is difficult or impossible to find elsewhere. The services mentioned above may be found on www.quackwatch.org.

Types of CAM

There are a number of conceptual organizational schemes for understanding CAM. I present one below.

There are six major types of CAM. They are alternative medical systems, mind/body interventions, biologically based therapies, manipulative and body-based systems, and energy therapies. Mind/body interventions are the most commonly used CAM (53%) when prayer is included. Alternative medical systems are complete systems of theory and practice developed by ancient cultures. They remain mostly unchanged and are independent from the conventional medical approaches used in the United States. A common goal of alternative medical systems is cultivating harmony of mind and body. While this concept is appealing, its underlying assumptions about how the body functions and how the disease process unfolds are not entirely supported by current scientific understanding. Examples of alternative medical systems include (1) ayurveda, (2) homeopathy, (3) naturopathy, (4) traditional Chinese medicine, (5) mind/body intervention, and (6) biologically based therapies.

Ayurvedic medicine has been practiced primarily in the Indian subcontinent for five thousand years. It classifies people into one of three body types, offering specific herbal remedies and dietary regimens to promote health and well-being for each. Ayurveda views a balanced consciousness as key to preventing and treating disease. It emphasizes techniques like yoga and meditation to maintain this balance. Few clinical studies of ayurveda have been conducted. The National Institute of Ayurvedic Medicine website is www.niam.com, and their phone number is 1-843-278-8700.

Homeopathic medicine originated in Germany during the eighteenth century, before the development of modern medicine and is based on the principal that like cures like. It uses small, highly diluted amounts of medicinal substances that would cause symptoms at higher, more concentrated doses to treat those same symptoms. The substances it uses to cure symptoms are derived from plants, minerals, or animals.

Systemic reviews and clinical trials have not found homeopathy to be a definitely proven treatment for any medical condition. Some researchers suggest homeopathy may help patients who believe the treatment is working, as a result of the placebo effect. Relying on this type of treatment alone when you have cancer may have severe and irreversible negative health consequences. For more information, visit the National Center for Homeopathy website at www.homeopathic.org, or call 1-877-624-0613.

Naturopathic medicine integrates various approaches to healing, including dietary modifications, massage, exercise, stress reduction, acupuncture, and conventional medicine. Practitioners believe the body will heal itself if a healthy internal environment is created. Many naturopathic remedies are also used in other types of CAM. There is no scientific evidence that naturopathic medicine cures cancer or any other disease. The effectiveness of different naturopathic methods varies. Though most methods are not harmful, some herbal preparations can be toxic. Methods like fasting, limiting the diet, and administering enemas can be dangerous if used excessively. Relying on this type of treatment alone may have profound and irreversible negative health consequences for the cancer patient. For more information, visit the American Association of Naturopathic Physicians website at www.naturopathic.org, or call 1-866-538-2267.

Traditional Chinese medicine (TCM) views the human body as an ecosystem; imbalances between opposing forces in this system and disruption in the flow of energy, or chi, produce illness. The goal of TCM treatments is to maintain and restore balance and energy flow. Specific treatment methods primarily consist of herbal remedies, acupuncture, diet, massage, and meditative physical exercise. Acupuncture, the most commonly used treatment in TCM, has been proven to reduce nausea related to chemotherapy in some patients. In addition, acupuncture has been found to be effective when combined with drugs in controlling postoperative pain for some patients. More research is needed to determine the effectiveness of the herbal remedies and other practices of TCM. While the anticancer effect may be limited, some practices have been found to reduce stress and side effects of cancer treatment. For more information, contact the National Institutes of Health National Center for Complementary and Alternative Medicine Clearing House. Information on acupuncture is available at the National Institutes of Health website: nccam.nih.gov. The NIH may also be contacted by telephone at 1-888-644-6226. The Society for Acupuncture Research website is www.acupunctureresearch.org.

Mind/body interventions use different techniques to enhance the mind's ability to affect bodily function and symptoms. Examples include prayer, meditation, guided imagery, and art, music, or dance therapy. Prayer for health reasons, when included as a mind/body intervention, is utilized by 43% of CAM users. The impact of prayer, spirituality, and religion on the well-being of cancer patients and their loved ones is an area of increasing study and interest. Meditation relaxes the body and calms the mind, often creating a feeling of well-being. There are different forms and methods of meditation, such as Zen, vipassana, and transcendental. It often involves sitting or standing in a quiet place and focusing on an object of meditation, such as the breath, a mantra, or the physical sensations of walking slowly. Meditation can be self-directed or guided.

There is no scientific evidence that meditation is effective in treating cancer or any other disease. Performed on a regular basis, however, it has been shown to have beneficial physiological and psychological effects. Clinical trials have found that meditation can reduce anxiety, stress, blood pressure, chronic pain, and insomnia. For more information, visit the Insight Meditation Society at www.dharma.org, or call 1-978-355-4378. The following article also contains good information on mind/body interventions: "NIH Consensus Development Program. NIH Panel Encourages Wider Acceptance of Behavioral Treatments for Chronic Pain and Insomnia. National Institutes of Health" (consensus.nih.gov/news/releases/017ta_release.htm).

Guided imagery practitioners help patients train the mind to produce a physiological goal. These goals allegedly can be self-taught with the aid of books or tapes, or practiced with the help of a trained professional. There is no scientific evidence that guided imagery can affect the progression of cancer. It has been proven effective in managing stress, anxiety, physical symptoms, side effects of chemotherapy, and pain. Imagery techniques are nonetheless viewed as safe, especially under the guidance of a trained professional, and numerous patients find them helpful as adjuncts in addition to standard therapy. For more information, visit the Natural Healers website at www.naturalhealers.com/qa/imagery.shtml. Also of interest is the following article:

Walker LG, Walker MG, Ogston K. et al and Psychological, "Clinical Pathological Effects of Relaxation Training and Guided Imagery during Primary Chemotherapy." Br J Cancer. 1999; 80:262–268.

Art, music, or dance therapy can be provided by professional artists, musicians, or dancers who are trained to deal with the psychosocial and medical issues that people—and, in some cases, cancer patients—face. Few rigorous clinical studies have been conducted for art or dance therapy, but anecdotal evidence suggests people find them helpful in reducing stress and enhancing coping skills. Randomized clinical trials have shown music therapy is effective for reducing anxiety, especially in a palliative care setting. For more information, contact the American Music Therapy Association (www.musictherapy.org, 1-301-589-3300), the American Art Therapy Association (www.arttherapy.org, 1-888-290-0878), or the American Dance Therapy Association (www.adta.org, 1-410-997-4040).

Also included in body manipulation are chiropractic and osteopathic manipulation and treatments. They do not treat cancer but can be helpful in relieving stress and, sometimes, pain. However, any patient at risk for bone fracture or with any other obvious reason to not undergo manipulations should steer very clear of this type of treatment. Bottom line—talk with your physician first.

Biologically based CAM therapies use substances that are found in nature, including herbs, certain foods or diets, and vitamins. Examples include dietary supplements, herbal products, and other natural, but unproven, therapies. Remember: a natural product is *not* necessarily a safe product! Please be aware of the following: An herbal product may keep other medicines from working. Herbal products and vitamins may keep other medicines, such as chemotherapy, from doing what they are supposed to do. For example, research on St. John's wort, sometimes taken for depression, has shown that it may cause certain anticancer drugs to *not* work well. A natural product may be harmful.

Dietary supplements may include vitamins, minerals, herbs or other botanicals, amino acids, and substances like enzymes, organ tissues, and metabolites. Dietary supplements come in many forms, including extracts, concentrates, tablets, capsules, gelcaps, liquids, and powders. They are considered foods, not drugs, so there are no regulations controlling their safety, content, quality, or dose recommendations. The FDA does not require manufacturers to print side effects on the labels of these products; nor does it require manufacturers to remove their products from the market unless it can *prove* they are unsafe.

Dietary supplements have different active substances, so their effectivenesses must be assessed individually. The American Cancer Society (www.cancer.org) has an extensive listing of dietary supplements on their website and offers guidance through advice given by supporters and critics.

The controversy of alternative diets still rages. Diet and vitamin cancer "cures" have not been found to be scientifically effective as cancer treatments. However, nutrition during and after cancer treatment is frequently a subject that concerns and interests people with cancer and their loved ones. It is hard to make sense of the abundance of information that is available related to anticancer diets. There are several popular approaches that are described below. Please remember that none of these approaches have been scientifically proven to prevent or eliminate cancer. People with cancer often find that a registered dietician can be helpful in improving their nutritional practices during cancer treatment and beyond.

- **Macrobiotic diet**: A vegetarian diet often cited is one consisting predominantly of whole grains and cereals (50–60%), cooked vegetables and organic fruits (20%–25%), and soups made with vegetables, seaweed, grains, beans, and miso (5%–10%). Proponents believe it can prevent and cure disease, including cancer, and enhance feelings of well-being. There have been no clinical trials to show that such a macrobiotic or vegetarian diet can prevent or cure cancer. Earlier forms of the diet (which involved restricting the diet to brown rice and water) were associated with severe nutritional deficiencies.

- **Fasting**: Fasting entails not eating any foods and drinking only water or fruit juice for two to five days, or sometimes longer. Practitioners believe fasting cleanses the body of toxins. This belief is not supported by scientific research. The body cannot distinguish between fasting and starvation, and cancer studies suggest fasting may promote tumors.

- **Gerson therapy**: This therapy involves using coffee enemas and a special diet with supplements to cleanse the body and stimulate metabolism. It is based on the theory that disease is caused by the accumulation of toxic substances. No well-designed scientific studies have supported the beliefs behind Gerson therapy. One critique of the therapy in a well-respected medical journal concluded that the explanation for how it is supposed to work does not align with established principles of nutrition, biology, and cancer immunology. For more information, contact the Office of Dietary Supplements, National Institutes of Health (ods.od.nih.gov, 1-301-435-2920).

- **Herbal products** are used in many different types of natural medicine. In the United States, herbal medicine generally refers to a system of medicine that uses European or North American plants. Ayurvedic medicine uses plants from India, and TCM uses plants from China. Modern herbalists often use plants from many different regions of the world. Because herbs and roots have different active substances, their effectiveness must be evaluated individually. The American Cancer Society (www.cancer.org) has an extensive listing of herbs, vitamins, and minerals on their website and offers guidance through advice given by supporters and critics. For more information, contact the American Cancer Society (www.cancer.org, 1-800-ACS-2345).

Other authorities categorize most of CAM into the following major categories:

1. Megavitamins and other essential meganutrients—especially calcium
2. Herbal products of every imaginable kind
3. Bioelectromagnetic-based therapies, such as such as energy healing, therapeutic touch, and magnets
4. Metabolic therapies, such as the Kelley, Gerson, and Rivici treatments
5. Manipulative and body-based systems, such as Reiki, mind/body medicine, support groups, relaxation therapy, guided imagery, and hypnosis (these I support in a complementary way, as they do not defer conventional therapy when I recommend them)
6. Unconventional chemotherapies, such as antineoplastons, hydrazine sulfate, Laetrile and 714-x
7. Unconventional immunomodulative therapy, such as immunoaugmentation therapy, MGN-3, and beta D-glucans (which are extracted from various mushrooms)
8. Others, such as thymus therapy

As you can well imagine, there are many more, but most fall into one of these categories or organizational descriptive categories.

What Is Really Going On

CAM is used all over the world by cancer patients irrespective of the sophistication of the patient or the nation. It is at least a $50-billion industry in the Unites States, but accurate estimates are very difficult to establish. There is no regulation. It is impossible to assess the cost of any toxicity caused and lost opportunity that could have occurred from more-conventional, proven approaches. Furthermore, it appears that the use of CAM is increasing worldwide, although the intrinsically slippery nature of the beast makes it difficult to be certain. Estimates in the United States are that somewhere around 40% of all patients will try CAM at some point. Research suggests that CAM users are usually young patients of high educational level and income. These studies are very difficult to do, but there are some recurring themes.

Most cancer patients use more than one CAM modality, often simultaneously. The use is greater among those with advanced disease and in those who feel they have exhausted conventional therapy and have a poor prognosis. In fairness, most studies state that utilizers of CAM did feel some measure of benefit was derived. In the United States, the most common CAM modalities employed are mind/body, diet alterations, megavitamins, herbs, meditation, relaxation, spirituality, and prayer, the latter four of which I wholeheartedly endorse.

Why

The general claim of CAM therapies is that they are effective in boosting the immune system, slowing the cancer, or affecting a cure. The primal driving force is to survive and deal with fear by doing something is powerful. History is replete with what now seem incredible and outrageous escapades of the millions who have tried to escape death. Thus there have been, and always will be, frantic pursuits of the next fountain of youth, magical cures, or forbidden secrets that the often maligned pharmaceutical companies and the universal demons (whether they be the government, big business, or conventional medicine) allegedly do not want you to know. The grand conspiracy theory is always lurking as a scapegoat. This is often a feeble attempt to avoid finality and any modicum of pain and suffering or, sadly, for proponents to exploit the desperate to see themselves as guardians and even saviors. Just as assuredly, there will always be those who see enormous profit in capitalizing on these fears. There are other reasons to seek CAM. There is the fear of recurrence and the uncertainty of response as well as the heartfelt desire to participate in the disease. The latter is a good thing that requires direction to proven therapies.

Of course, I am *not* advocating giving up hope for alternative effective approaches. I celebrate thoughtful, rigorous, and judicious inquiry. The fact of the matter is that there are superb, safe mechanisms in place to welcome, encourage, and fund the study of the next better mousetraps, no matter how initially incredible or unlikely they seem, remembering that irrationality spawns only one offspring: irrationality. In the world of oncology, the only dividend of reckless disinterest and deviation from thoughtful inquiry is death, sooner or later. I implore all patients to read the section on self-talk, as *that* is a reliable alternative medicine I know will complement your treatment.

Sacred Cow Killing

I am not going to get into every reference that has discredited most, but not all, of the therapies I have enumerated. The references are easy enough to find through the NIH office and on the web at Pubmed, Medline, MD Consult, Medscape, and numerous other reputable sources that reference peer-reviewed literature. Acknowledged experts, in whatever their field of endeavor may be, have subjected these publications to intense scrutiny and question. Such a system has enormous checks and balances to ensure intellectual honesty as well as provide a forum for widespread public and rigorous debate. Rather, to really drive the point home, I wish to roll through some of the more notorious and outrageous therapies, as well as the more common. Some of these have a counter-culture elite status and need to be exposed.

There is hardly *any* corroborated (by worldwide conventional modality of study) high-level evidence for the effectiveness of *most* modalities of CAM therapy. In some cases, the "clinical trial" often touted as proof by the supporters of the treatment was precisely *not* a clinical trial. In general, ranging from the Mayo Clinic study of Linus Pauling's claims of the benefits of vitamin C megadoses to raw shark cartilage, there is nothing to support their use as a standard of care.

Nonetheless, a good deal of our armamentarium of drug therapies, as well as clues for development of future therapies, comes from the plant and animal kingdom. However, promising agents have and always will be subjected to rigorous scientific scrutiny in the form of irrefutable methodologies. Think about this: Were you a purveyor of potions of dubious merit, would you spend the time and hundreds of millions of dollars it takes to develop a promising drug if all you probably had was snake oil? Furthermore, would you do it *if the law did not require it*? As was explained previously, it is very easy to offer what *may* be active therapies, supplements, and alternative treatments and in no way be practicing medicine without a license. Remember, it is dubiously motivated individuals and patients, often desperate or made so by irresponsible claims, that sustain all this. After all, who does not want to hear of an almost instantly accessible treatment with glowing testimonials when they are either ill or, more often, deathly afraid of becoming so?

Some of the more notorious therapies have been either studied or attempted to be studied in clinical trials. For example, there have been the somewhat secretive promises of antineoplastins; they went the way of Laetrile and vitamin C. Studies by the NIH showed *no* benefit beyond placebo. The Gerson coffee bean enema therapy "trials" used retrospective, historical, uncontrolled data without access to authenticated records. In other words, fatal flaws in the study made all data irrelevant and highly suspect. Macrobiotic diet studies have been unable to develop a consensus that any of the evidence is compelling.

The Kelley-Gonzalez regimen for treatment of pancreatic cancer, in terms of clinical scrutiny, is a prime example of how *not* to do studies. However, there was enough of a hint of a possible response that Columbia University began a controlled clinical trial against our best therapy. It failed to show any benefit. Once again, this demonstrates that in reality, conventional medicine wants new therapies but demands careful study. It is the CAM advocates that issue the hue and cry, wailing that there's enormous arrogance and conspiracy by an establishment that is determined to see CAM fail.

What is the solution? A search for truth in a truthful way and a demand that CAM advocates be forced, through legislation, to either go the route of the FDA or require third-party independent scientific review of all claims as well as clinical trials to show safety and efficacy. There needs to be a clear declaration if no effectiveness is found or if there are toxicities. There also must be immediate study as outlined in this book if hope or promise is shown.

The bovine and shark cartilage stories are precise examples of this. The work done to date has been, at times, shoddy and has led to painfully difficult questions because some responses have been seen, but not in a properly administered trial. The value of what seemed to be promising substances contained therein did lead to research. Matrix metalloproteinases and antiangiogenesis factors are present in these types of cartilage. There is a wealth of research ongoing with these compounds, as they are pivotal substances used by our bodies in attempting to block tumors from gaining a foothold through the formation of new blood vessels that facilitate their survival and spread. I discuss them in "The Future." MD Anderson Cancer Center, as well as other international institutions, forged a path rapidly in the study of these types of compounds. However, simply because the raw substance has the tiny molecule of promise within it does *not* mean that ingestion of the raw product will deliver the molecule in an effective way and at an effective dose. It is thus easy to see the damage that can be done by not adhering to the enormous benefit reaped by following the scientific method.

Essiac is perhaps one of the most common herbal therapies; some of its constituents have been shown in the laboratory to have some antitumor activity. Yet there have been no clinical trials. Why? Money. There is already a market—largely free marketing by word of mouth by the uninformed and somewhat desperate—propelling its use. Furthermore, no regulations regarding the manufacture, sale, safety, or effectiveness exist; thus, there is every motivation to press forward. This is enormous medical irresponsibility that I feel borders on the criminal, at least ethically. It could be my or your tumor someday that responds to the correctly isolated and purified molecules if appropriate controls are in place and scientific scrutiny has been applied.

Mistletoe, marketed under many different names, the most well-studied being Helixor, has shown promising effects in the laboratory, and results in a few clinical trials have been promising, but only minimally. One can only hope in such instances that, based on the data, funding will continue to see if a new drug has indeed been found.

PC-SPES, which is probably no more than an antitestosterone compound (a well-known conventional method to treat prostate cancer), has shown some promise. But again, it has not been tested in head-to-head trials correctly done among similar patients. Such work is being done. Preliminarily, it looks as if we perhaps have another weak treatment for certain stages of prostate cancer but *not* a better modality. It is not without estrogenlike effects either.

Hydrazine gained so much notoriety in the lay press that the largely negative trials done by the NIH were criticized as flawed and the General Accounting Office was called in to audit them. No errors were found. The substance is, at best, controversial.

Complementary Exercises for People with Cancer

Yoga is a form of exercise, usually nonaerobic, that involves a sequence of postures and breathing activities. It can relieve some symptoms associated with cancer and other chronic diseases. A system of personal development from the Hindu tradition, it combines dietary guidelines, physical exercise, and meditation to create *prana*, or vital energy. Research has found yoga to be beneficial to control bodily functions like blood pressure, heart rate, respiration, and perhaps metabolism. It can lead to improved physical fitness and lower levels of stress.

Tai chi is an ancient Chinese martial art form. It is a mind/body system that uses movement, meditation, and breathing to improve health and well-being. Research has shown that tai chi is useful for improving posture, balance, muscle mass and tone, flexibility, stamina, and strength in older adults. Tai chi is also an effective method for reducing stress.

I am a great supporter of some *complementary* approaches, such as spirituality, some forms of self-help (self-talk), support groups, hypnosis, guided imagery, relaxation techniques, and acupuncture. These all have a well-proven record of accomplishment in the treatment of emotional, intellectual, bodily, and spiritual distress. They are not a substitute for conventional anticancer therapy, however.

Once again, allopathic physicians do not pooh-pooh research into CAM out of hand. There is an enormous amount of work being done. The Oshner Center at the University of California–San Francisco, Memorial Sloan Kettering Cancer Center in New York, and the University of Texas–Houston all have well-funded NIH-supported centers dedicated to CAM research. The National Cancer Institute Office of Cancer Complementary and Alternative Medicine and the Best Case Series Program have been dedicated since 1998 to focus and extend the research efforts of the institute into investigation of the most promising CAM therapies. They work in close collaboration with the NIH Cancer Advisory Panel for Complementary and Alternative Medicine to assure identification and research into promising modalities of CAM. Some of the more front-burner modalities studied in the recent past are black cohosh, soy, ginseng, over-the-counter antiandrogens, and a bevy of antioxidants.

Physician–Patient Communication

I believe physicians are mandated to act for the benefit of (in beneficence of) their patients. As such, it is essential that allopathic physicians become familiar with the over-the-counter and CAM world. It is easy to do, and it is reality that the majority of patients have at least considered looking. A balanced approach, when warranted, is wise. Patients must not be humiliated. Rather, I suggest they be advised to read this book and others, gain an understanding of the need for clinical trials, and learn the meanings of the words "anecdote" and "placebo effect."

Furthermore, physicians should explain what happens when the hands of the FDA, Congress and the AMA are tied. Patients should be assured of the great work being done in dedicated centers. However, there will come a time to fish or cut bait wherein the patient must be candid regarding whatever he or she is doing or taking and relate this to the oncologist, after which the two may decide which way they are going to proceed. An oncologist cannot possibly guess all of what his or her patients are ingesting or subjecting themselves to. Patients have a responsibility to not only inquire with their physician regarding recommended and alternative therapies, but also to inform the treating physician if they intend to try alternative therapy *before* they actually try it.

Fortunately, there are excellent unbiased, reputable resources available to help the treating physician learn about compounds patients wish to try or may have already tried. The PDR Network publishes a very thorough and well-referenced guide, *The Physicians' Desk Reference*. In addition, http://www.pitt.edu~cbw/altm.html is a very useful website.

Actually, frequent sources of information for patients are other patients, well-meaning family and friends, herbalists in malls, and, not surprisingly, weekend and late-night television and radio shows. The claims can be outrageous, and the proof, as science defines "proof," is usually nonexistent. What is sad is the degree of authority with which non-board-certified folks both diagnose and prescribe advice over the phone to folks who call in to these shows.

Perhaps the best source for scholarly and comprehensive information regarding alternative and complementary therapies is the Office of Technology Assessment at the NIH. The address of their website is http://www.ota.nap.edu/pdf/1990idx.html. In addition, the American Cancer Society has summaries of various CAM modalities at www.cancer.org. The dedicated CAM office at the NIH is at http://nccam.nih.gov. Summaries of CAM therapies can also be obtained from the National Cancer Institutes information service at www.cancernet.nci.nih.gov and the direct CAM office at http://www.cancer.gov/cam.

The consequence of dabbling in the "black arts" of complementary and alternative medicine can range from missing the benefits of conventional therapy to toxicities from the therapy or its interaction with conventional medication to potentially disastrous outcomes either directly or by removing oneself from the possibility of benefit from proven treatments. A diagnosis of cancer and the experience of pain and suffering hold enormous power to seduce us into leaving our intellects at the door. I implore patients not to do that. The greatest antidote to anxiety has always been, and will remain, knowledge. I prescribe heaping helpings for all.

THE FUTURE

Understanding Cutting-Edge Therapies

Understanding what the future of cancer care may hold can leave one absolutely awestruck by the enormous complexity, mystery, and genius of normal life at the most fundamental levels. Such is the stuff of genetics and the intricacies of our immune system, which miraculously protects us in a hostile world. For example, how did our toe know—yes, our toe; let's say the middle one on the left foot—how did it know when it had reached completion? How did it know when it was just right in only what a toe knows: size, shape, function, nail formation, maybe a little hair? Why is it not three feet long, shaped like a finger, or fundamentally not very much like it should be? Why did our liver stop forming at the point it did, and why are there not liver cells sitting in our kidneys, building up bile or, for that matter, making urine? Moreover, why did our kidney not end up in our spleen or large intestine? What directed these cells to the right location and honed them to the right and normal function? What is behind all this?

It seems everything in our bodies has its place and function. Although all tissues grow as we grow from a toddler, they know when to stop and say, "Okay, I am done now, and I am ready to be an adult organ." The answer is that it is all in the genes.

We have twenty-three pairs of chromosomes—thin strands of the building blocks of proteins called amino acids that are strung like rungs on a ladder on a sugar backbone in duplicate pairs called nucleotides. We also have one set of sex chromosomes, XX for female and XY for male.

All that genetic material is our DNA. Furthermore, that DNA holds the architect's blueprint, the magic key to each of us. Although I am not the same as you, I have largely 99% the same DNA in the same structure, right down to the atomic level, but I do not look, think, feel, act, age, or get diseases just like you. It is all in our genes. Is this not amazing? How did this all happen? Returning to our toe analogy, it would be correct, although simplistic, to say that in that very toe only the "toeness" part of the DNA was turned on. However, what happens to the non-toe DNA? Does not our toe have the same DNA as our cornea? Indeed it does, but it is not read or written into being something more.

In addition, every day thousands of foreign viruses, bacteria, and other foreign agents attack us; why do we not succumb? It is not only because of better hygiene and new vaccines. Let us look at simple acne. What is the pus in a pimple? It is nothing less than an army of specific cells from our immune system. This system is marvelously complex and integrates both a surveillance function as well as a "seek and destroy" capability that rivals the best military strategists' plans. Our immune system even has what are similar to marines—cells that hit the beach first and are early casualties in the cause of defense. We have grenadiers (cells that kill from a distance) and cells with lifetime memories once they are formed. There are ways for our cells to talk to each other over distances ranging from shorter than the width of a cell to as far as the length of one's body. Messages can be sent by touch or as chemical messengers with or without myriad intermediaries falling in place like dominoes.

The story complex and wondrous. We know self as self. We know it is *our* spleen and *someone else's* transplanted kidney. We have much more individuality than the singularity of fingerprints. We have millions of molecules as numerous as the stars in the heavens that mark our self as self. One of the recent Nobel prizes was given to a physician from Seattle who helped us discover this mystery in our bone marrow, where some of the most primitive of all cells live. Understanding this, he started to crack the code and matched patients sufficiently enough to accept a transplant of another's bone marrow.

Internationally, there have been and will remain thousands of investigators working on how the immune system performs surveillance, how it suppresses and fights things that are foreign invaders, and how all the while it knows us as uniquely ourselves. It follows that if the same DNA is in all cells, there must be some cells with more of it turned on than turned off. These cells would then have the potential to be the Adam and Eve (of Genesis) cells—the stem of the vine. Yes, we have found these cells, and of course, they are in both our bone marrow and human embryos. They are stem cells.

All other cells, such as those in the tissues of our toes, liver, nose, kidneys, and other organs, migrate in the growing embryo to their normal adult locations. There they mature, slowing turning off that DNA which is not needed and turning on that DNA which is needed to become the adult form of the toe, liver, nose, or kidney cells. Thus, it is easy to understand the enormous excitement and controversy over stem cell research, as these are cells with a complete package of chromosomes in one cell, ready to become whatever they wish. These are omniscient, multitasking cells with DNA scintillatingly active and harmonically resonating to whatever triggers the call for them to develop into a normal adult cell of a specific type.

All of these cells must have nutrition to live. Thus, there must be the birth of rivulets of blood in minute capillaries. This blood brings sustenance in just the right amount and carries away waste. Science has long been fascinated with trying to decipher how the signals are sent to create these new vessels. Furthermore, how do new cells know to go to the liver to be a liver and to the spleen to be a spleen? Why can some cells replenish themselves to some degree, whereas others appear unable to do so, such as skin cells and nerve cells, respectively? The human vessel we inhabit, this marvelous body of ours, determines it all fundamentally at the molecular level.

So what are we to make of all of this, and what of cancer treatment in the future? We are barely scratching the surface as we garner this knowledge faster than it can be published. It has long been clear to science that when armed by the discovery of just what is normal, one can begin to unravel what the clever and insidious enemy, cancer, does. Through understanding the norm and its unraveling, science is designing atom-specific attacks rather than medieval battering rams against cancer. Soon the days of chemotherapy will be ended and biologic, immunologic, and intelligent singular customized attacks will characterize our armamentarium. Clearly, we are at an embryonic level of questions and are not yet mature in our answers. Now with marvelously fast computer software and hardware, phenomenal abilities to detect and dissect proteins to the atomic level, and the human genetic code "cracked," the very building blocks are in place for unfathomable progress in our fight against cancer.

This is not to dismiss advances like finer microscopic surgical techniques, twice and thrice a day three-dimensional radiotherapy, or the focusing of radiation beams stereotactically with computer-aided precision. They are important as well, but they are not at the core genetic or immune level, where the unraveling of what makes cancer and normal unique will lead to cancer cell–specific therapies. I am talking about cracking the "code" for cancers at the genetic and protein level. We have entered into a new world—a world filled with the technologies of monoclonal antibodies, radioimmunoconjugates, farnestryltransferase inhibitors, small-molecule rationally designed drugs, tumor vaccines, proteasome technology, nonsense oligonucleotides, growth-factor inhibitors, and heat-shock proteins. We are cracking the code, the Achilles' heel of these evil killing clones, by understanding and manipulating cyclooxygenase inhibitors, matrix metalloproteinase inhibitors, anticytokines, anti–epidermal growth factor receptors and hormone receptor down-regulators and destroyers. These novel approaches are breaking the secret code of human malignancy, and they are entering the armamentarium of the clinic at warp speed.

So where do we start? Let us look at the beginning of the life of a cell by looking at the cell's DNA. This thousand-meter-long molecule is magically coiled, twisted, recoiled, and twisted again. It is *the* architects' code for all of life. Imagine a fire ladder from a huge hook-and-ladder truck. Imagine that the ladder was remarkably unbreakable and pliable and a mile or two long. Envision the legs, the backbone of the ladder, as a seemingly random sequence of four different colors. It is always just these four colors, abbreviated A, T, C, and G. They must always match their partner on the other rung: A with T and G with C, ad infinitum. That is the code of life. Some areas of the ladder are housekeeping blueprint sections, and some are time bombs set to trigger cell death. Some determine the color of our eyes. These sequences of varying lengths are the blueprint and the code for everything we are, down to every minute detail. This is the magic decoder ring, the secret handshake. This is our DNA.

What is the purpose of this divine code? It codes for proteins, millions and millions of proteins. Just think of the interactions. Some of it is code for building bigger proteins, some is code to send signals, some makes receptors to receive the signals, some codes for toxins against things that would hurt us, and some determines our cells' and organs' identities. Some of the code is for monitoring functions; other code is for molecules that will carry energy locked in chemical bonds. Some helps us digest the food we eat and rebuild it into more protein or fat, or the storage form of sugar. Some of the proteins are coded to signal for danger, and some trigger allergic reactions. Regardless of what the proteins are coded for, they all come from the secret messages in our DNA. Almost all of this is done with signals we have only just begun to discern in a constant and tumultuous barrage of information. The elegancy and precision is overwhelming. Imagine DNA being the command center for any one of a million tasks all occurring at once. All this is precisely timed, with a billion atoms fitting a billion times on the end of a gnat's eyelash and even then not being crowded for space.

This is life, this is living tissue, *and this is you and me*. This DNA sends and receives signals for self-regulation and survival out to the protein factories in the cell all because we need precisely that balance to live at that moment. All the while, red blood cells, moving like the treads on a tank, roll through tiny capillary rivulets and deliver oxygen to help this divine engine work. Myriad pumps are constantly maintaining the right pressure and water content. The very energy of life makes heat; we warm-blooded beings are reaping the benefit of a billion furnaces sustained by the very food and water we eat and drink. Moreover, each cell knows exactly what it is and what it is not—a spleen cell, a kidney cell, a neuron. Each has a very exact role and a very exact lifespan, and each is always talking to its neighbors near and far. This is the greatest of all designs.

All the while, the grandest supercomputer of them all, our brain, runs thermostatically over the whole enterprise. We call the amazing smoothness of it all homeostasis, and for the longest time, all is well. Cells are on feedback loops more elegant than that of the most finely tuned, modern, energy-efficient dream home now or ever. The thoughts in our minds drive our feelings, and our feelings drive us. Think of the symphony of events that must take place simply to smile in wonder. Ponder the intricacies of how our thoughts choreograph the enormous complexity of the muscles and nerves in our face, the feeling of joy, the subtle fluctuations in pulse and blood pressure associated with the symphony called a smile.

Just as our minds have enormous influence over this magnificent machine, so do genetic errors, and they come in all manners. Some may be lurking and insidious, needing our unknowing help; others may be more overt, à la cigarettes, obesity, diet, alcohol, or other toxins. Our environment may also conspire against us. We do not live in Eden. We are assaulted every day. The years of bad habits and the stresses of simply living take their toll. Systems do break down; the machine is magnificent but not immortal.

Cancer is precisely the unraveling of the norm. There is a perverse genius by which cell-to-cell boundaries are made, held, and then, with cancer, broken. There is a sinister brilliance, foretold by many Nobel laureates, to the viperous whisper of the cancer cell to blood vessel factories, telling them to build new roads to carry the cancer cells and their babies to wherever they please. Thus, understanding the norm allows us to peer into the future, when we will beat the beast at its own game, for its game is literally the perversion of our own.

Cancer cells have genes that hold the key—the blueprint to make proteins, just like normal cells. However, many of these proteins are crucially different in degree or kind from those made by normal cells. One of these proteins is the epidermal growth factor receptor (EGFR), which is made in great excess in many cancers, especially our most common killer, lung cancer. This overproduction occurs in a wide range of tumors and has been linked to poor prognosis and increased risk of tumors being able to metastasize. Once the receptor is activated, it can increase the tendency of the cancer cell to multiply and become immortal. An activated receptor can also promote the production of new blood vessels to bring essential nutrients to the cancer cell to sustain it and increase the odds that the cancer cell or its children will spread to other parts of the body. The gene that holds the blueprint for EGFR is called *ErbB-1*. Two strategies directed against this receptor have been investigated in the clinical setting. They include monoclonal antibodies (mAbs), which we have discussed, which block the ability of the receptor to receive vital messengers and thus confer their evil intent to the cancer cell and small molecules that compete at the receptor with "normal molecules" and thus indirectly block the receptor.

Through the marriage of molecular genetics, computer-assisted rational drug design, and small-molecule therapy, we can inhibit the signal from an activated EGFR. Thus, we can attempt to block the signal that helps tell a cancer cell to spread, divide, and make new cancer cells; we can even potentially block the cancer cell's attempt to recruit blood vessel factories. An oral pill that can do this is now FDA approved and is seeing clinical use with some success in constantly increasing ways. This is indeed clever stuff—exploiting what the enemy thinks is an advantage and using that aspect against it.

Earlier, the highly specific identity of cells was discussed. The key to that identity, the fingerprint of sorts, is found in a dazzling array of proteins functioning as antigens—unique fingerprints on the surfaces of these cells. A few years ago, the Nobel Prize in Physiology or Medicine was awarded to those who in 1975 developed the technology to make immortal sterile factories for customized monoclonal antibodies.

The idea was for these monoclonal antibodies to recognize, on an almost atom-for-atom basis, those very specific protein antigens discussed above on the cancer cell surface. These protein antibodies directed against tumor antigens would then function as highly specific homing devices seeking out what were hoped to be tumor-specific antigens. The theory was that either the locking on to these tumor antigens by monoclonal antibodies per se, or the use of the antibodies to deliver a radiation or chemotherapy payload to which they were coupled, would kill individual cancer cells but spare normal cells that did not share the same antigens as the tumor cell. Think of it as a minuscule, molecular, laser-guided cruise missile.

The hope has become reality, as seen with the monoclonal antibody Rituxan, a billion-dollar drug taking advantage of the CD20 protein antigen on the surface of non-Hodgkin's lymphomas. Other monoclonal antibody treatments now exist for the treatment of inflammatory bowel disease and rheumatoid arthritis, as well as other forms of cancer and other diseases. It was only thirty years ago when leading news magazines spoke with awe of the theoretical promise of what were then called magic bullets. The bullets are now in the armory of the oncologist.

Let us delve deeper into small molecule therapy. Molecular therapy agents are specifically targeted against proteins made by tumors that confer their ability to thrive as well as molecules against receptors that function as a type of combination lock that, when opened, again give the tumor some survival advantage. Routine nonsteroidal anti-inflammatory drugs, such as Advil, Naprosyn, etc., inhibit the enzyme cyclooxygenase (cox), and this helps them have analgesic and anti-inflammatory properties. Cox is present in more than the usual amount in cells that have a mutated form of the gene *P53*. This first-of-its-kind gene is normally present in many cells and is essential as a safeguard against the cell turning malignant. It puts the brakes on this process, in a genetic sense. Thus, having a normal gene is a good thing. A mutated gene may mean increased risks for a cell becoming malignant, like a runaway car having no brakes.

Some cancers may activate a form of cox called COX-2. Thus, inhibiting COX-2 may have a good impact in fighting tumors and cells trying to become tumors. Furthermore, it also turns out that COX-2 has a role in helping potential cancer-causing agents become more active, as well as possibly helping tumors create their own new blood supply. Furthermore, COX-2 is found in higher concentration in some of the most common cancers of the GI tract, as well as lung, bladder, head and neck, cervix, and skin cancers. Thus, many of your cancer research dollars are being used to look into exploiting COX-2 inhibitors. The lessons learned are being applied to increasingly clever and elegant techniques to rationally design small molecules, attempting to exploit or inhibit some process or substance tumor cells depend on more or use to survive more than normal cells. This is the gist of small-molecule-therapy research. The key is to intervene at earlier and earlier and cancer cell–specific stages to prevent further advancement of the malignancy, as well as to combine these agents with presently known effective therapy.

The singular uniqueness of a portion of any antigen (remember them as fingerprints) is called the hypervariable portion of an antigen. We call this the idiotype of the protein antigen—its unique calling card, immunologically speaking. In some cancers much more than others, such as lymphomas and, to some degree, melanomas, cancer-specific idiotypic proteins clearly exist and can be identified. Thus, similar to the process of making a flu vaccine, the road for development of vaccine-like treatments against the idiotype has opened. Furthermore, if one can make an anti-idiotype antibody and marry it with a payload of deadly poisons, one then theoretically has a type of laser-guided stealth missile that will seek and destroy only the tumor cells that bear the idiotype and spare normal tissues. This work is well underway, with promising results. Imagine custom-made killer vaccines for just your tumor. We are now trying to aid this process by administering cells of the immune system, recently described and known as dendritic cells, that seem to help identify the tumor cells in a manner that marks them for attack by one's immune system.

Some may recall the drug thalidomide, which was touted as a sleeping aid but resulted in deformed children without fully formed limbs. It was reasoned that this might have occurred because the drug was inhibiting the normal new formation of blood vessels necessary as a crucial step in creating new tissues, such as limbs. As we discussed, new blood vessel formation is essential for tumors to thrive and spread. It was reasoned that inhibiting this process, which is exaggerated in cancers, may help fight the cancer, as cancer cells may be well be more susceptible to inhibition than normal cells and organs of the body. Thalidomide is now showing promise for multiple myeloma and is finding a role against other cancers. Furthermore, its effects are widespread. It is may also activate protein molecules that facilitate cancer cell death or recruit antibodies and cells of the immune system to help.

The entire field of preventing new blood vessel growth in tumors—antiangiogenesis—is rapidly growing. New vessels form largely as a result of stimulation by a growth factor called vascular endothelial growth factor (VEG-F), which requires cells it targets (largely cells with the genetic ability to make new vessel walls) to have a receptor for VEG-F. "Neutralizing" this hormone of sorts can block the development of new vessels, and after a while, the tumor starves. There are now FDA-approved angiostatins—drugs that pharmaceutical firms are racing to perfect to arrest the development of new blood vessels by tumors.

The tool called the polymerase chain reaction (PCR) has revolutionized enormous aspects of medicine and science in general. It is essential in DNA testing. This technique is able to amplify one copy in a million of the smallest identifying units of DNA. If a disease is caused by a reproducible genetic flaw, then it would be wise to amplify that gene enough to have sufficient quantities to study and discover just what it does for the tumor. The next step is to attempt to confound or block its function directly or block the proteins it makes, which carry its code.

The metaphor has been around for eons; knowing what the enemy does that is unique or essential for its survival puts one very close to exploiting that knowledge to fight the enemy. One might think of it as undercover genetic spying. Once researchers have the information, computers assist them in designing custom-made strategies and drugs that exploit the knowledge.

Dr. Peter Drucker and others did just that. The oral drug Gleevec blocks a binding site on an aberrant critical protein in some cancers that is created solely because the cancer has a highly specific genetic flaw. Patients with chronic myelogenous leukemia who take this drug are having unheard-of responses, as the drug actually suppresses not only the product of the aberrant gene but also, apparently, the gene itself. Furthermore, if the Gleevec stops working, we probably have the tools to quickly find out why and redesign our approach to outwit the cancer cell.

As it turns out, Gleevec also blocks the c-Kit protein in a rare, previously incurable stomach tumor. This is another tumor-specific substance that is intimately related to the rare cancer's ability to survive and thrive. I treated a walnut farmer who had multiple pounds of the tumor spread throughout his body. Now he is a new man. He is seventy-six years young and is in a multiyear complete remission.

There is another enormously famous example of a big breakthrough of directly blocking a gene product with a billion-dollar blockbuster drug. It is used in breast cancer and can extend survival in some patients. The drug is Herceptin. Those breast cancer cells that are vulnerable to this treatment have millions of receptors, known as Her-2/neu, on their surface. Similar to the concept in chronic myelogenous leukemia, these receptors, are there because of a fundamental genetic flaw unique to the cancer cells that make those breast cancer cells more aggressive than breast cancer cells without the flaw. Once the drug Herceptin finds its receptor site, it locks the receptor down and a signal is sent that tells the breast cancer cell to die.

What about the ability of a cancer cell to insidiously invade its neighbor's yard and dissolve away tissue in its way. Much of this is accomplished by molecules known as matrix metalloproteinase inhibitors, and they are an area of intense research. As one might suspect, there may be great benefit if there is a way to unravel exactly how tumors use these substances to their advantage in facilitating their spread and invasion. As we have seen before, if we understand how a tumor gains any of its unique survival advantages, therapies can theoretically be designed to capitalize on that knowledge and block a tumor's ability to spread and invade.

Proteosome inhibitors are a very recent and extraordinary area of future promise. The first such FDA-approved drug, Velcade, has found use in the second most common primary cancer of the bone marrow, multiple myeloma. Proteasomes are enormously important housekeeping and "refuse maintenance" enzymes that digest and cleave proteins no longer neither needed or desired, and they are required for healthy cell maintenance. When these are blocked, there is a buildup of cellular garbage that is usually toxic to the cell. Normal cells have their own biological clock that generally determines their maximum life span. Skin cells have a short life cycle, and nerves, by contrast, live much longer. Thus, there is a preprogrammed, genetically determined life expectancy.

Proteasomes have a major role in the aging of a cell in that the more proteasomes there are with more functions and more activity, the better the cell can fend off the potential toxic effects of accumulated by-products and excess biochemical baggage that is produced during the course of normal cell life. Cancer cells have more of these proteasome "sanitation engineers," which confer an advantage of increased life span of the tumor cell as compared to normal cells. Thus, inhibitors of proteasomes in cancer cells might shorten the life span of the cancer cell.

As we have discussed, genetic differences in cancer cells are the code that serve as the blueprint for the many molecules that play a role in giving the cancer cell an advantage over normal cells in terms of survival as well as the ability of the cancer cell to resist therapy, multiply, invade, and spread. The genes of a cancer cell are made of DNA. DNA is what chromosomes are made of, this was previously described as a ladder with millions of rungs. The ladder twists and coils repeatedly upon itself, allowing for an enormous amount of rungs in a comparatively small space. The rungs are composed of a mandatory code of just two possibilities, using building blocks of molecules known as amino acids. There are only four amino acids possible in the rungs; these are represented by the letters A, T, C, and G. The letter A must always be paired with T, and C must always be paired with G. Sequences of all different lengths, varying from tens of rungs to thousands of rungs on the ladder backbone, are codes for specific proteins or instructions. These sequences are what we call genes.

These small sequences are known as oligonucleotides (from "oligo-" [few] and "nucleotide" [the unit made when an amino acid on a ladder backbone connects with its paired amino acid]). These oligonucleotides are thus very specific secret combinations for each protein and substance that makes up the tumor cell—and, for that matter, all substances of human life. These oligonucleotides can be thought of as being zipped together at the level of each rung. In order for the oligonucleotides to tell the cell's machinery to make new substances, they must "unzip" and be "read" by other key mechanisms for making all molecules in the cell. Once this is done, they are then "rezipped."

All cells must have a full set of chromosomes from their parent cell to survive. Doing this requires the parent cell to double its DNA and give an identical copy to each offspring. This doubling is done by the DNA unzipping right down the rungs and the parent cell then using each half-ladder as a template (mirror) to build up an identical half-ladder with which it can combine to make a whole ladder of a new chromosome, always following the A–T and G–C rule. Thus, the two half-ladders of all oligonucleotides, all genes, all DNA, and all chromosomes are complementary. Thus, both the making of all substances needed for the tumor cell to live *and* the creation of new offspring tumor cells require unzipping the parent DNA, complementary oligonucleotide by complementary oligonucleotide.

Researchers thus reasoned that since all the various molecules that a tumor cell uses in some way to survive, spread, multiply, and invade must be coded for by various oligonucleotides, and since these oligonucleotides are made of two complementary half-ladders, it should be possible to catch the tumor cell with its genes vulnerable, in a manner of speaking. Using the PCR technique we discussed above, scientists are now making oligonucleotides complementary to tumor cell oligonucleotides that the tumor cell uses to make substances crucial to its survival.

The trickery, however, is both brilliant and simple in its design. Researchers create oligonucleotides sufficiently similar to the correct sequence needed but with fatal flaws; once bound to the parent tumor DNA, they cannot be read correctly. Even better, these oligonucleotides may instruct the parent tumor cell to stop some vital function and possibly even to die. Since these oligonucleotides made in the laboratory make no sense to the tumor cell, they are called nonsense oligonucleotides. The concept is both elegant and simple, but the implementation has many hurdles to pass.

One of the biggest challenges to fighting cancer through the immune system is that your body may not sufficiently recognize the cancer as foreign either at all or in a timely manner. Thus, cancer cells frequently do not die; they multiply into tumors right under the not-so-watchful eye of your own immune system. The most powerful carriers or transmitters of the message that there is trouble afoot from your cells to your immune system may well be heat shock proteins (HSPs). HSPs are released when a cell dies. They are, in a sense, your cell's version of an autopsy report. HSPs deliver an antigen to your immune system.

As you may recall, an antigen is a molecular fingerprint of whatever is attacking your cells. It is a protein capable of eliciting an immune response. Antigens are how your immune system recognizes what is attacking your body. However, one of the ways cancers escape destruction, multiply, and spread unchecked is that they have various ways of escaping detection by the immune system, and thus their presence may not trigger an immune response; at best, they trigger a weak and inadequate one. Thus, they may spread unchecked by natural defenses. About ten years ago, it was discovered that HSPs could be isolated from cancerous cells. Such HSPs would ideally be specific and customized to your tumor and infused to you as an outpatient. They would function as nontoxic vaccines, alerting your immune system to a highly specific fingerprint of the tumor and thus allowing it to recognize the threat and mount a response. There have already been some dramatic responses in patients with very advanced disease.

Farnesylation is a key regulatory process performed on many crucial molecules that allows them to tether to a cell's membrane and in so doing to be active and perform their function. Thus, one form of therapy may be to compete and possibly block this tethering, perhaps blocking the function of crucial molecules that confer the ability of cancer cells to survive, multiply, spread, and invade. Up to 30% of lung cancer cells possess key proteins that require farnesylation. Presently, there are a number of so-called competing or blocking molecules in development.

Finally, let us take a brief look at the possibility of using a type of stem cell to fight cancer. Researchers in Texas at the MD Anderson Cancer Center have gotten some exciting preliminary results with fighting human tumors implanted in mice by employing human stem cells. These cells are used to deliver cancer treatment directly into the tumor and bypass normal cells. These researchers manipulated certain types of stem cells, known as mesenchymal stem cells, that come from bone marrow and help maintain normal connective tissue that holds tissues and cells together. These types of cells grow and mature rapidly when new tissue is needed to help heal wounds or form scars.

Even though cancers are malignant tumors, they act, in a manner, as wounds that never heal, thus beckoning such stem cells into them. These researchers have devised a way to turn on the necessary genetic codes in these stem cells for making beta interferon, a potent naturally occurring molecule that is one of the many interferons made by the human immune system to fight various infections and foreign cells. Beta interferon can kill cancer cells, but in practice, simply administering the protein itself has exhibited problems with toxicity and with its effect disappearing moments after administration. These stem cells, however act as guided missiles, targeting tumors while producing high concentrations of therapeutic beta interferon within the tumor. In early tests in mice, researchers observed that the new approach tamed many of the adverse side effects and that the beta interferon affected the tumor for a much longer period of time. As a result, mice with implanted human breast cancers and melanoma that received the treatment had a markedly longer survival. Investigators are now designing very preliminary trials to begin shortly on a limited basis.

Other fascinating areas of research include putting chemotherapy wafers in brains, freezing tumors, overheating and killing tumors with microwaves, and infusing tumors with alcohol to the point of lethal toxicity.

New Diagnostic Tools

It is widely known today that early detection of cancer can dramatically increase the rate of survival. Along with treatment advances, another branch of cancer research involves finding new tools to diagnose the disease. These new tools help detect cancer earlier, determine the stages of the disease, monitor the progression of cancer, and select the most effective therapies. Current research is concentrating on cellular and gene-based testing to help accomplish these goals.

Some cellular tests are being used to detect and count circulating tumor cells (CTCs) in a blood sample. Gene-based testing (also called molecular testing) determines the presence and tissue origin of cancer cells to establish disease staging and will most likely help in prognosis and therapy selection. Molecular tests offer the potential for greater accuracy and more patient-specific information. Many tests are still in the investigative phase and are not yet approved for widespread use. It is hoped that someday a test will be discovered that does not just detect cancer once it occurs but will also detect it as a precancerous condition at the very earliest cellular level.

In the section "The Enemy," I illuminated the unmistakable recurring theme of infernal mimicry of what is normal as the hallmark of the clever mechanisms that a tumor cell uses. As every brilliant military strategist and geopolitical leader has observed since antiquity, one must keep one's friends close but one's enemies closer. The metaphor for cancer clinicians and researchers is clear. The key to fighting this dreaded disease is to understand it at the most basic genetic level. We must discern and uncover every trick and technique unique tumor genes use to create molecules that empower cancer to hide from our immune system, survive, multiply, spread, invade, and make its own blood supply. Science is up for the fight, and with your help—through healthy lifestyles and perhaps a deeper understanding that it will take years and trillions of dollars to uncover all this—this fight can be won.

I close with a recurring theme of this book: understanding and progress will only come from knowledge. Perhaps put more poetically, in our lifetime, our time of life will determine our lives time and the time we spend studying the timings of life, the better the time spent.

SPIRITUAL CARE

Patients have a soul. So do their doctors. We all struggle with "Why am I here?" "Why did this or another thing happen to me?" and "What is my purpose?" Humans will always have moments when they will languish in existential angst, and not only cancer patients long for a connection of the most intimate kind. Not only cancer patients are afraid in an unfair world. It is indeed quite common for the patient and loved ones to face despair and battle some form of overt or cloaked depression or anxiety.

There is a nature to being human, and no one is exempt. There are no original emotions, just individualized styling on personal dramas and routines. There is a spirituality to us all, and the prospect of facing a life-threatening diagnosis magnifies and focuses it. Woody Allen quipped about not minding dying as long as he was not there when it happened. Many cancer patients will die, and when they do, they will be there body and soul. The skilled provider knows all of this and either personally or through consultation, which may or may not be pastoral care, addresses the spiritual longings of the patient faced with a diagnosis of cancer.

In a sense, patients fighting the diagnosis have been both burdened and blessed on a spiritual plane with fighting the good and noble fight, striving until the prize is won and the race is done, continuing until weary. They cannot do it without invoking the powers that the creator has given them. Never is the soul more present, and perhaps never is it more willing to receive love. As Neil Young mused, "To give a love, you've got to live a love; to live a love, you've got to be part of." I plead with cancer team clinicians to, as much as possible, be "part of" with their patients. Touch a hand and hold a heart.

Many physicians could address spirituality better. Addressing spirituality is not synonymous with praying, as that is only one of innumerable ways to embrace that which is felt but not as easily seen. As regards praying however, many are embarrassed or uncomfortable praying either alone for their patients or along with them, which may be appropriate. It is quite true that God does not need doctors' or patients' prayers, but the doctor and patient need them, as prayers are largely for the benefit of those who say them. God knows the weight of the responsibility of the healer, as he is in the business. He knows suffering.

Physicians in postgraduate training and young attending physicians are frequently not as appreciative of the spiritual realities of the practice of medicine as they could be. Perhaps time has not yet doled out enough up-close and personal hurt in their patients. In this regard oncology stands alone.

Physicians are in the top 5% of their age group in so many secular measures, with the mighty sword of science to brandish while smiting disease and driving away pestilence. However, the spiritual aspects of the clinician's calling and the tools available to clinicians are in a very real sense powerful components of the world of cancer medicine. Our patients need us to be both human and humane. I am not evangelizing intense metaphysical discussions, probing spiritual interviews, or losing the necessary level of clinical distance and objectivity required to shoulder the responsibility of being the doctor. I am talking about being a *complete* physician, which means being a *complete human* in your practice. Perhaps clinicians could try this: First thing on greeting a patient, make your best guess as to the patient's comfortable personal space and then shake his or her hand, and perhaps hold his or her forearm. Then gaze into, not at, the patient's eyes and give him or her your best "I just learned I got into medical school" smile, and hold it. If you can master the transition, close with the unmistakably supportive look of someone who knows another is scared. See if they do not smile back. *That* is spiritual medicine.

Medical school curriculums would do well to pay more attention to the whole being, and in particular the notion of man being a spiritual being. It is so often paid lip service. I am not referring to religion. This is about spirituality and perhaps theology, but it is not about rites, rituals, and practices within theologies that religions are defined by. Religion has a narrower focus as a ritualized communal system of beliefs, very frequently with strong cultural overtones. However, a significant portion of us consider ourselves religious in some manner, particularly when our lives are threatened. Thus it behooves the clinical practitioner to have a sense of familiarity with the topic.

Inquiring about religious affiliation serves two roles, one of which is pragmatic as to what type of ministry is most appropriate, but second, and most importantly, the patient's responses to the clinician's simple inquiry may reveal a much deeper problem smoldering within. Just like a couch on fire, the smoldering never ends; the same is true with most of us when grappling with fundamentally spiritual issues. Thus, when a patient is clearly not at peace with the topic of religion, it may be a guiding light for the physician, their team and consultants, and family to approach this topic with sensitivity and flexibility.

In addition, the physician who is theological or religious must remember that many terminal patients are not. Although many religions call on their followers to evangelize, one must walk a fine line. I have seen hospice, which is a wonderfully caring program, unwittingly show its Christian roots a little inappropriately for some patients. On the other hand, not all patients realize how uncomfortable and, in some cases, ill-prepared their physician may be toward religion. Thus, a patient may find himself or herself on the side of the issue opposite his or her physician. The spiritual scalpel cuts both ways.

Commitment of the physician, the patient, and family to attend to spiritual as well as purely physical issues is necessary and a key component of the very essence of palliation. Once again, this is not about religious issues. That is the domain of the chaplain, except in the hands of the exceptionally well-heeled religious physician. Yet many physicians have largely abdicated their role to these messengers of mercy. The spiritual dimension is infinitely broader than the religious, and as I have stressed, it emphasizes the search for the meaning of life and true values. People facing cancer become keenly aware of a need to make some sense of meaning or purpose out of their life and illness. The future becomes a precious jewel whose promise they long for to be realized. Patients need their spirituality to face their current illness.

Traditional religious practices are often very important for coping with death, dying, grieving, and loss. Even those who do not regularly attend any church may find great solace in a return to previous expressions of belief and practices. It may rekindle fond childhood memories. Unfortunately, many practitioners feel that if they are not knowledgeable in the patient's particular religion, they will be inept at being of any assistance. In-depth knowledge is not necessary and causes far too many staff to hold back from saying or doing something that may offend. In reality, this fear is usually groundless. Patients can be guides to help advise their caretakers about any special spiritual or cultural needs. The key for clinicians is to be sensitive and open, gently asking questions rather than allowing anxiety, fear, and ignorance to impede the relationship and the patient's progress.

The importance of prayer cannot be understated. Some patients appreciate the offer if they sense it is from a heart of compassion and not religious fervor, which is often a very quick way to turn off a patient and other staff. There is no magical formula. Prayer is, once again, for physician and patient alike, not God. There is no magic set of words or incantations; just settle in on what feels right. Formal rituals and prayer are best left to trained and experienced clergy. However, most patients welcome simple addressing of their possible pastoral needs and the assurance that they will be met. Some patients may wish to listen to biblical readings or tapes. Others may wish to hear recorded Buddhist chants on a self-rewinding Walkman or digital media player. The assets are out there; all one need do is be aware and ask. My advice to clinicians is to be ingenious in addressing your patients' hearts and not just their heads. My advice to patients is to help your physicians with the journey.

Religion will define the rites associated with death and burial, and some knowledge of these is helpful. This is often the realm of the most adept spiritual advisors. Other rites and sacraments, if existent, should be offered and acknowledged.

We need to stress again that patients may cope with the facts of the illness and yet be in horrific spiritual pain regarding a desperate search for meaning: "What did I do wrong?" and so forth. Another certain indicator of spiritual pain is guilt and regret. This can concern all manners of past and present events and interactions, lost opportunities, and unfinished business. The clinician's gentle probing relieves some patients. It does not take much on the part of the doctor if he or she has ears to hear and eyes to see. Simply talking releases and such relieves many. Other patients may adhere to religions that practice formal sacraments of reconciliation. Sadly, there are those who are never reached, and the anguish can be mortifying. I can assure you that I hold fast to the opinion that such an outcome is largely preventable. Death scares us all, as does all manner of terminal suffering. Physicians are fix-it people, and their reality is often somewhere between the more immediate and concrete outlook of an orthopedic surgeon to the warm and fuzzy bosom of the family practitioner. All physicians are by no means the same.

Clinicians and family members should look for agitation, insomnia, and fear of sleeping. Rapid changes in narcotic requirements, especially at night, can all be a tip-off to growing spiritual anguish. Remember, if the grist of man is his soul, then there is no limit to soul ache; it has no bounds. Sometimes patients will deny the very existence of their anguish, but not for long. It has no bounds, this soul ache, and eventually the energy used to suppress it will wither and a sudden release of enormous angst will come. Remember, for those who feel that this is all there is, they will believe the "never and forever" lie: it will never change and the suffering will forever be. Furthermore, suffering is intensely personal in nature, and the cause is often perceived to be out of control, leaving the patient feeling helpless. Add the risk of personal disintegration to this, and you explode the intensity of these perceptions.

We have grown flippant with the words "soul" and "suffering," with the latter often referring to some sort of measurable entity in balance with our belief of the severity of an ailment. Cancer patients are people suffering a loss in capability, identity, future, purpose, meaning, and connections to loved ones, as well as the loss of body functions, which can be extremely embarrassing. Physicians may inadvertently aggravate all this by the quantifying of the pain a bit too easily with a morphine mindset and thus treating what is truly spiritual with only an opiate, which patients may also well need. That is only one aspect of what the cancer patient needs, because of the ephemeral, spiritual aspect associated with pain and its representation that one is now less than what one once was.

Physicians must be wary to focus not only on the cancer, which can diminish focus on the overall patient. Frankly, in my opinion, I believe God may hang his head in sadness and weep for those who suffer and are ignored in this way. Many factors make it difficult for providers to recognize and treat spiritual suffering. Physicians tend to have limited personal experience with suffering, with younger staff particularly inexperienced with the suffering life doles out. In most cases for the younger physicians, both the parents and grandparents are still alive, so there is nothing personal to draw from. Thus, without this avenue for empathy, it must be taught.

Health-care providers are also people—people who fear death at a subconscious level and harbor a hidden aversion to death and dying. One common concept that research has revealed is referred to as relabeling the problem, which allows one to avoid seeing it as the problem of suffering that it is. Clinicians may diagnose suffering as anxiety, depression, or adjustment disorder. A transition occurs wherein the patient and his or her cancer becomes the problem, not the pain or suffering.

Scientific training conspires, to some degree, against doctors being as adept as they could be in dealing with suffering. Their methodology is dispassionate; they are didactic, regarding diseases as entities unto themselves. The very frequent embellishments patients add when giving their history are totally missed as the cues needed to reach an understanding of the whole patient and his or her hidden concerns. Enormous cues, both verbal and otherwise, regarding patient suffering can be missed, as we have neither the life experience nor the formal training to recognize them. Multiple surveys of medical school curricula have shown that training on the treatment of pain as well as death and dying has been inadequate. Fortunately, however, it is improving every year. We train young doctors not to say "I don't know." Think of the impact; can you see how this may lead that very same budding physician to be encouraged to develop strategies for walking past the room of a dying patient on ward rounds? The training of nurses is clearly superior as regards addressing these special needs, but alas, if the doctor does not listen with his or her heart and ears, he or she will not hear the patient's spiritual pain calling to him or her from the heart of the nurse who feels it from the patient.

When I went for a few rotations of training in England years ago, I saw senior physicians routinely actually talk with their patients and truly examine them, including spiritually. Moreover, they listened with all their senses for all the cues and clues that are always there. However, back in the United States, I realized there was a tendency to use verbal and nonverbal methods to avoid the stress of patient contacts. I saw, on occasion, staff finding the pressure of unfinished work undermining communication skills. Thus I learned to use open-ended questions rather than closed-ended questions, such as "So, I am sure you understand all of what I have told you now?" Physicians also may frequently stand during the interview, cross their arms, look aside to avoid eye contact, or stay near the door, all of which indicate impatience to the patient. Sadly, physicians that are more senior may reinforce these strategies.

Adding to this is the very real fact that cancer patients want to please their doctor. Thus, there are many personal and professional reasons that providers find it difficult to recognize and deal with suffering. Many wish to avoid distressing situations, especially if they lack the experience, knowledge, and skills to handle them.

So how do we manage suffering? A team approach is how. Patients will typically not say things to upset physicians, but patients will talk to the nurse or the office staff. Although all team members have different professional skills to be brought to bear, the main necessity is to be human, to be present. Cancer treatment team members must not reinforce a patient's feeling of isolation by staying away or avoiding the patient. Conversely, a physician is not a never-ending well of consolation, and the burden can grow overwhelming at times. Sometimes all that is needed is for the doctor to be there, listen and acknowledge the pain and the unanswerable questions. Affirmation of the suffering is a confirmation of the spiritual aspects of the diagnosis.

Sometimes it is wise to venture headlong into patients' worst fears by asking what they are. Many are future-based and rarely will happen as patients envision them. This may be an opportunity for a doctor to allay some fears and bring enormous relief. In addition, we must remember that families are often dysfunctional to some degree, and the very ill or dying loved one will uncover this. Family members may often project their own distress and needs. Remember that we are, by definition, self-centered beings. Thus, again, family conferences are stressed. Patients, in turn, often worry enormously about becoming a burden and seldom express these fears to their physicians and thus become increasingly anguished, which can also adversely affect the family. Open addressing of these worries can be truly liberating.

Patient support groups can be enormously helpful. People with similar experiences can very quickly help develop an atmosphere of understanding and mutual support. There can be an enormous therapeutic effect from feeling that you are not alone. Most of these groups work best with a professional facilitator.

Suffering can also be associated with intense anger. Many individuals with such anger issues have problems expressing their rage. The family, staff, and even physicians may be subjected to outbursts. The distress increases if an easygoing front is maintained with visitors that are kept distant. We often also hurt the ones we love, and we love to "kick the cat" when something goes wrong. Patients must have this second spiritual cancer ferreted out or they will most assuredly do poorly. I have shocked more than one intern with my seeming bravado by almost antagonizing a patient until he or she finally broke and, in so doing, went well on the way to spiritual healing, as the demon was then released and the patient knew we all still cared for him or her. This is tricky business, and there is no substitute for experience.

Most patients are not actually looking for an answer; rather, they feel the need to express the conflict of distress and fears and all the personal vagaries regarding their situation. Physicians would be wise to be wary of letting too many issues remain covered. In general, I have found that after I lifted up the rocks and cleared out the snakes, there was usually less venom eating at a patient's heart. Interestingly, most patients are not wishing to die the "good" death in pacific serenity. Studies have confirmed they want to fight and die while struggling to live as ordinary a life as possible. The point is that if a physician's goal is to ease all the suffering by merely covering it, he or she will usually make it worse.

When suffering is not relieved, it is often time to bring in a palliative care specialist and psychiatrist for formal evaluation and possible drug therapy. There is no place at this point for professional pride. Unfortunately, many psychiatrists know less than the oncologist about death and dying per se unless they specifically have long-term experience. Above all, the team must be kept tight so there is mutual support and respite time and so no one individual gets overwhelmed.

Occasionally, patients become so distressed that intervention with drugs is required. This requires specialized knowledge. Sedatives and tranquilizers may be needed in significant doses, and family may struggle with the resulting dulled senses and seeming emotional or intellectual absence of the patient. However, cessation of the drugs may be a dark sentence for the immediate and profound return of symptoms and suffering of the patient.

There are those who unswervingly support euthanasia for the dying and suffering patient. There is a great deal of data gathered on this topic, and as is the case with most zealots of any cause, data-derived decision making and evidence-based conclusions are not their typical strong suit. It is rare for a patient to ask to be euthanized in the first place, and it is rarer when appropriate palliative care has been given. On the rare times it occurs (I have had thousands of patients and have been asked twice), it usually is a call for help. In Holland, with its liberalized approach, it is important to note that there are almost no specialist palliative-care services. The response to suffering should not be to play God, but to encourage better training and greater availability of palliative care.

Teaching about suffering and symptom control should be among the top five of all topics in medical school. Strong role models need to be developed in teaching hospitals. There should be specialist advisory palliative-care hospital teams or hospital-based palliative units. Training must address the enormous fears and discomfort of the caregivers. Issues ranging from unaware racism to sexual discrimination to relabeling should all be addressed. Students must be exposed to as many colors of the rainbow of suffering man as possible. Speakers from various ethnic groups and religious affiliations should be part of our medical curriculum. No one should be allowed to stay in all his or her rotations in the comfortable suburbs of Hollywood. Inner-city training is necessary, as is Veterans Administration training, if possible. Suffering is not a respecter of persons and has many faces.

SELF-TALK

I have had my turn with cancer. In my fellowship, I had a mole taken off that was diagnosed as early-stage malignant melanoma. I did not talk to anyone about it, but I should have. It was very thin and early, but in the mind of the oncologist racing at warp speed, I struggled a bit. I did not tell my family; I just mustered on. Therefore, although I cannot say I know what many cancer patients are going through completely, I had my little episode twenty-five years ago, and I have been taught by those with cancer for over thirty. There are common themes that occur, and I have seen some beautiful solutions to the rush of emotions when the diagnosis is made.

It has been said, "So as a man thinks, he feels." You may think or feel the opposite is true, but overwhelming evidence indicates that this is how the species operates. Our thoughts drive our emotions, and to a large degree, that forebodes a lot of hope for psychological well-being, as we can exert some control over those thoughts.

Why Me?

First, why not? Were you born with some blue-ribbon guarantee and a free pass? No one is. Cancer is no respecter of persons and never will be. You may have been obese, smoked, drank too much, or had a horrendous diet high in fat with no fiber or fruits. Yet even then, the point is that you now have cancer; it is for real, and you have to deal with it. Dwelling on what may be the worst event in your life will only compound your woes. I hereby give the cancer patient permission to be scared witless, *temporarily*. Permission is now granted to cry, feel out of control, and lose control of some basic bodily functions for a while. There are those of us who will withdraw; okay, permission granted for that too—*for a while*. Then, enough. I have said it multiple times; none of us gets out of this alive, and the mere diagnosis is not synonymous with a death sentence.

Second, you are not alone. There are millions of us out there, and you most likely have a family that will be with you. You are probably in a first-world nation. Think about that. In the majority of the world, cancers are not found as early as here; nor are there as many treatments so readily and widely available from so many expert facilities and practitioners. So why you? Because God is not a puppet master and he has given us free will, because disease and infirmity is a natural part of the mortal coil, because to understand light you must know dark, and because it was your turn.

Laughter and Beauty

Yes, it is time to talk of laughter and beauty—and not in spite of how ugly things seem right now, but because of it. Read Matthew chapter 6—the second half, which is about worry. Worry is ugly. It is a plain fact that creation around you abounds with beauty. Now is when I urge you to simply open your eyes at all we have taken for granted. Grass is green, trees still arch skyward, the rip and roar of the oceans and the lapping of the lakes as they strike shore continues, and life will not stop living because of you. Is that a testimonial to the callousness of the world to those who suffer or a blazing reminder that we are all connected in the circle of life with stops along the way at pain and suffering? Yet the circle remains unbroken and the cycle keeps turning. It does not ignore you; it wishes to embrace you, especially in your suffering.

Watch the Nature Channel—no, I am not getting fashionably touchy-feely. Look at how much you have as a human and how beautifully life goes on with or without you. Stare at the mirror and study your face for a long time. Then, whether you feel like it or not, smile—smile the broadest smile of the fondest remembrance you have. You will feel the glow. Smile at everyone you meet. Call waiters by their name and greet the world with that smile. Fake it until you make it, but smile, and soon it will be part of you, and the laughter and beauty of a smile returned will brighten the world and lighten your day. Pick a flower or two, put them in your house, and—although you may accused of being an idiot—study them millimeter by millimeter. That is beauty, and creation sees you as more beautiful than the flower. Study a colony of ants and be amazed at their communion and communication. They pull together, and so can you—are you not more than an ant? Remember, you are precious and loved in your creator's sight, and we are to proclaim it with laughter. You have a choice; choose to live with laughter and beauty.

Baby Steps

I have never seen a baby in the Olympic triple jump, have you? Have you seen them in the pole vault or maybe clearing hurdles? I think not. Moreover, you will not. Those gleaming athletic gladiators were babies once and trained from day one. So shall you. Set small, realistic goals of all we have talked about, and take them one baby step at a time. Rent the movie *What About Bob?* with Bill Murray and Richard Dreyfuss. You will be laughing, but the message of baby steps is on the money. It may be emotionally agonizing for you to just leave the house. Fine, then open the door and at least put a foot out there.

You have not left society. You are in the heart of it, and the integrity of a society is measured by how it deals with its young, its aged, and its ill. Soon those little baby tasks will become adventures. If you can, take a piano lesson, rent a trombone, and go to a gardening class. Enroll in anything you damn well please in the local junior college. Shop for a wig with a friend and imitate old-time actors when you do. Take the step, and you will be a baby in this journey no longer.

Daily Affirmations

First, affirm that you have a pulse and blood pressure and a respiratory rate. You have vital signs that say you are alive! *Believe* them. Tell yourself they are for real. Think about how magically your life still goes on, and affirm that you will *not* be a bystander and let the parade pass you by. Strengthen your spiritual walk and read the promises of God to you. He will always be with you. Did you know that there are 366 admonitions to "fear not" in the Bible? There is one for every day in a leap year. Go to the local bookstores, secular and spiritual. They are teeming with life and stories of conquest.

You are not doomed; you are not dead. You are not a murderer or crook. You *deserve* to think healthy thoughts. You are probably a parent or someone's child and are probably not alone. Journal every day as to what you feel and see how it tells you what you're thinking. Then try thinking positive thoughts before you journal your feelings, and note the changes that come. Let us get practical also; your survival depends on a positive attitude. You have a complex immune system with billions of soldiers counting on you to fight, *not lie down.* Talk to your immune system and focus on how it will help you. No, this is not voodoo. Those who pray and maintain a positive outlook do tend to fare better than others in clinical trials. Most of all, affirm to the heavens, to those around you, to those you love, and to yourself that you are alive and you will *not* quit.

Toxic Stress

You know this one. Toxic stress is the presence of stress in your life that you really do not need. It includes those people who, quite simply put, bum you out. Beware of those who say they know how you feel. Do they? Have they gone through it? Good—if their attitude is positive. You deserve a break each day from simple BS. BS can come in many forms. It may wear the cloak of well-wishers who are falling over their own pity, simple bad-attitude players, tedious chores that can be delegated, or negative feelings you are harboring (that is a big one). If you want toxic stress, then go to the dark side with all of this and you will fertilize your cancer. Do not make that mistake.

Perhaps a leave of absence to simply take it easy, play, and do things for *just you* is in order. I guarantee you that a healthy perspective will come on you, unrestrained as to what really matters, as opposed to the "nit noid" minutiae about which we worry. Get away from it. As bizarre as it may sound, you have been given a pause during an important part of life, the real grist of it all. Make the most of it. Go to the Internet, write down your questions, and leave little room for anxiety—fear of the unknown—to scoot in because you are not participating in your disease. Trust me, you will know what counts, and it is neither martyrdom nor messiahship. It is living the simpler life. Thoreau wrote to Emerson, "Simplify, simplify, simplify," in response to which Ralph Waldo Emerson brilliantly quipped, "One simplify would have sufficed."

Live the Moment

Live the moment. Do not just exist in it. Live it. Feel with all your senses. Blindfold yourself in a familiar area and listen for hours. You will be amazed as to what you hear. Go to the local children's museums, especially those featuring science and discovery, and be wowed at all you lost and glossed over. Live each step you take, feel the floor under you, and think of the construction around you—who built it, their lives. Look at amazement at a bird in flight and then look for that behemoth plane overhead that you just simply ignored. Look at the gadgets and gizmos in your kitchen. Are they not fabulous? A mere century ago, you would have had none of these.

Although I am not a global advocate of TV, think of the medium sent on invisible signals passing through buildings and even you to bring the world to your door. You are surrounded by wonder, both man- and God-made, but nothing matches the perfection of the latter. Grasp the visceral essence of existence by the throat and hang on for the ride of your life. Go to an amusement park. Do at least one silly thing a day. Most of all, end each day knowing that your pulse is there and that you had millions of moments to live.

Honor Your Thoughts

You are the highest order of life, and God expects you to use the gift of reason he gave you. Be as the Bereans in your discernment. Furthermore, you will have dark thoughts. They are to be honored no less than the light and bright ones in terms of their presence being part of the process and your right to experience them. This is all about actively choosing how you feel and think and not letting the darkness choose you.

You will not have a truly original emotion, and thus you are not alone. You have permission to cry, to pound sand, and to brag about minor achievements that seem to others as no big deal. Honor those thoughts in terms of not just your right to have them but also the power they have over your feelings. They, not feelings, are the driving engines. Respect and understand that. There must be self-talk when oppressive times come that this, too, shall pass and you can handle it as millions have. As much as I say I could never handle what I see heroes go through daily, my mind knows I am I am wrong. We all can handle it, but it starts with your mind. It is an amazing thing, the power to think, and it can completely control you in a positive or negative manner. The choice is yours. Nevertheless, honor your power of thought, and you will take one more step toward walking through this episode in your journey. One of the key ways to honor your positive thoughts is to give them fuel—the fuel of knowledge—and turn that anxiety into action.

Conspire against Your Emotions

Panic, fear, anxiety, loneliness, isolation, hopelessness—these are all driven by emotions derived from negative thoughts. *You must conspire against them.* They are your enemy, and they will seek you out. Fight back with thoughts of what you have learned about your situation that you did not know—affirmations such as the power you hold as a result of the knowledge you possess because of participating in your disease as this book recommends. Conspire against allowing them to slip in, and when they do, acknowledge that they are real as feelings but *not* as the final reality. You can create your thought reality, and succumbing to a mind filled with anxiety is a recipe for disaster. It is classic paralysis by analysis. You must look at the facts. Yes, you have cancer. Yes, this may be the toughest road yet to travel. Yes, it may even be incurable, but are you to play God and simply die to your fear? Who do you think you are? You have an obligation with the life that was given you, and that is to live it. No, you will not be the bravest. No, you may not be a swashbuckler, but you can sure pull up those bootstraps, take those baby steps, and get moving with honoring the power of positive thought and people. It does sound so glorious and easy. No, it is not. However, the alternative is worse, and although extremely rare, I have seen patients with both curable and incurable cancers be reduced to no more than a walking corpse by living to die and not dying to live. That is an insult to you, God, and all your loved ones. *We* need you to pull, even if feebly, on the oar of your raft of life. So conspire against those negative emotions.

Set Goals

We were built with eyes in the front of our head for a reason. We share a will to love for a reason. We dream and have hopes for a reason, and the reason is that such stuff is the warp and woof of being human. You may feel stripped of lost opportunities. Life plans may have gone awry with an inescapable sense of loss of your golden retirement years or the rape of young innocence. All of these are, to some extent, possibly true and very reasonable, but they are not conclusions.

Conclusions are too frequently the place where we smugly or comfortably arrive when we stop thinking. Therefore, what are your choices? Fester and stew in disconsolate depression or set new goals. Your goal may be just getting to the car without a wheelchair, or it may be winning the Tour de France. It matters not what your goals are; it matters only *that* they are. Goals motivate us to press on for the prize, and my friends, it is the passion of the pursuit that is the real prize, not the attained goal. There will be others prizes more glorious or more humble, depending on your course, to come. Goals empower the will and imagination, and armed with that, you can climb your Everest, if need be. Look at Jake in "Snow Job" later in the book when you get to his story. The impossible today may the possible tomorrow. The possibilities may narrow, but if there is still a life, then there is still the power of the will to strive for them. Goals are one of the many gifts God gave us in making us truly human. Be truly human; set them, and *never* stop.

Support Groups

Regarding joining a support group, I have heard so many say, "Oh, that is not for me," or some other such poppycock. Maybe that is your pride sensing "Nobody knows the trouble [you've] seen," or perhaps your fear of disclosure is talking. Sorry, kiddo, you and your situation are not that original. There is enormous value in knowing that another knows what you have gone through and may go through in the future. Support groups may provide relief and an enormous release of toxic stress for those who participate. Yet still, as humans do, we hide and frequently suffer privately. This is potentially a big mistake no matter what you think. We were designed as communal beings, and we benefit from the corporate sharing of our pain and darker moods. There is also fun to be had and a celebration of life. Victories will happen in the group, and you can be part of the celebration. Who really does not like a party when the underdog wins? It will prepare you for the future, as will those with less fortunate fates. Yes, this will sadden you, but like it or not, knowing them and what they went through is a veritable gold mine of experience. You have no unique anxieties that others have not dealt with, and in short order, you will be the teacher and the consoler. What greater gift than that can you give?

When you give to another suffering and grappling with the diagnosis you receive beyond all measure. The definition of "support" says it all: "to bear the weight especially from below, to hold in position especially to keep from falling, slipping or sinking, to keep from falling or yielding during stress." It is from the Latin "*supportare,*" which means "to carry." Look at its synonyms: "uphold," "sustain," "maintain," "advocate," and "champion." As the flying buttresses support the vaulted ceilings of cathedrals of worship, your hands may reach out and hold another hand, while another heart holds you. *Do not pass this up.*

Forgiveness, Gratitude, and Unconditional Love

Many patients with cancer carry some measure of guilt as to why they have the malignancy, and in some measure, this guilt is justifiable. However, who among us is perfect? Who can cast that first stone? None! The same principle applies when looking at a delay in diagnosis or other perceptions of suboptimal attention to your needs. Speak up and make it known. The overwhelming majority of providers respond appropriately when confronted. Do not sow the seeds of bitterness in your heart. They sprout and strangle all with whom you interact. Gratitude, however, is a never-filling cup. You can never receive or give quite enough. It is magic to your health care team and, in a manner, magic to you. The art of creatively thanking those who strive to help you is an exponential one. It grows your relationship with your team almost ballistically, like a skyrocket on July 4.

On what may seem an initially unusual and incongruous note, I have seen the cancer diagnosis cultivate gratitude by the forgiving of past hurts in families, the changing of attitudes and lifestyles, and the helping of those who were merely getting by in life to truly live to fight a fuller life. I have seen it invariably pull marriages together. Sometimes a mighty hammer is needed on those thick skulls of ours. You do not need harsh judgments, ominous proclamations, worries of inconveniences, or complaints. Therefore, you have my permission to talk to yourself, your heart, and your God and listen and watch how your world improves.

BUT WHAT DO I SAY?

Those of us who are not diagnosed with cancer will most assuredly interact with those who are. Little in life, and in particular in our Western culture, prepares us to deal comfortably, intimately, and competently with the understandable challenges presented in relating to one we know or love who has been diagnosed with cancer.

I can think of no better way to guide us down the road of what I have learned from thousands of patients and families and friends than to use an e-mail from my mom wherein she struggled with how to talk with her niece, who was diagnosed with a particularly ominous type and stage of lung cancer. In a manner, she asks, "But what do I say to the dying, seriously ill, and perhaps terminal patient?"

She wrote,

> I have been very intent in reading your book to enable me to give support to not only ——— but also to others. Again, I shall seek your help. Will there be a section that will tell me how to respond to the patient who is becoming irritable, impatient, and angry at the lifestyle she has been placed in? Her day is filled with medications, doctors, and tests that have taken away her independence. I do not know if I am doing the right thing. I lend her my ears and allow her to vent her anger and frustration on me. I merely say I understand and do not offer any platitudes. I just become her sounding board. Thanks, Love Mom.

This is my response to my mom and the millions who may be in her shoes. What I have learned is that being *real* is what counts. A patient venting anger and frustration or expressing whatever emotions is not something one "allows" another person to do. This is perhaps just semantics for some, but the point is crucial. "Allow" sounds like getting permission from somebody with authority for approval before doing something. We who are merely witnesses to those suffering do not have the authority to give permission; nor are we an authority on someone else's suffering. Although some of us may once have been a cancer patient or been the close relative or friend of one with cancer, the experience is nonetheless very personal; it was your experience, not someone else's. As was the case then, the lesson that rings the truest is always the same: the patient is the one with the disease. The patient will do what he or she chooses to do with or without your permission. However, being *present* when they do something is an active choice.

Patients are extremely sensitive to a number of classic missteps when it comes to the behaviors of those who are not the patient. Thinking that you fully understand all the personal nuances and aspects of others suffering is but one of them. There is also the pious platitude syndrome, which is really a ruse to avoid dealing with the reality of the situation and displace it all into ethereal and impersonal terms. This is when folks use statements like "This, too, shall pass," "Oh, it was meant to be," "It is God's will," or "It will all work out."

Alternatively, there is the "I really do not want to hear it" dodge, which is largely a reflection of self-absorption. When folks do this, they are really putting a premium on their own neediness or concerns and not the patient's. This is not too dissimilar to the denial syndrome, in which friends and family downplay or even outright deny the severity, urgency, and suffering of the patient. This can be so severe that it may even show up as admonishment, anger, and impatience with the patient. Again, this is all about self-absorption and is often just another face of the anger we feel when looking at a loved one's or friend's situation. There are other missteps, but those are the most common.

Fortunately, there are a number of role models in history that can help us gain insight into dealing with those who are suffering and give us a

Fill a Bag. Help Feed Families.

Place healthy nonperishable food donations near your mailbox

Donations Stay in your Community

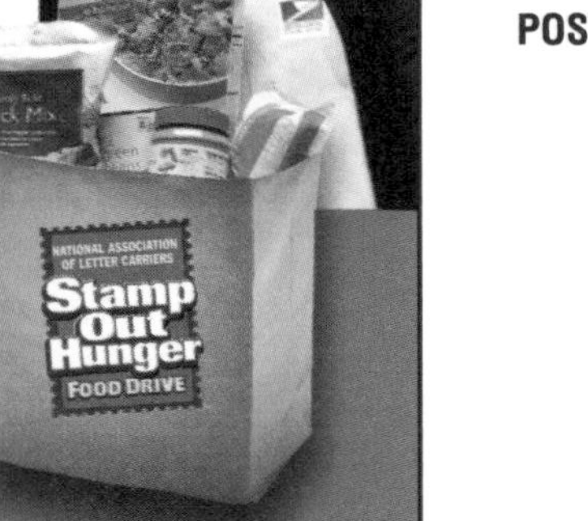

Saturday, May 13, 2017

Help Us Stamp Out Hunger,
Spread the Word.

Facebook.com/StampOutHunger @StampOutHunger

stampouthungerfooddrive.us

PRESORT STANDARD
POSTAGE & FEES PAID
USPS
PERMIT NO. G-10

POSTAL CUSTOMER

Fill a Bag. Help Feed Families.

Saturday, May 13

1. Collect and bag HEALTHY nonperishable* food items
*Coloque los alimentos **saludables** no perecederos en una bolsa junto a su buzón de correo*

2. Place by mailbox for letter carrier to deliver to a local food bank or pantry
El cartero las entregará a un banco de alimentos local

* Donate healthy, low-sodium, low-sugar items such as beans, canned tuna in water, peanut butter, soup, vegetables, pasta, pasta sauce, cereal, oatmeal and other whole grains, canned fruit, canola or olive oil and canned meats. Please do not donate items that have expired or are in glass containers.

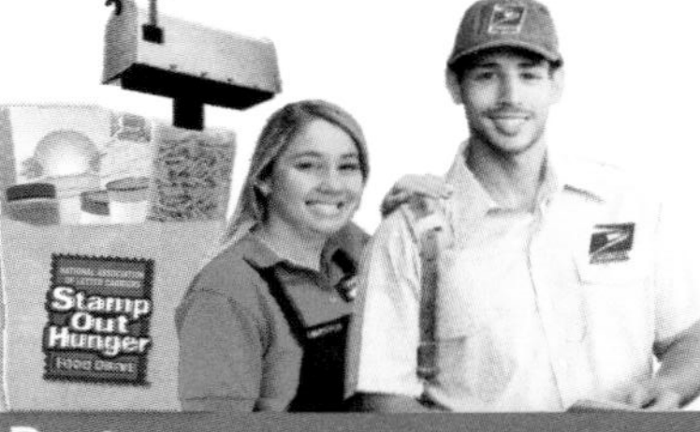

NALC Thanks Its National Partners

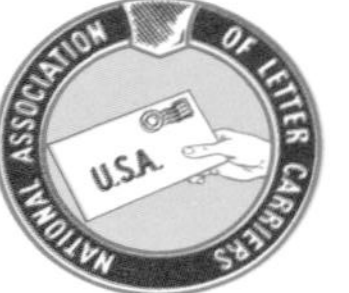

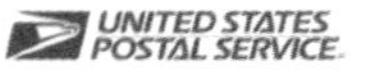

AFL-CIO

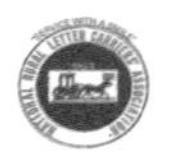

AARP Foundation

valpak

LOCAL FOOD PANTRIES

Valassis

Premiere Partner

UFCW
a VOICE for working America

From your bagger to your butcher, we're the hardworking men and women of your neighborhood grocery union. Together, we are proud to put the food on America's tables.

better understanding of, what to say. Without any intent to be evangelical, I can think of no better example of how to answer the question "But what do I say?" than to point to what history tells us Christ reportedly did when dealing with great suffering.

There have been countless interpretations of Christ's reported interpersonal skills, but some very basic techniques clearly come to the forefront. He was *real*, and he was emotionally available. He did not own the suffering of others while he ministered to their needs. He was present. He acknowledged that bad is bad, happy is happy, bad hair days are real, and people can be asses. He laughed with all and cried with many. He did not tiptoe around suffering and the enormous conflicted feelings it evokes. He was ready and quick with grace, which, unlike mercy, is something you do not earn or deserve. He understood fear but always shunned and destroyed anxiety.

Christ took action. He did not obsess on avoiding fearful events. He took them in stride as part of the pursuit and passion of living. No topic was unmentionable. He was not gingerly with the truth that life is not a collage and a rainbow of colors. Life is not some two-dimensional box crafted only from the intersecting lines of "should" or "ought," or painted with only happy or sad tones. The same is true of human emotion. Christ knew that anger was not only okay but also important and necessary. He taught that indignation may indeed be righteous and that impatience is natural, normal, and often necessary.

The problem of communication with the suffering or terminally ill is compounded in our nation and culture, where we have grown accustomed to the fact that most of us will spend the end of our days out of our home, in some form of institution. This only enhances the discomfort of friends and families, as they have so little experience with being intimate with dying that it somewhat distances the experience both literally and figuratively. How sad, as it is one appointment all of us must keep and virtually no one wishes to do it alone. This entire topic receives an excellent treatment by Dr. Robert Bruckman, a medical oncologist at the University of Toronto, in his book *I Don't Know What to Say: How to Help Someone Who Is Dying*. A seminal point correctly made by Dr. Bruckman is that "one of the biggest problems faced by terminally ill patients is that people won't talk to them and the feelings of isolation add a great deal to the burden."

Earlier in the section on anxiety and fear, I discussed how anxiety is fear of the unknown, a sort of paralysis by analysis. In my metaphor about the two clans of cavemen, the anxiety-ridden caveman clan died by taking no action, by not facing their fears. Failure to engage anxiety magnifies it enormously, and patients left alone with their thoughts frequently prefer to have an expedited death, as in many ways they are already living in a "thought hell." Far too frequently, uncomfortable family and friends fall prey to this fear-based conspiracy of silence, causing far more harm than they realize.

The formula is *normalcy*. What works with a healthy, good friend will not fail with the sick and dying. Pull up a chair, get comfortable, listen, and maintain eye contact. The cancer is not contagious, but the fear and discomfort will be.

As in any conversation, although everyone's favorite topic is himself, visitors should focus on the other person. The patient is the one with the disease. Once again, remember the behavior of Christ and other great spiritual leaders and philosophers. The world grows enormously when we make welcome room for the presence of another. This is *their* show. Keep it simple and ask, "What do you want to talk about?" This is the time for active listening, paying attention to body language, tone of voice, and general demeanor. Paraphrase and return what the patient says, which instantly makes it clear that what the patient says is important and that you want to convey genuine interest by getting what the patient said right—to his or her satisfaction, not yours.

Inevitably, there will be points where the patient will talk about unpleasant topics such as pain, suffering, remorse, last wishes, and dying. This is holy ground, and you have a ringside seat at one of life's great constancies: facing our mortality. It does not get more intimate than this. Encourage such conversations if they are initiated, and ask open-ended questions. Do not ask closed-ended questions with preconceived conclusions, allowing only yes or no answers that cut off any desire for anyone to answer, and limit all risk of hearing something you do not want to hear but perhaps should. Essentially, make yourself available as a listener.

Visitors must remember that they are not gurus, "Dear" Abby, or Heloise. As emphasized previously in this book, patients are individuals, and visitors are not their doctors. This is not the time to inundate the patient with stories of wondrous cures from some Kickapoo joy juice or miracle medic read of or heard of at the club or beauty parlor. Just as a car has only one unique vehicle identification number, the patient is an individual.

These wounded pups respond to a gift that keeps giving to senders and receiver alike: strokes and positive feedback about things that are valid to give them for. Strokes are not platitudes; they are positive feedback that is given when warranted. The person with a life-threatening or terminal disease will be making all kinds of decisions and choices. Many may be pretty darn admirable or worthy of praise, whatever they may be. It can be very reassuring for those who are suffering to be given "attaboys" when they have done something that was difficult for them. Remember, it may be nothing for you to brush your hair, get out of bed, walk to the patio, or tell someone you might see again how you really feel. The scope is irrelevant as long as the feedback and the strokes are proportional, not overblown. I can think of no greater gift a loved one can give than encouraging the suffering one to embark on *dying to live, not living to die.*

A personal story comes to mind. A woman dying of small-cell lung cancer called her cousin. She did not call expecting empathy or in-depth discussion, as they had never been close. However, that cousin's eighty-six-year-old mother (the patient's aunt) was a trusted and intimate confidant for the patient. That aunt had an older sister whom the patient did not want to be involved. The patient knew that if the older aunt knew of her sister's closeness to the patient, there would hell to pay. The patient also knew that her cousin kept in touch with the older aunt. That is why, despite her own immense suffering, she called her cousin and instructed her not to let the older aunt know much of anything. The patient's motivation was to spare the younger aunt from being emotionally beaten up.

Ponder this for a moment. The patient did not call because her favored aunt was under attack, but rather because her aunt might come under attack at some unknown time. This is preemptive empathy. This is human nobility at its best. That is placing one's own very real and pressing issues as secondary to the welfare of another *in anticipation*, rather than in reaction or response. This is selflessness. Such nobility is a virtue that suffering may bring. It is also certainly cause for any aware of it to take pause and give credit and emulate it when dealing with the dying or severely ill patient.

Another common error is what I call the "hide-the-peanut game" of not sharing information. This is as asinine as trying to hide the peanut from a determined African elephant. Once again, it is time to get real. What is the worst that can possibly happen by focusing on facts and not fantasy and fears? The patient could die. Well, that may already be in the cards. We are no longer children who can successfully disappear from a scary world by placing our hands over our own eyes and triumphantly declaring, "You can't see me!" Supporters and loved ones are well advised to never deny or try to cover up the seriousness of a situation.

If something is clearly funny, then it is. Humor is one of life's greatest opiates, antidepressants, and aphrodisiacs. Engage it. Conversely, this is a sad time, and crying is one of the things normal people do when they are sad. Welcome tears. Frequently the patient may be angry. Fine, as there is good reason to be miffed. The problem will arise when visitors mistakenly assume some sort of responsibility or blame if they *appear* to be the object of a patient's anger. This is silliness; understandable, but silliness. The anger is directed at the disease and the situation the patient finds himself or herself in. Once again, I implore family and friends to remember that *this is not about you.*

Rarely, patients will hold to fervent denial to the end while still quite competent. Frankly, this is largely overplayed both in our imaginations and in fictitious Hollywood death scenes. As a visitor, as well as family member, you have no responsibility to engage, accept, or refute any patient's denial. It will pass, and if not, a useful approach is to simply defer to the health-care team and whatever they have told the patient.

As has often been said, nothing tells a tale better than real life. A friend shared with me her reflections on how she came to be intimately involved in the dying process of a previously somewhat more distant relative. My friend had experienced the loss of a long-term spouse from the same disease as her relative fourteen years earlier. Her spouse died less than a week after being diagnosed. She took great pains to make it clear to me that she did not know much about the journey she was about to go on in support of her dying relative when the journey began. Below, in her intimate experience with dying, I hear the celebration of life. Do you?

> After speaking with [the dying relative] at great length, these are my thoughts. I want to preface all this by stating I have had no experience caring for a terminally-ill loved one for an unknown length of time. Mine was only of a week's duration, and that was in a hospital setting. Over the years, I have been exposed to many dear friends who have succumbed to a terminal illness.
>
> I have learned these things. When faced with the news that a family member or a dear friend has been diagnosed with a terminal illness, one is immediately faced with a deep concern as to what should they say or not say. You want to help, but you fear you will say or do something that will further upset the loved one. We seem to forget that *dying people have the same physical, emotional, and spiritual needs as everyone else.* In addition to these needs, people who are dying are very often concerned with being abandoned, losing control over their bodies and lives, and are very often in excruciating pain or distress.
>
> The physician can meet these special needs, such as with painkillers and prescriptions. I feel that all other needs for the dying can be met by anyone. Through the guidance of the doctor, caretakers can be trained to lessen the affliction by being taught about pain management.
>
> Psychological care is equally important. The patient very often will exhibit negative feelings, such as anger, anxiety, and fear. These very real emotions need to be identified and acknowledged and, above all, expressed.

Many would-be helpers are uncomfortable, wondering again what they should say or do. I guess there is no universal thing to do or say, but I feel several things could be helpful. These things include *being present, speaking the truth, and most important listen, listen, listen—not passively, but actively.* Acceptance of the impending death is key! The patient is not stupid. Let them talk about it. A gentle touch, hug, or just holding their hand seems to heal psychologically.

[The Patient's Name] ***has been disempowered when unknowingly, caretakers have taken over the work of the dying person.*** They are telling her what to do, telling her to get dressed, put her teeth in, get out of the house, etc. They mean well, but instead of providing a joyful atmosphere, they are generating an atmosphere of gloom and depression that evokes anger, apathy, and hopelessness within the family unit. The family is striving so hard to appease her with these suggestions, never realizing that on the contrary it makes her more depressed. *Telling her what to do is discouraging.* She is fully aware that she has no control over the impending death.

Control of how she wishes to fill her remaining time should be totally within her one and only control. Frivolous as this may sound, if she wishes to don a clown's hat, let her! If she wishes to remain in the house with a housecoat, so be it. She can control these mundane things. Only she knows whether she has the stamina to get out. To spare her "supporters," she has not revealed to them the horrible torture she is in just to place one foot ahead of the other.

Seems to me the roles have been reversed. ***The supporters have become the supported.*** Very sad all around. As for me, I shall sing the song "What Lola wants Lola gets." Love, Mom.

I answered, "Thanks, Mom. You get it. Love, Kev."

So what do you say? Although the singular moment of death is experienced when we are most alone, the journey need not be. We are in this boat of life together, and when it is time to dock for some, hold fast to their hand, steady the craft, and help them lovingly ashore, because those who are dying teach us much about life, especially that left which we cannot predict but can fully experience.

So to Mom and everyone else who will ask, "But what do I say?" I tell you, say, "Thank you."

FRONT OFFICE

I know if you were to look in the dictionary under "oncology front office," it is dubious that you would find the entry I wish I could sneak into the *Oxford English Dictionary* (the mother of all English dictionaries). It would say, "See courage, patience tolerance, kindness, gentle spirit, humility, trust, friendship, and instincts for illness and faith." That is exactly what front-office staff should be when a patient calls, just stops by on the way to another appointment, receives a visit if admitted, or arrives for his or her own appointment. These are the cherubim and seraphim of the clinic. At times, I have not been sure whether they or the winged wonders they emulate inhabit the front office.

I certainly can only speak of my personal experiences, although I suspect there are countless examples of wonderful front offices. Thus, I will use them as my realizable ideal that I wish for all offices to emulate and the qualities all patients should demand. Front-office staff invariably know, as closely as they can, without being the patient, what being a patient is.

In every staff meeting, we talked of patients as a type of family, a precious cargo with special needs or pressures. All of my staff have always wanted to know everything they can about what is going on with the patients. They understand the importance of the tone of their voice in person or on the phone, as well as their body language. They are vigilant regarding it. I have never—and I do mean never—had a complaint, but I have been inundated by compliments from the patients. They know that just greeting the patient and family is a huge part of the patients' world, as so much may be riding on that day's news. The office staff is crestfallen when patients are smitten with difficult news, and they rejoice when a patient is lifted up. Cancer care is a team endeavor and, at times, an extended family of sorts.

The job of getting the appointments straight, working with individual social and clinical needs, and assisting with "administrivia" is no small task, and they are usually flawless. If ever there is a misstep, no worry; they will assume the blame, which on one level is probably not theirs. On another, perhaps they feel they forgot to remind a patient of their appointment. It is all about attitude. That is something you not only cannot hide but also is readable in seconds, and they know it.

Even though many offices are largely paperless, documentation is crucial in my business. A great front-office staff attends to detail better than a Quaker planning his daughter's wedding. Nothing fails to be filed, signed, dated, or stamped. Nothing is lost. Records are to be timeless and are recognized as the irreplaceable crucial documentation of a human life that they are.

They are responsible for keeping the patient literature well stocked and the waiting room a positive, happy place. They never simply *react* to a patient who may be upset for any number of understandable reasons. They *respond*, even if it means getting me or one of the nurse specialists out of a room, as all our patients know that people in trouble always come first.

We all understand the absolute joy of receiving messages that have complete names, appropriate identifications, correct phone numbers, and thorough, legible, comprehensible messages. That alone must save ten hours a week. The staff understands that the deferred dividend of lack of attention to detail is a disaster for the doctor, the nursing staff, and, most of all, the patient and family. If this is not handled correctly every time, the clinical staff can become buried in lost and misfiled reports and, most importantly, may fall behind in picking up on symptoms that may be heralding more ominous times ahead.

Yet this is not where they excel. It is the small talk, the banter during the taking of vital signs. It is their remembering little details about the other person's life to spark a pleasant conversation. I can tell you this; come Christmas, Santa brings an extra sled just for the presents these folks receive. Yet, Christmas is year-round for them. They are always receiving gifts, as they are always giving the gift of their time, attention, and concern. They are always as their namesakes—the seraphim and the cherubim.

In a teaching facility, our young doctors learn enormous lessons from front-office staff and the records they provide. Oncology is frequently responsible for a large share of the admissions to the hospital, and thus the quality of what a front-office staff provides and prepares has an immediate impact on the quality and timeliness of care that patients receive. First impressions are everything in oncology. Great staff know that and take pains to be sure every possible fact that is relevant is known by all who will next touch the life of the wounded. As I have said so often, after these many years, the easy part is the science; the hard part is the human art of being a part of a team and understanding what it is to suffer, to have anxieties and very genuine fears of very real threats—day after day. The front-office staff touches the lives of all patients and their families deeply and alters the lives of patients yet to come.

I have seen the glow of patients, having been in the tail of their comet. It enriches all of us on the team, and we gain by the patients passing through it. Many of the patients are helped in their quest and fight for peace because of this staff. There may be less fear, less concern about ignored pain, and far less worry over everything else because of the front-office staff's enormous concern for others. This staff can help patients feel, in a sense, that they are at home, and that is where the heart truly is.

So often I am asked how I do this job, as if I were some fountainhead of courage or unfathomable knowledge. *I do not do this job. A team does.* When it is my turn, dear God, give me just a pinch of the class, the sheer humanity, and the professionalism steeped with compassion of a great front-office staff. Oh, and, one more thing, God, while I have you on the line: give the patients—no, help the patients demand that they have the staff they deserve to serve them. If not, help them find another office. Oh yes, and thank you, God, for the family of friends I have been blessed to work with.

NURSES

I can best express the enormity of impact nurses rightfully have by relating a story—a parable of sorts. I had not been back about the business of boxing with God very long when, scurrying about, I peered at an object that caught my eye and caused me to ponder. I failed to understand what I truly saw. It gave me pause to think why such a thing would be here. It was a feather—soft, floating, and yielding to invisible currents, seemingly buoyed by an imperceptible force cradling it in a most improbable manner just above the cold, sterile clinic floor. I rationalized that it must have been left there by housekeeping. Thinking nothing more of what it truly must be that I saw (a trait that is all too common as we become adults), I placed it thoughtlessly in my regal robe—the doctor's white coat—and went off onto my rounds.

I was blessed to work with angels every day—men and woman who, for a God-given reason, have sought to be not only nurses but also oncology-certified nurses. This is another thing patients should look into: whether their nurses are Oncology Nursing Society members and officially credentialed as oncology nurse specialists. Be wary otherwise.

These nurses are the winged wonders of love. They greet patients after the diagnosis, arrange for a venous access port to deliver chemotherapy if one is necessary, and explain all that is involved in their upcoming journey. They address and ease fears of patients by taking as long as it takes to teach the patient and family all about the drugs, their effects, and the need for frequent blood tests. They teach the effects on taste, appetite, daily living, and risk of infection. They address issues regarding nails, bowels, the mouth, and the skin. They address everything. Then they teach it again. They explain each drug and sit with patients, carefully building a calendar so that all of the drugs can be given on time and all blood and diagnostic tests are understood. They anticipate fears, as they have so closely walked this razor's edge before, and they give patients permission and time to be scared. Oncology care is not a commodity. It is, at its best, a grace-imbued art of loving to fight a treacherous foe as bravely as a human can—and never alone. These nurses are the master artists.

Oncology nurses are an enormous aspect of every visit and are the ones who frequently answer all patient and family questions. They are not there to shield the patient from "occupying" the oncologist but are rather there, in part, to embrace the patients and family with their knowledge and assess intelligently and lovingly if the issue needs escalation. If so, they can be a Joan of Arc.

They will pierce skin and draw blood. They will often relay the message of anxiously awaited test results. They will administer cancer chemotherapy after giving medications to prevent nausea and vomiting. They are expertly trained to recognize any adverse reaction calmly and swiftly intervene. Yet, even more importantly, they will take and give a hand, give a hug, hold a heart, and share a life or a photo or two. Patient downslides are theirs, and patient victories are heralded and trumpeted by them as only angels can do.

They are the backstop that catches whatever they think perhaps the doctor is not aware of, such as a certain test result or a new clinical complaint. They are both an advocate and spokesperson for the patient. They are a key ingredient needed to turn paralyzing anxiety into action-provoking fear and, finally, acceptance. They are there to keep morale high and even play with patients with wigs and prostheses—yes, play. It can get downright silly sometimes. They are there to calm fears and touch the soul. My advice to patients is simple: If you do not feel the glow, and if the angelic breeze does not gently caress you as the nurses pass closely, you are not home. Do not stay; find another place for care.

Therefore, what of the feather on the clinic floor I thoughtlessly put in my pocket? I have often scurried about my clinic, occupied with the crisis of the day, ignorant and oblivious of what may be occurring under my nose. Yet there are times when, while grousing about in the pockets of my imperious robe—untarnished, unblemished—I finally "see." Look! It is a feather from an angel's wing.

INPATIENT CARE

Perhaps a few introductory remarks are necessary for the future patient. At a teaching institution, attending physicians are fully privileged and credentialed physicians who are legally responsible for the interns one year out of med school and second- and third-year residents. It is the policy of the governing body in a very closely regulated system that the patient is the interns' primary responsibility. The intern is in the charge of the resident and the resident is in the charge of the attending, who is ultimately responsible for all that transpires. There is immense supervision but also significant delegated authority. The American Board of Internal Medicine has very strict guidelines to protect patients and ensure the very best in care. As a word of advice to patients, it is wise to have every attending physician be board certified.

"Roundsmanship," as used here, refers to the rules of engagement, if you will, while being a physician in training or in a supervisory position on an inpatient hospital ward. In this chapter, I will discuss the secrets of the magic decoder ring and secret handshake of the guild in practicing inpatient medicine on a medicine ward. These are the adages I tell my charges when it is my turn at the helm as the attending physician. Some are amusing, some profound, and all have a powerful lesson patients would be wise to know. This is the inside scoop that will help the patient be active in his or her care and prevent some of the deification of the regal white coat.

Precept 1: If caught sleeping on rounds, try saying, "They told me at the blood bank that this might happen" or "In Jesus's name, amen."

The practice of inpatient medicine is particularly tiring work, and although there are laws (not guidelines) as to how many hours and how many patients an intern and resident can be responsible for, it is still tiring work. The law now limits the workweek to eighty hours per week with one weekend day off per month. Not all are compliant with this, however. This is exhausting work. Thus, fatigue must be watched for very carefully. Working longer, as I did during my years, can cause one to fall prey to possibly ineffective medical care.

Precept 2: Read the PDR for every drug, and check orders vs. Kardex.

The PDR is a compendium of all the FDA-approved drugs. If a student of medicine gets in the habit of reading about every drug he or she prescribes, redundancy alone will make them brilliant, and medical misadventures will all but disappear from the drug side of the equation. Polypharmacy, whereby especially the aged are on numerous drugs with many interactions, occurs in over 30% of all nursing-home patients. Furthermore, almost 20% of ER visits are related to medications in some manner. Drugs do not have front, back, or side effects. They have *effects*. My advice to patients is to ask your intern if he or she has read the PDR on all the drugs he or she is giving you. They will be ultimately grateful. Ask you intern or resident if the doctor's orders, the nursing flow sheet, the records (the Kardex), and what you received are all the same, as well as whether the right drugs have been prescribed or administered at the right dose. Furthermore, ask them if they check that regularly, because I said so. I have done this for decades. Trust me. When a human hits the equation, it is time to do checking.

Precept 3: Remember: 47.5 % of all statistics are made up on the spot.

Get the point: people are individuals, and statistics refer to what has already happened to a group similar to you, *not you yourself*. They are used in an attempt to offer odds of probability of specific outcomes from past scenarios regarding patients that are sufficiently similar to a present patient. Correctly applied, they *may* have a 95% or 97.5% chance of accurately predicting your outcome. Remember, that is only if all the factors and variables are known and extremely similar; *that is not always reality.* I again advise patients to enlighten themselves when they hear physicians cite statistics (which may be very appropriate) by asking what confidence interval they can state with the statistics in question. Namely, ask for the range of confidence they have that the statistics apply to you.

Of course, you really do not want or need to know all about confidence intervals other than to think of them as tools that can tell us literally how powerfully accurate a statistic, when applied to you, may be. Using a ruler marked in inches to measure millimeters is not a wise idea. That is where confidence intervals come in. It really is just asking for straight shooting. You want to know to what degree, and based on what evidence and information, your team can assess *your* odds of response to treatment. Once again, there is no substitute for information, and nothing quite as valuable, after a skilled physician, as an informed and involved patient. Everyone wins.

Precept 4: Always communicate, using whatever means are available, effectively, timely, securely, and agreeably to all with everyone who is involved and approved by the patient. The more you can document what was said to whom, where it was said, and when it was said, the better.

Communication is key. This is basic stuff and a common mistake. Everyone needs to be on the same page at the same time to their limit of their intellectual, educational, and emotional abilities. This is not a secret guild. Secrets can kill patients, disrupt families, inflame other consultants, and require remembering what you are trying to hide from whom rather than what you are sharing appropriately.

Precept 5: Although notes and records have a key role, they complement intimacy with the situation and do not substitute for it.

Although this is largely my style, it builds strong minds and verbal skills for all. It drills into the young doctors that patients are people in need and that they should know all that should be known about their patients, *in their minds* and not only in their notes. This directly improves communication with the patient and other consultants, as well as general patient care. As a patient, you feel a lot more secure when your doctor does not have to rely on notes to take care of you. We remember vastly better that which we understand and forget quickly what is not truly of great importance or misunderstood. That is how the human mind works. How can your physician help you as well if he or she does not have a full grasp of at least the most important information? I am sorry, but there is no excuse for that, and if we teach doctors to rely too heavily on a piece of paper, they will never develop their minds or learn to think well on their feet. Of course, documentation is key and repositories of detailed data are essential, but they must not be a crutch or the primary intellectual tool. This is painful for some but a universal blessing in time for all.

Precept 6: Do *not* put off until tomorrow—etc., etc.

The old adage "Out of sight, out of mind" is true. Medical documentation must be contemporary to the events it documents. This applies to daily progress notes or the summary of care when discharged. Memory does not improve with time or age. I have seen patients' health directly compromised because of shoddy and tardy record keeping or transmittal of clinical information. This is unacceptable and threatens patients' care. The record is the treating physician and institution's property, but the information in it is the patient's. This simply means that patients are always entitled to a copy. These copies are invaluable not only if there is a permanent change of residence but also when a patient with a medical history of problems that could persist or recur is traveling away from home.

It is an excellent idea to have some simple laminated cards that list all of one's medications. These should be in every wallet, in every glove compartment, and on every refrigerator. Patients and families would be wise to tell their physicians and hospitals that upon discharge they want a copy of the detailed summary of care that is always dictated, not just an overview that may be lacking in crucial details. This is of enormous potential benefit if illness strikes in an unfamiliar location or at an unpredictable time. Finally, I advise patients to insist that their treating physicians always immediately send copies of their summary of care to the patient's primary and referring physicians. This is fortunately largely routinely done in this country.

Precept 7: Focus on books, manuals, and communication; do not sweat the journals in lieu of horse sense.

Of course, all physicians must be familiar with the most up-to-date information regarding patient's diseases, diagnostic techniques, and treatments. However, all must be wary of addictive technocracy, whereby there is an unnecessary and unrealistic zeal and belief that if you are not being treated at some world-famous institute, your fate will certainly be compromised. This is *not* usually the case. Certainly, rare diseases require institutions and clinicians with experience. Certainly, new techniques and information that may be cutting-edge and as yet not widely available or known come forth all the time and may be available only at certain teaching institutes. However, beware of inappropriate grandeur and pomp holding too large a sway against one of my personal favorite adages of all in the practice of medicine: Common manifestations of common diseases and uncommon manifestations of common diseases are more common than uncommon diseases in any manifestation.

As one of the fathers of modern medicine, Sir William Osler, put it, "When you hear hoofbeats on the cobblestones of London, think of horses, not zebras." This is rather similar to the timeworn admonition of not losing sight of the forest for the trees. The correct recipe is a balance struck after clinicians are rock solid on common manifestations of common diseases and uncommon manifestations of common diseases. Yes, we all must be constantly learning and up-to-date, but we must always be practical and master the basics for advances in the field to be in perspective. "Young and brilliant," as describes a physician, is a state of mind from perpetual learning and experience, *not* a chronological phenomenon.

Precept 8: Address spirituality and do-not-resuscitate orders.

Numerous dedicated patient advocates from all walks struggled successfully for years to develop a patient's bill of rights, which is now law and addresses what a patient wishes to be done if his or her demise appears probable or imminent. There is no understating the disastrous consequences emotionally—and, at times, financially and legally—if this is not attended to in advance.

Nevertheless, it is foolhardy as well as perhaps unintentionally abusive, albeit not rare, for clinicians to fail to address the spiritual aspect of care. Spirituality may be unaddressed, but it is always present. It transcends from the physician and patient's first handshake to their final goodbye. This is why, in this book, there is an entire chapter devoted to it and it is a powerful theme throughout. The patient is not his or her disease. Patients are more than flesh and blood, and saying so is practical and not ethereal, in-vogue whimsy. It has enormously pressing and urgent implications.

Spirituality may encompass religion, theology, or simply worldview, but we all know far better than that. It is the bastion where hope resides, and it suffers when we despair in the merely physical realm. Muscle and bone do not alone shoulder the burden of the walk of life; it is the spiritual heart and skeleton that truly support us. Failure to address the whole patient in this regard, especially if the stakes are high and the situation serious, is a failure to address the whole disease. Of course, not all physicians are equally suited for this task for every patient every time, and not all patients require the same level of care. Furthermore, the spiritual aspects of all diseases are not the same and are intimately tied to the level of discomfort, the prognosis, and any associated disability. Nonetheless, this is a pivotal aspect of caring for the seriously ill and their families. We all suffer more, immediately or cumulatively, when we stay in what some irreverently call the material world. Perhaps we doctors could on occasion hold a heart with the same reverence with which we hold the metaphorical test tube.

Precept 9: No pissing contests are to be allowed, overtly or otherwise.

Every good leader, manager, or coach of any team knows this as well as his or her name. Medicine is not a contest among "magnificent demagogues." Doctors must never compete with their patients. Patients must never compete with their doctors, and doctors must never compete with each other. Patients and doctors together should never tolerate or engage in sly, slick, between-the-lines, or overt castigating of a colleague or patient in the chart, the hall, the nursing station, or in front of the patient or another doctor. Never! It is a recipe for courting disaster and akin to swearing in the Sistine chapel. Furthermore, if a physician wants to scare the living daylights out of a patient, all he or she has to do is question the competency of another physician within earshot of a patient. In like manner, how wise is it for a patient to editorialize irresponsibly regarding the professional staff? The key word is "irresponsibly." There are many appropriate forums and avenues for this, and it has no role in the sacred professional and personal relationship between doctor and patient. My advice to all is to keep the contest where it belongs—in adolescence, which all of us should have long since grown out of. We all stay happier that way.

Precept 10: Tribal councils or tribal warfare: choose.

The family, which is whomever the patient identifies as such, must be in communication with each other and the professional staff as a matter of routine—not by special engagement, unless that is the patient's desire and direction, which is uncommon but not unheard of. This is pivotal. Ancient familial pathology and dysfunction always finds a way to exhibit itself when any member, especially a parent, is seriously ill. In like fashion, the beautiful harmonies of a family bound by love and fueled by a steady stream of information and knowledge can play more sweetly than a Brahms lullaby. The goal of the maestro medic is to not entertain the former and exalt the latter.

Clarity is also crucial: clarity as to who the spokespersons are if not the patient, clarity regarding the laws of the state in which care is being rendered, and clarity among all the family members that the patient is the one with the disease. Clarity must rule the "tribe" so there will no decision-making or decision-influencing conversations or "powwows" in the absence of the competent "chief"—the patient. Failure to do this will cloud rather than clarify, and tribal warfare, covert or otherwise, will be sure to follow soon.

Precept 11: Your mother was right; God gave you ears to listen, so clean them out and pay attention.

Yes, our mothers are right. Just as it is true that one cannot hold anything with a closed fist, it is true in like manner that one cannot listen if one is talking. This cuts both ways. Physicians have been told for centuries that the lion's share of many clinical diagnoses is the history. Similarly, the lion's share of antianxiety therapy is best delivered through knowledge. Both require the art of active listening by clinician and patient alike.

Active listening is the process whereby distractions of all manners are minimized as one individual relates information. Then it is time for the other to paraphrase, restate, summarize—anything that lets the speaker know that what he or she said is what was heard. This is in no way to suggest agreement or disagreement. It is simply the first crucial step—and often one done poorly, thus dooming all further effective communication. Once done, clarification can occur quickly when the listener and speaker check in with each other as to the exact nature of what was said. This is a repetitive process as each new piece of information is relayed. The stakes are enormous if this is done poorly. An entire diagnosis may be missed.

It does not stop there. Physicians need to hear the nonverbal communication that may be easy for some to hear and inaudible to others. Clinicians must also be wary of the nonverbal communications they are sending. Doctors must have their spiritual (some call it emotional or psychological) ears on and tuned in; otherwise the real grist of what ails the patient now, or will ail him or her in the future, may be missed.

Listening also involves manners. Eye contact, patience, understandable language from the patient's perspective, and a friendly tone of voice with a welcoming attitude are paramount. Some physicians stand during the interview, stay near the door, or pepper the interview or visits on rounds with verbal or nonverbal messages that seem to telegraph impatience, a hurried demeanor, or simply no emotion at all. In addition, too many patents fall prey to either anxiety, deification of the white coat, embarrassment, or feeling they are an imposition, and thus they do not "come clean" with disclosing and forthright statements about their complaints and concerns.

The astute physician always listens for the "Oh, by the way" as he or she heads out the door. This is often the big-money moment as to what is really going on. Although Americans are more effusive and communicative than many other first-world cultures, we often get an acute attack of muteness, shyness, or I-don't-want-to-whine-or-bother-the-busy-doctor-itis, both in the doctor's office or when the doctor is on rounds. In contrast, there are those patients who struggle to focus or prioritize their complaints or "gunnysack" enumerable issues into one visit where the reality, let alone importance, of any one complaint, let alone all of them, is tough for the doctor to discern. I urge all patients to write down their thoughts, questions, or issues literally as soon as they think them, wherever they may be. Then they should organize them before the visit. Doing so not only has an immensely positive impact on the clinical visit, but it also, in many cases, facilitates making the right diagnosis, beginning therapy, or scheduling other tests much more quickly and efficiently.

There is often so much mysticism in seeing the physician on rounds that communication frequently breaks down on both sides of the equation. Yes, it is tough to "joke with the pope," so to speak, but the doctor puts his or her holy vestments on one appendage at a time. Physicians cannot read minds if patients do not speak them, and patients cannot be read if physicians do not use their ears—both literal and psychological.

Precept 12: "Alleged" means just that.

So much of life is hearsay. This is sad and potentially dangerous. Passion, pain, and pleasure are never truly experienced by proxy. Physicians frequently first learn of a new patient or a new problem over the phone or in some other secondhand manner. As is the case in our legal system, until one knows that a certain allegation is a fact based on evidence and driven by data, it is not a fact. It may be probable. All of one's experience may suggest certainty, but it is not fact. Although certainly one does not always have the time or opportunity to get the evidence or be driven by the data, in reality that is usually not the case. In an emergent situation, one must do the best one can with all the data one can gather quickly without losing the window of opportunity to act. However, the vast majority of clinical decisions in oncology and most of medicine are not emergent situations that clearly do not afford a reasonable chance at better information.

The game of "he said, she said" can kill in oncology. That is why this precept is actually a battle cry: "'Alleged' means just that." It is alleged until proven otherwise. Unless you know with certainty that a particular laboratory value, test result value, scan, or initial opinion is true or overwhelmingly likely to mean what you think based on experience and the preponderance of the evidence, all concerned may painfully spend the greatest amount of dollars that they cannot afford to spend—emotional dollars. Possession of the truth in a timely manner is the prize. Certainly, the entire team must move swiftly, but speed is never to be substituted for due diligence and getting firsthand evidence from a primary source when good clinical judgment warrants.

There is a nature to being human, and one of the potential darker sides of that nature is jumping to conclusions and hasty generalizations. The haste with which we may jump in oncology can land the entire clinical enterprise in a wasteland ranging from disinterest to despair and even death. For example, the latter can occur when a finding seemingly close to normal is presumed to be normal. "Normal" is a statistical term in medicine. It is reminiscent of the well-known bell-shaped curve that many of us remember our teachers using to grade us. The vast majority of folks getting the Bs to the high Ds are under the arch of the curve, with the peak representing about where half of everyone can be found. The two far ends of the bell-shaped curve are short and leave little room. These are the failing grades and the As.

Statistically, when many laboratory values are reported, there is given a normal range, meaning that whatever the result was did not occur by chance and really is a normal result in the usual, commonplace meaning of the term. It means the result is within the range that healthy normal people would have for that test. The probability of the result really being normal is well over 97%. However, if the test is outside the normal range, even a smidgen over, there is the same greater-than-97% chance that the result really is abnormal and is not occurring by chance. Of course, this principle applies to tests that have objective findings with clearly established normal ranges, such as laboratory tests and some types of radiology tests, as well as biopsies. There are some tests that, by their very nature must be interpreted in the clinical context they are occurring in and are thus both objective and, to some degree, subjective.

The consequences of not understanding the validity, accuracy, and precision of diagnostic testing and the concept of normalcy can be enormous. The following is a story that illuminates the importance of attention to detail and understanding what "normal" may or may not mean. One of the many internists I respect enormously pursued a platelet count (a test that is part of a routine blood count that measures the amount of platelets—small fragments of cells that help blood clot normally) that was repeatedly just 3% above the upper limit of normal. A request for consultation was made, and we pursued it. The elevated count was the earliest manifestation of the most common form of chronic and, previous to the recent development of breakthrough drug, often lethal leukemia, chronic myelogenous leukemia. At the time, clinical trials were just opening up for an oral wonder drug. The patient was promptly treated on one of the initial trials of the drug before there was any other damage from this disorder of the bone marrow and is now in a complete remission.

As is the case with passion, pleasure, and pain, disease and death are not experienced by proxy. They are not something alleged. They *are.*

Precept 13: What did you spend?

I am never in favor of cutting corners, but we all need to exhibit discretion and common sense in terms of ordering tests that are able to produce results that, even when negative, will have a material impact. It is worth noting that the alleviation of emotional suffering by test ordering can have a material impact, but the ordering of tests should not be reduced to pandering to paranoia and running up expenses. There is a deeper danger besides fiscal issues. Tests ordered in this manner are just as subject as appropriate tests to yield false positive results (i.e., stating that something is amiss when in fact there is nothing wrong). This can lead not only to the path of craziness but also to the path of medical misadventures and potential physical harm, as not all tests are risk free and some require more direct interventions.

I once consulted on a patient swearing her urine was red. In a measured, stepwise approach, we were about to begin an evaluation. To the credit of one clever resident, before invasive and expensive procedures were embarked on, he discovered it was only red at home, in the master bedroom bathroom, when the infrared heating light was on. It was illuminating one of the metabolites of her hefty drug regimen that was being excreted in her urine. Fortunately, no harm came from this, as good detective work was done and the basics were kept in focus. It is too easy, in our nation in particular, to become addicted to medical technology in a manner that interferes rather than assists. Technology is to be our slave, not the converse. The price paid for overexuberant care may not only be financial.

Precept 14: What did they hear—nonverbally?

Silence, as well as the many forms of nonverbal communication, may be defeating. Doctors must not make the mistake of assuming that the only message they relay is the one they convey through words. Their words might not be the message the patient and family hear loudest and most clearly and remember longest. The impact of body language, demeanor, mannerisms, and time spent can be enormous. Clinicians usually do quite well at thinking about what they are saying, but all of us humans tend to fall short in saying, both verbally and nonverbally, only what we are thinking and wish to convey, no more and no less. Furthermore, repetition—unlike the aforementioned quip by the great thinker Ralph Waldo Emerson, whom I suspect would exempt oncology physicians—is not the bugaboo of little minds until it is clear that everyone is on the same proverbial page. Repetition is a major rhetorical strategy for producing emphasis, clarity, amplification, or emotional effect.

The darkness of failed communication does not need to be your "old friend." The visions of bad first impressions and unspoken words will plant seeds and linger. The silence of a failed connection resulting from the noisy pandemonium of nonverbal communication will make the emotional cancer grow.

Precept 15: Speed is a drug.

"He who laughs last thinks slowest." Humorous and profound, this not necessarily true precept speaks to the deepest core of the physician. "Slow" does not mean "dumb." It may mean measured, deliberate, methodical, and considered. Physicians are weaned and suckled in a competitive environment. Early on, we embark on lifelong programming to be the first, the fastest, and the quickest to squirm in our seats with our hand up with the right answer for the teacher. Scorecards, evaluations, grades, judging, and measuring, as well as measuring up, dominate our world. The positive side of such intellectual exuberance—coupled with a sincere desire to please, to discover, and to fix—is apparent and essential. We all benefit enormously from these traits.

However, thank God for the pragmatic dreamers, the intellectual clinical entrepreneurs, the scientists, the egalitarians who endeavor for the greater good for all. It is good to have zeal to understand the incredible mystery of visceral existence and harbor an insatiable lust for knowledge.

However, there is a darker side that can take center stage *if* the pressure to perform grows out of balance and the unspoken admonition that medicine has zero tolerance for defects is heeded too closely. This darker side can be seen when there is almost an addiction to being the speediest physician. The early bird may get the worm, but it is the second mouse that gets the cheese. Can it be said more clearly? Rarely in medicine does being first translate into better care. Being fast, especially too fast, ranges from damned annoying to dangerous There is a darker side that looms on the horizon if egos soar unfettered and the delusion of grandeur that "MD" really does mean "magnificent demagogue" no longer flickers but strongly illuminates the sky in which these eagles soar.

In ancient Greek mythology, Prometheus (whose name means forethought) was one of the Titans and was known as the friend and benefactor of humanity. Prometheus was given the task of creating humanity and providing humans and all the animals on earth with the endowments they would need to survive. Prometheus took over the task of creation. To make humans superior to the animals, he fashioned them in nobler form than the animals and enabled them to walk upright. He then went up to heaven and lit a torch with fire from the sun. The gift of fire that Prometheus bestowed upon humanity was more valuable than any of the gifts the animals had received. The sun was the source of power and light and a symbol of ultimate divinity and strength.

Later in mythology, King Minos of Crete imprisoned Daedalus and his son Icarus in a labyrinth as punishment for revealing the key to slaying the half-bull, half-man Minotaur. Although the prisoners could not find the exit, Daedalus made wax wings so that they could both fly out. Icarus, however, flew too near the sun; his wings melted, and he fell into the sea. Daedalus flew to Sicily, where King Cocalus welcomed him. Some regard the labyrinth as a metaphor for the treacherous journey of life with its ample share of human pain and suffering owing to our inherent imperfections, as symbolized by the Minotaur. *Knowledge* was the key that freed the prisoners from themselves. This book attempts to provide a key for the cancer patient to conquer his or her labyrinth, just as every physician struggles with the Minotaur of disease and the mazelike job of negotiating the labyrinth of diagnostic tests and difficult treatment decisions. Yet when we soar too high—when the air becomes thin and we see our place as one with the sun—our wings will melt. This is true for all of us in any profession, but in medicine, the consequences can be disastrous.

These comments are warnings, not broad-sweeping generalizations or condemnations regarding either the individual physician or the practitioners of the craft as a whole. I am not as much a preaching proselyte as I am battle-wizened regarding the dangers inherent with any form of power. The more the power is tied to another's survival and relief and release from pain, the more potentially intoxicating and the more on guard we all must be. Thus, blindly soaring in an attempt to be first to the sun (the right answer) can have very bad consequences.

Eagles may soar, but ferrets are not sucked into jet engines. Consider the ferret, who locates something by persistent searching, who forces something out of hiding by diligence. Oh, how I wish I could pluck more than a few flight feathers from some self-appointed soaring eagles. The ferret, from whom we get the phrase "ferreting out information," survives. Enough said.

Precept 16: Nothing is foolproof to a talented fool.

We physicians are talented fools, and we have immense power to overthink, overtreat, and overcompensate, owing to a pressing urgency that "*something must be done.*" We must remember that sometimes it is wisest to wait. Although in oncology there are not many second chances and your first shot must often be your best, I have found it wise, when issues are not truly emergent, to remind myself at times, "Do not do something; just stand there." Although any thought-filled craft can witness its practitioners suffering from paralysis by analysis or inactivity, it is not the rule in medicine. That is literally contrary to much of the training and basic personality of the clinical doctor.

Precept 17: A conclusion should not be the place you reach when you grow tired of thinking.

I consider this primarily one of the key mantras of adolescence. How true. Adolescents, as often as not, reach conclusions without thinking. There is a very long adolescence in medicine, and as we have been discussing, there is always lurking that squirming, eager third grader frantically waiting to be called on. The same holds true for the patient and family. Once again, mommies are right. It is often wise to hold your horses and keep your pants on. Rarely is there such urgency. Frequently when there is pain, suffering, and fear fueled by ignorance and dread of an ominous outcome, patient and families leap to conclusions without the guy-wires, net, and welcoming arms of knowledge to break their fall into outright panic. In short, no one wants to be a talented fool. Give me a thoughtful ferret any day. Emergencies are clear enough and warrant emergent and thoughtful intervention; They are just not that common where only moments exist to intervene without an irreversible or avoidable disaster being sure to occur.

Precept 20: Mercy is not that hard; shoot for grace.

This goes both ways. Mercy is deserved favor, pity, empathy, and sympathy. Grace is unmerited mercy. This is *not* to say that it is something that one should not give. Simply *being* is reason enough to be extended grace as a patient. I suggest we stick to the message of Mother Theresa on this, as well as others throughout antiquity. The message is as old as antiquity, as espoused in Hammurabi's ancient Babylonian code of the eighteenth century BC, through the time of Jesus, and beyond Gandhi. It is easy to feel sorry when everyone would. Shoot for grace.

The Bible tells a tale of the hatred with which the Jewish populace regarded the tax collectors in the time of Jesus. These were individuals who were confidants of the ruling Romans and had been given the task of collecting at least the already burdensome taxes mandated by Rome, as well as whatever else they could squeeze from their frightened fellow Jews who knew that the tax collector had not only protection but the ear of the occupying armies of Rome. The collectors were seen not only as despicable traitors who took advantage of the poor while hiding behind the Jews' most hated nonbelieving enemies, but also as graven sinners.

As the story relates, Jesus had gathered a considerable following owing to rumors of miraculous words and deeds, as well as his having begun to be regarded as possessing some level of holiness possibly beyond measure. Zaccheaus, the local tax collector, was a little man; thus, on hearing of the Rabbi's approach and surrounding pandemonium, he scurried up a sycamore fig tree to sneak a better view. While surrounded by teeming throngs, Jesus looked to the tree in the distance and saw what few (perhaps none) could see. He saw an opportunity for grace, and that evening, shocking all, he dined with the hated tax collector. Throughout our lives, we will have a Zaccheaus—a hated tax collector up a tree. If you can muster it, show your Zaccheaus grace. You will grow as a result, and perhaps so will your Zaccheaus.

PSYCHOSOCIAL/HOSPICE/ END-OF-LIFE ISSUES

Psychosocial Issues

The area of psychosocial issues is an art. Before I actually get into hospice, per se, and the most common and difficult scenarios at home for the patient and family of the terminally ill, let us strive to see some of the psychosocial issues not already discussed and some possible approaches. There is no way around it; the care of imminently dying is one of the most difficult roles a human can continuously bear. This section has value for all of us, as our mortality rate is 100%, and as I said, care of the dying or severely ill can be profoundly difficult for all involved. It is largely written in a tone whereby I am speaking to physicians and the health-care team but inviting the patients and families to carefully listen in, as ultimately it is all about them receiving the best of care.

The force and fight of life is part of the warp and woof of being human, and understanding it is essential to being humane. Yet the price is high for the theist and nonbeliever alike. The scope is broad: the technicians, the nurses, the physicians, the family, and the world, the last of which is diminished in one sense, and appended in its warehouse of legacies in another, when one of us passes. This is difficult for the veteran as well as the novice. Both are uncomfortable, sometimes to the extreme of avoiding verbal involvement and even physical connection with those who are likely to die.

Each patient dies individually and yet not truly uniquely. The semantics matter not, as the fears are individual but the phases, not their order or mixture, are not. Through the work of Elisabeth Kübler-Ross and others, we have learned of the phases in the dying patient of denial: fear of isolation, anger, bargaining, depression, and, in some, acceptance. Yet these are a blend, not a current that flows longitudinally. However, the blend does occur, often with fluctuation and blend being expectable features. As the caregiver, your role is to minimize discomfort and to support patient defenses that aid and abet that pursuit. However, you also must strive to counteract harmful defenses, such as inappropriate anger, manipulation, and passive aggression. We must strive to avoid isolation of both caregiver and patient alike. We are social beings and are made to be so. I have been to too many bedsides, the listener of too many tales. It is isolation that is dreaded, and we will talk of it.

We fight this isolation with a multipronged approach. It is wise to be well versed in the clinical scenario and progress to date but unwise to perseverate, hang hopes, and agonize over every test, scan, and lab result received or pending. All must see the forest despite the trees and understand what is important, while also knowing where things stand. Progress reports should be timely, honest, and compassionately delivered. Although discussions of death are best not forced by the caring, they should be brought to bear with all the parties concerned, following the guidance of those most experienced in general and with the patient. Sometimes simply a gesture and hints of the direction are enough. Then actively listen.

Sometimes a more directed approach is warranted. Look out for the demon of guilt when the news is bad. It is astounding, but not surprising, how quickly we can go to this. It can be as if things went wrong because the patient failed. Applaud the good and noble fight, and honor the warrior. Tell him or her the truth of how being scared has its places, such as when the journey begins, at each major turn, and when news turns toward discussion of palliative and terminal care. I always suggest to the medical students to consider holding a hand, touching a heart, and letting patients feel the presence and press of shared humanity, while also letting patients, to some degree, touch inside them. It may be the time to talk of acupuncture or guided imagery, massage and therapeutic touch, hospice and living wills, and family concerns. It is definitely time to embrace spirituality and the soul in the willing patient.

Hope is a challenging notion. It is said to not be method, although I have seen it as a means to travel the journey to acceptance. Realistic hope for attainable goals never lies when it is focused. Hopeful patients absolutely think more of living than dying. The meat of the matter is what is the truth of the hope. Is it the fantasy of one more experimental approach, a miracle of healing, while ignoring the inevitability of death and absence of further antitumor therapies, which is not synonymous with therapeutic intervention in the suffering and dying patient. Is it hope of an afterlife? Is hope a sense of completion, an end to pain? Is it the finishing of things undone, the glorious gain in perspective of embracing the miracle of what life has been? Is it the union and communion with distant friends and family? Is it knowing they did make a difference in this mortal coil and they will be remembered? Is it hope that you will not prolong death or expedite it?

It can be some time before the need of hospice, when multiple phases—in particular, anger—arise. What of the manipulative patient who pursues one more angle, one more play of one staff member against another, once more sense of being able to control. That is it, is it not? Control to rage against a beast that is no respecter of persons Do you, as the physician, then grow angry and then ashamed and angered at your anger, or do you remind sufferers that you know of their suffering, that you are there to help, that their behavior is not helping, and that their right to swing their fist ends at your nose. It can be challenging, especially if the genesis of the anger is not correctly recognized.

Is psychological counseling needed if the only way their anguish can be vented is through hate or unpleasantness? Sadly, there are those rare times when the fear is so overpowering—for that is the engine that runs the anger—that a technical, sterile approach is all that is effective. This can ultimately lead to a failure of the therapeutic relationship and the search for a new physician.

The deadly word "I" is isolation. This will kill and sap the life strength faster than any potion or pill. It must be avoided, and it must be recognized in any of its more uncommon forms.

On the other extreme is the verbose or garrulous patient. This patient's behavior is often caused by fear in one of its many forms. If the patient is insightful, or the family is, explain it to them. However, you must set limits, or the patient will talk until their death, *not about it.*

Seek out depression aggressively. This was mentioned earlier; it can be treated, and causes for reactive depression can often be found. Most importantly, directly approach fear and anxiety as noted earlier. These will eat away at your patient and pull down those around him or her. Address fear and abolish anxiety with both medications and talk therapy. Be sure to actively listen or solicit consultation from professionals whose job is to work with such issues.

Never lie when it seems there is nothing left to say. Physicians must not harm patients by their typical need to not just stand there but do something. Sometimes the opposite is best. Sometimes expectant vigilance and watchful waiting, merely being actively present, is interaction enough while letting the patient and events that cannot be changed take the lead. Set new goals of palliation, treatment of pain, realistic expectations of functions, necessity of tests, venue of care, family roles, family issues, and even the occasional use of placebo in the most needy. All of that is very much therapy and " doing something". A placebo is not medical chicanery; it is a timeworn poultice for many ailments—tapping the power of the patient to believe when there is so little to believe in. Be present and in the moment when important news comes. Understand appropriate touch as we discussed, and keep eye contact; the eyes are often windows to the soul.

Moreover, address the soul, as I have discussed so many times. If you are speechless or see no need for words, indicate so. You are not God. If the patient is frightened, words may not help enough at that exact moment, but the right dosage of sedatives or hypnotics or pain relief may bring everyone back to earth and not to some drug-induced stupor. That should be rare and never a goal.

The key will be teamwork. Clergy, family, friends, and other physicians are there to help. Be watchful as physicians. Look for the feelings of helplessness, hopelessness, and guilt that is not based in fact, remorse on loss of time, or inappropriate optimism. Look for the physicians buffering themselves from the toil.

And now directly to the patients: patients should be encouraged to look at the legacy they have left, which invariably has much good to it. People do leave a mark on the hearts and souls of family and friends, and they must be told that. This is not just in the healthy life, but in the process and course of their disease. The house staff, the younger physicians and nurses and techs, will undoubtedly not forget you but take lessons from you that will invariably help others yet to come. This is how they learn; you teach. You have aided in the care of thousands of those yet to walk their path to the other side. You may have, God willing, moved the heart of the atheist or the agnostic or secular humanist or moral relativist or just someone confused about what really matters in this life.

You may have reached out to your family, finally and not futilely. You may have left an understanding of death—that it is not an ogre to be feared, but a passing. You may have given courage to the meek in their first steps in caring for those with terminal disease. You may have touched more hearts than you know and probably made a difference bigger than you will ever know, and you must be told that.

I have urged all of my dying patients to take make a video and tell their story, alone and to be seen over the ages by the survivors. You had a childhood, adolescence, fell in love, fought despair and disappointment, felt joy, perhaps parented or mentored. You lived. There may be those whom you wish to finally tell off or let the cat out of the bag to. What is the worst they can do? This has proven, over my decades of practice, to be one of the most cherished gifts to give to the survivors. You will be amazed what you will say in private to a machine that you won't be there to see later that you would never do while conversant or in person You are never in this alone; do not go out that way. Give them what they need: your solace, your dreams for them, your love, your happier moments, your unconditional forgiveness. Truly connect with your thoughts and feelings, and they will have a memory to cherish forever. We all have a tale to tell; none are alike, and no one has your perspective as you do.

Children especially can benefit by seeing you speak of the most enormous responsibility in the world—being a parent. Let them hear it from your side, and let them know there was no manual. If there is a need, ask for forgiveness, no matter how great you think the transgression may be. Reach out from a place that scares them so, and tell them where you are and that you will be in their hearts and minds and on tapes they can ceremoniously or simply play ad hoc when they need you. Why should there only be Hollywood movies, largely fictional, starring dead actors that help us reminisce? Your stage was life, and no one acted your part better than you did. Trust me; it is a little miracle maker and a gift that keeps giving.

Hospice Care

> You matter because you are, you matter to the last
> moment of your life, and we will do all we can not only
> to help you die peacefully but to live until you die.
>
> —Cicely Saunders, MD

Hospice is a special team-oriented approach to caring for patients with terminal or incurable diseases and assisting the patient, family, and caregivers. It does not necessarily mean a patient is no longer seeing his or her doctor or receiving palliative chemotherapy. It is a philosophy of care, not a "place to die." The venues of care can vary greatly, from home to skilled nursing facilities to inpatient settings.

The Sisters of Charity in Ireland first began hospice in the middle of the nineteenth century, owing to the horrendous conditions that the terminally ill were finding themselves in. By the 1960s, through the help of philanthropists and national health funds, there were soon over twenty-five places where the terminally ill could be compassionately cared for.

Cicely Saunders was a nurse in England caring for a terminally ill patient who described to her just what he thought a hospice should be like. He bequeathed funds to the hospital on his death. Cecily went to medical school, and after graduation, she opened St Christopher's Hospice in 1967. It was renowned for its homey atmosphere and activities, its sense of life, and the absence of any heroic measures for the dying. Within two years, a home hospice program was initiated. Saunders came to Yale in 1974, and the first American hospice opened shortly thereafter. In 1979, the National Hospice Organization was formed in the United States, and in 1983, the Health Care Finance Administration established the Medicare hospice benefit. In 1987, palliative medicine was recognized as a specialty in Britain, and the International Hospice Institute helped form the Academy of Hospice physicians, now known as the American Academy of Hospice and Palliative Medicine.

The team concept is critical. There is a hospice medical director, registered nurses, social workers, chaplains, health aides, and volunteers. The focus is the family, not just the patient, and the patient is ultimately in charge. Team members meet frequently to assure interdisciplinary input, and they usually meet monthly for mutual support.

The roles are as you would imagine, with the medical director attending to the diagnosis and treatment in a palliative mode regarding patient complaints and symptoms. They usually are not the primary physician and are available twenty-four hours a day, seven days a week. Think of the registered nurse as the empath—the eyes and ears for the physician and the one who usually administers palliative therapies and suggests them. She is also a teacher of the patients and the families on care issues. She will do an assessment and develop a care plan with the physician and the family. Such items as air mattresses, walkers, wheelchairs, types of pharmacological agents needed, and the need for oxygen or hospitalization and such often are in her realm of expertise. She monitors the ship of life as it travels and helps the medical director trim the sails as required by symptoms.

An individual with a master's in social work trained in hospice does a great deal of the psychosocial work. She addresses a great deal of the support and grief counseling, especially complicated issues, as well as mental status assessments and life reviews by the patient. She is there to teach appropriate coping skills and, in part, assure respite is available for family and caregivers. She facilitates discussions of death and dying from many perspectives, including spiritual, funereal, financial, and legal. She also acts as a facilitator if special levels of care are needed.

The chaplain provides spiritual support to the patient and family. This is key, as great anger with God can occur, as well as acquiescence that this is all simply retribution or God's will. These chaplains are ecumenical and nondenominational unless specifically requested otherwise. The chaplain can offer memorial services for the patient, the family, and those that cared for them.

The home health aides are like cherubim. These are certified nurse's aides with specific hospice training who directly physically assist with the activities of daily living of the patient. They also teach this to family members and reassure them regarding their common fears of inadequacy. Both the golden gift of common physical touch and often the closest relationship with the patient are the specialties of the aide.

Hospice volunteers first go through a rigorous screening and then extensive training. There is a lot to learn about dying with dignity and safety. Patient and family needs, proper roles for all involved, and the overall hospice philosophy must be known and addressed. Hospice volunteers are to be physically there as a compassionate manpower pool, taking care of tasks like cooking meals, taking walks with the family, running small errands, or just providing brief respite care. They often come in a close second in intimacy to the nurse's aide. Finally there is a role for visits from other allied health personnel, such as physical therapists, physiatrists, occupational therapists, music therapists, healing therapists, pet therapists, and even art therapists and aroma therapists—whatever helps.

So when is a patient eligible for hospice, and when is it appropriate? This can be one of the most daunting decisions for a treating physician, as it may send all the wrong signals. Many are referred too late—far more than the opposite—and suffer needlessly. However, some patients and families are not ready to discuss hospice until such a point. Under Medicare, Medicaid, and most private insurance plans, a patient is eligible if his physician and the hospice medical director certify that the patient has less than six months to live. Furthermore, there must be concurrence with the philosophy of hospice by the patient and family. This means that the focus is on comfort, palliation of distressing symptoms, and management without the use of heroic or life-prolonging measures. A plan must be made for twenty-four-hour coverage, which can be accomplished in many ways we have already mentioned, in different venues and with different levels of skilled personnel. It is important to note, however, that Medicare will not pay for a skilled nursing facility but will cover visits by the staff we mentioned, as well as medications for pain and symptom relief, and medical supplies. There are provisions that allow, for as brief as necessary, inpatient care covered by Medicare. This includes temporary respite for caregivers who are exhausted or ready to break, and for medical conditions, such as seizures or intractable pain or bleeding, whose amelioration is best sought in an inpatient facility. Furthermore, the primary physician must have the approval of not only the patient but also the hospice medical director if he or she feels that certain palliative procedures are not needed, such as draining excess chest fluid to assist breathing, draining excess abdominal fluid, or administering intravenous hydration or feeding. The latter two procedures have scores of legal texts written about them. Suffice it to say that most medical directors of hospice and the team have probably made it very clear to the family and patient that these are often unwise decisions, as they are seen as a lifeline and can cause a whirlwind of often panic-ridden interventions.

We will discuss the possible role of hydration later, but it is generally accepted that such an intervention is one of the last things to ever consider and is usually best reserved strictly to administer a palliative drug. Feeding intravenously or with various tubes into the GI tract, other than what the patient takes orally, is a slippery slope and is not really ethically defendable.

One final and very humane coverage by Medicare under hospice is that of bereavement assistance, which is available for up to a year after death for family members and can include phone calls, home visits, or an annual memorial service. More extended needs can be sought in the community.

End-of-Life Care

As has already been mentioned, when treatment with intent to cure or induce a prolonged remission is no longer possible, we enter the sanctuary of end-of-life care. This means an acceptance and awareness of the futility of further treatment and a shift in focus to palliation of symptoms and care by family and friends. It may be carried out in the setting of hospice, which I recommend and have described above. Some may choose another path.

The "good death" is achievable and is a holistic approach that addresses the four dimensions of the physical, emotional, spiritual, and emotional. The first step is open and honest communication with the patient and the family that death is eminent and reassurance that the family and the patient will not be abandoned.

I will make some general comments on some of the most common physical symptoms. The good death consists of dying without pain. It is the knowledge that physicians and nurses with a positive attitude will address distressing symptoms promptly. There must be clear acknowledgment that the patient will remain in control as long as possible and that his or her wishes will be respected by a team that is truthful and open to communication.

There is to be a clear understanding that the physician will not make decisions that, albeit well intended, put a burden on the patient or family or create ethical dilemmas. A common mistake is the routine installation of intravenous lines. This is to be avoided. There are oral, rectal, transdermal, and vaginal approaches that should always be considered first. The less invasive the route, the better.

The issue of hydration and nutrition is an emotional slippery slope. Frequently, personal and religious beliefs will conflict with medical knowledge. There is a natural stage of dying when the patient ceases to eat or drink. It is sadly at this point that some physicians, often at the urging of family members, place intravenous devices and begin hydrating or nutrition. This is prolonging death, not extending meaningful life. Furthermore, such interventions often increase the emotional distance between the family and the patient. Hunger is usually gone in forty-eight hours and is rarely a source of discomfort. There is even some literature that suggests a euphoric state like that induced by fasting may occur. In addition, hydration often only makes discomfort worse. Dehydration in the terminal phase decreases pulmonary secretions that decrease shortness of breath, and it also decreases episodes of vomiting and urinary incontinence.

The most frequently asked question by family is "How long will it be?" The best approach is a simple, gentle explanation of the changes in breathing and mental status, skin color, weakening pulse, and such. These simple guides can help the family to come together when it is time.

Some specific common syndromes bear addressing for the practitioner and family and patient. First is bowel obstruction, which occurs in 3–15% of hospice patients. Functional bowel obstruction tends to have overflow vomiting, distention, and diffuse, constant pain. This usually occurs in ovarian, colorectal, pancreas, stomach, endometrium, and bladder, and prostate cancer patients. The pain is colicky and continuous. The higher the obstruction is, the more pain, nausea, constipation, or overflow diarrhea and abdominal distention. There is both mechanical and functional obstruction, such as tumor-related obstruction, in the former, and some medications, such as opiates, can cause functional obstruction.

If a patient can tolerate surgery and has a life expectancy of at least two months, operative approaches can be considered to bypass the obstruction or vent it with a gastrostomy tube leading to the outside. Patients with a poor prognosis, diffuse intra-abdominal cancer, marked fluid accumulation, a bad liver, or many other sites of disease, or those who are elderly or wasted, are not good candidates for operative modalities for palliation. The physician is then left with medical therapy to try to rule out treatable obstruction and treat it. Often drugs known as anticholinergics, such as atropine and scopolamine and its cousins, will decrease gut motility and secretions. Often Decadron in significant doses does wonders. Laxatives should be stopped, as should all drugs given other than orally, if possible. In some cases, the drug octreotide is used to markedly slow the gut down. An initial approach, such as a nasogastric tube and suction, may be somewhat invasive and should not be viewed as a long-term measure.

Thirst and a sensation of a dry mouth are common; it is usually the latter. Sponge swabs can be of great assistance. Do not start to intravenously feed a patient to treat thirst, as noted above. If fluid must be given, one can use the subcutaneous route called hypodermoclysis.

Confusion, delirium, dementia, and restlessness are exceedingly common and will eventually occur. Delirium is when perception, thinking, memory, orientation, recognition, attention, concentration, wakefulness, communication, and mood are seriously impaired. It occurs in up to half of terminal patients in the last forty-eight hours. Dementia is more of a loss of memory and worsening confusion, and it worsens over time. Restlessness is frequent, nonpurposeful motor activities and irritability. It is an inability to focus or relax. Sleep and rest are disturbed with fluctuating levels of consciousness.

Anxiety is frequently present. There is general cognitive failure and a frequent progression to agitation. This is many times much more bothersome to the family than it is to the patient. A good rule is to take measures to avoid self-harm, but this is very hard on the family, as it can be their last memory. This can be understood as the multiple metabolic problems that are working themselves out, possibly causing the encephalopathy. If a patient cannot rest, intervention may be needed to obtain peace for the patient and, very likely, the family in close attendance. This is a frequent cause for hospitalization. There are highly effective drugs, such as Haldol, Compazine, opiates, Ativan, Valium, Nembutal, and risperidone, that will always eventually work to calm and sedate a patient. One should remember to always consider use of the laxative lactulose if there is the possibility of liver failure inducing a state of confusion. There may be also urinary retention with or without kidney failure, or expanding tumor in the brain, requiring more Decadron.

In delirium, there are moments of interspersed clarity and lucidity. There may be delusions or hallucinations, hypoactivity or hyperactivity, and lethargy or withdrawal. There is no need to break a harmless delusion or hallucination. This state will occur in over 80% of the terminally ill. Nonetheless, we must be mindful that it may also be due to a treatable simple infection, untreated tumor in the brain, nicotine or alcohol withdrawal, low oxygen, or the drug regimen, and appropriate steps can be taken. Therapy is usually a soft, calm, quiet, relaxing atmosphere, perhaps with music. Drugs like Haldol or Ativan, or a rotation of pain medications, may be used.

Dyspnea is the sensation of breathlessness, severe shortness of breath, or uncomfortable breathing. This is one of the most disturbing symptoms and occurs in 70% of the terminally ill. It may be caused by the weakness brought on by the terminal cancer, fluid in the lungs and abdomen, a failing heart, fluid around the heart, bad heart valves, anemia, anxiety, fear, or neurovascular causes, such as myasthenia gravis or other disorders. Sadly, many will not respond to supplemental oxygen, and invasive procedures to drain fluid may be needed. The best therapy is bronchodilators, steroids, opiates, and antianxiety medications.

The so-called death rattle is caused by a failure to control terminal secretions and is one of the reasons to avoid hydration. It is often more important to find out who it is bothering, as it is not a sign of suffocating. It is usually a close family member who is most bothered by it. You may try to dry secretions with transdermal scopolamine, or even administer diluted atropine eyedrops into the mouth. It is rarely necessary to be more aggressive.

The last issue is nausea and vomiting, and the former is usually much more disturbing to the patient than the latter. There is a long list of causes of nausea and vomiting: failure of every organ, medications, bowel obstructions, radiation therapy, and opiates. However, the armamentarium against these symptoms is large. The first action is to review the clinical situation of the patient for reversible causes and act accordingly. Once again, Decadron given twice or thrice a day with some of the newer antinausea medications is excellent at bringing relief, as are a number of other available agents.

Finally, it is worthwhile to mention that the American Society of Clinical Oncology has developed a CD-ROM curriculum: *Optimizing Cancer Care: The Importance of Symptom Management.* It is available at 1-800-338-8290, and I strongly encourage all oncologists and health-care team members to consider subscribing. It covers what to do and how to do it with scenarios, algorithms, and tables with invaluable data on palliative medications. It assesses both the physical and the psychological.

ETHICS

Principles

The literature regarding oncology and ethics is just over a decade old. There can be inherent conflicts in the goals of oncologists while treating patients. On one hand, there is the goal to preserve life, which is often not possible. Then there is the relief of pain and suffering, which may not be completely possible. Thus a gentle compromise must be reached. Critical to this is an understanding of the law, ethics, and the wishes of the patient.

First, we must understand the major principles of ethics in medicine. Perhaps the most important is autonomy. This was covered in the beginning of this book as perhaps the single most important notion and take-home lesson for patients and families. Autonomy is the patient's freedom to make personal choices. Physicians may participate in choices, but the final decision is the patient's. Difficulties can arise when the decision of the patient goes against the moral precepts of the physician, such as in the matters of euthanasia, physician-assisted suicide, and suicide. When such a conflict arises, the physician may withdraw as long as a competent substitute is arranged.

The second principle is beneficence. This is where the caretaker is charged to remove harm and promote good—the so-called "goods versus the harms" concept. Physicians must strive to promote the good.

The third principle is justice. This largely refers to the fair allocation of medical resources, which are often limited. Sadly, rationing is an unpleasant fact. There are many faces of rationing, including inconveniencing the patient, hassling the physician, or denying insurance coverage. Probably the most affected are the working poor—about thirty million—as the wealthy are usually covered and Medicare and Medicaid provide some level of care. We will see how well the new health-care law addresses these issues.

Managed Care

There is a burgeoning industry of managed care. It attempts to reduce costs by reducing waste, utilizing case management, emphasizing prevention, and imposing quality measures. Yet with it comes rationing in some form or another, such as budgetary allowances for certain tests or medications, economic profiling of physicians, or actual incentive payments made to physicians to keep costs down. This is obviously dangerous from the patient's point of view; patients should ask if such is the case with their provider. There are even "gag rules" whereby physicians can maintain their participation with a payer as long as they essentially put the interests of the payer first when it comes to tests that are expensive or not easily available but necessary. Any priority other than making the patient the priority is unethical. Patients are ill-served when physicians are treated as economic cost centers, moved about, scrutinized, or simply excluded from a managed-care organization's panel of preferred providers. Again, we will see how the new federal health care law impacts the managed-care industry.

Hospitals feel the restrictions of managed care also. They are often forced to deal with the realities of managing costs, and this often puts them at loggerheads with the best in patient care. There are defined durations of inpatient stays, selected drug use, rules of what is required for an inpatient stay, and the discharge of more permanent staff, such as pathologists, anesthesiologists, and radiologists. There may also be an emphasis on marketing or outsourcing their services to the least-expensive vendor. Important capital improvements that could affect care may be delayed.

Truth-Telling

Fortunately, there has been a metamorphosis in the last few decades whereby physicians have become far less paternalistic and withholding of all the truth from a patient. This is essential to avoid blowups with the family and to obtain informed consent from the patient as to what further therapy entails (both good and bad), alternatives, risks, and things that could happen if no therapy is undertaken. This is pretty much firmly embedded in our legal system. We have previously discussed the method of telling the cancer diagnosis, and once again, it is best not done with just the patient in attendance.

Patients are at the mercy of the cancer, and sometimes the system, and are suffering. As such, it will be difficult for them to say no to whatever is proposed as a clinical plan and therapy. Thus, the World Medical Assembly recommendations for informed consent state the following:

1. There should be an explanation of the proposed treatment in words the patient obviously understands.
2. The risks and benefits of the treatment should be clearly stated.
3. Any alternatives should be included in the discussion.
4. Adequate time should be given for questions to be asked.
5. The patient should be aware of the option to withdraw temporarily or permanently at any time while knowing he or she will continue to receive support from the health-care professionals.

There is an implied contract whereby the patient places his or her life in the physician's hands; this must never be forgotten. The goal of a researcher is to find new knowledge, whereas the goal of the physician is the beneficence of the patient. These may or may not be the same.

Living Wills

Sadly, one of the more frequent complaints by patients toward oncologists and surgeons is that, despite carefully worded living wills and powers of attorney, they end up with IVs, other lines, or even intubation against their wishes. This, I believe, does not happen to keep hospital beds and wallets full, but rather it is testament to the powerful drive of the physician and health-care team to save lives. Death can be a symbolic failure for the physician. As I stated earlier, most have difficulty dealing with death and find it hard to let go.

Not all of those closely involved always know when the war is over or when there are no meaningful battles to be won and further efforts are prolonging death rather than life. This is the time when all the talking beforehand, the living will, and the work with the family can pay enormous emotional dividends to all and care can be focused strictly on alleviation of suffering. Documentation is key at times like these, as is full communication and attention to spiritual needs.

Discontinuing Care

Discontinuing care is difficult. First, it is hard to stop a functioning IV line; it is easier to maintain one if you need it to deliver medication for the alleviation of pain and suffering. It can be difficult not to restart one but not to remove one that is inflamed. Nutrition is the next most difficult issue. It is hard to embark on intravenous or enteral (intestinal feeding or NG tube) feeding in the terminally-ill patient. There are some guidelines, but the law is not very clear. This is a major emotional issue for families and providers alike. Some guidelines are as follows:

1. If the patient is emotionally and legally competent, it is best to follow the patient's wishes and constantly check in with him or her on this.
2. If the patient is incompetent, follow the guidance of the living will or the next of kin if he or she knows the patient's wishes.
3. If the patient is comatose and there is no living will, physicians should be guided by the rule of goods versus harms and look to the next of kin of the family.

We have mentioned advanced directives a number of times. Soliciting patients' desires when they come into the hospital became federal law in 1991. The types of advanced directives that state patients' desires if they become gravely ill are the living will, appointment of a health-care agent, and durable power of attorney. The living will is a document in which a patient specifies what he or she will allow. It can be revoked or revised at any time. The health-care agent is an individual empowered to state a patient's wishes if the patient is unable to do so. A durable power of attorney allows a designated individual to make health-care decisions for the incapacitated or incompetent patient. It is very unwise to ignore these measures as a health-care provider and unwise as a patient to not address them.

Physician-assisted suicide is a tough issue, and I have no answers, just some facts to relay. At least half of physicians in most surveys have said they have been asked at least once by a patient to assist the patient in dying. In one survey, one-third of physicians said they had complied. I personally do not believe this is representative data.

This is *not* death by secondary intent or double effect, by which, for example, the amount of a narcotic needed to relieve pain also puts the patient into a respiratory coma. In such a situation, there is a primary act of beneficence by the physician to treat pain, and not a veiled attempt to kill the patient. There are many pitfalls. For example, this nation predominantly adheres to the Judeo-Christian ethic that condemns such acts, as it contends that only God can give and take life. Although the five suicides in the Bible—Samson, Saul and his armor bearer, Judas, and Achitophel—are never criticized in the Bible, one of the origins of the doctrine against it is clearly biblical. Suicide has clearly now found its way into common law as illegal. My answer is prayer and expert techniques at relieving pain and suffering, which usually are very effective. Two states, Oregon and Washington, allow physician-assisted suicide.

Sadly, there are other less savory arguments against physician-assisted suicide, such as that it can be done for family convenience to save money or to get rid of an annoying patient whose suffering is tearing a family apart. I have seen this in action and, it is the darker side of what hospice proponents call the slippery slope of euthanasia.

Sedation and Symptom Control

Our goal as oncologists is often primarily to relieve symptoms, improve quality of life, and, as some say, ease patients toward a good death. When medications are used, there is always the very serious potential tradeoff that, especially in the mentally frail or those with impaired liver, kidney, or respiratory function, a patient might poorly metabolize drugs or succumb to their effect on suppressing respiration. Drugs do not have front, side, back, top, or bottom effects; they have *effects*. One of those effects may be grogginess, which may be particularly distressing to the patient and the family alike. A classic example is using morphine for pain control, as in my short story "The Flood." Although rare, the sedation can be so severe with necessary narcotics that impaired ventilation leads to pneumonia or respiratory depression and an expedited death. The medication successfully relieves the patient's duress while expediting his or her demise. This dilemma has long been studied by theologians and ethicists, and once again the principle of beneficence comes to bear where relieving the agonizing suffering is the ethically correct thing to do, even though it may hasten death. This is known as the so-called double effect of medication.

Extremely agitated and confused patients are another area that can frequently evoke the principle of double effect. Although some patients may have lucid intervals, it does frequently happen that they are continuously confused and require regular medication. In most of these cases, the agitation is sadly largely relieved only at the price of sedation. Once again, clear family education and input that such prolonged sedation may expedite death is paramount. They must know that a delicate balance between alertness and symptom control of such patients without sedation is not always achieved.

The art and science of the principal relief of pain and suffering is known as palliative care. This is a relatively new field that has undergone a slow start since the first Hospice was founded in England at St Christopher's. It demands a holistic team approach and an understanding of ethics and its principles. It interweaves the social and spiritual needs of the family and the patient. There is more that can be done than most doctors think, and families and physicians are urged to aggressively seek out and, in fact, form such palliative-care teams. It must become so integral to the fabric of health care that all aspects of the care delivered are affected, not just people with advanced cancer.

Legal Aspects of Oncology

Insurance awards and defensive medicine account for *at least* 10% of per-capita health-care dollars. Physicians "win" 80% of those cases that go to trial, and more so if they are jury trials. Statistics from the Physician Insurers Association of America indicate that cancer of the colon, breast, and lung are consistently in the top twenty by award. The top five missed diagnoses are cancer of the breast, cancer of the lung, appendicitis, heart attack, and ectopic pregnancy. Remember, this is business to attorneys and liability carriers. Probably the most common mistake physicians make when deposed is to be emotional. They would be wise not to rent free space in their mind to the plaintiff by being defensive or angry. The opposite is equally true for the patient. The patient may or may not have realistic expectations; the treating physician has a lot to do with that. Physicians must simply and clearly tell the truth and be sure the patient hears it; they must *never* assume that patients understand without asking.

Patients frequently have very understandable misperceptions regarding the polar opposites of medical breakthroughs and a diagnosis being a death sentence. A pivotal element of a malpractice claim is whether there was a breached duty or injury due to breach in the standards of care, which can be regional or national standards and can be quite tricky. National guidelines for defense-only experts may not be what all oncologists agree to. The concept of timely diagnosis and lost chance of survival, no matter how small, is crucial in oncology litigation. It can become a veritable statistical battleground. Another battleground besides physical damage is mental anguish—for example, in the case of a diagnosis of cancer without basis.

Prevention is key for all concerned, as time spent on legal ramifications is sharply reduced if we understand the law. Physicians must become very clear as to whether they have established a doctor/patient relationship, and they must appropriately document it. This comes into play when a physician thinks he or she is just doing a passing-moment "curbside consult." Casual encounters with patients are *not* equal between physicians and patients. Furthermore, physicians must remember when overseeing care in a training center that they are still the legally responsible attending physician; it is *not* the resident in training, who may misstep in thought, word, or deed.

Another area of intense potential litigation that was touched on earlier is the decision to terminate care. Oncologists are under contract to render care. A good rule of thumb for all is to stabilize the situation first, be mutually clear, arrange referral, and provide records. This is critical in oncology, as follow-up care may last throughout the patient's remaining life.

Do not make the mistake as physician or patient in thinking that an informed consent document alone is sufficient. This is merely a paper that is meant to document something far more profound. There are many mitigating factors, such as how much information patients with incurable disease really want to know or can grasp (often a surprisingly great deal). Was there a dismal prognosis disclosure, statistical data on suffering and mortality, or disclosure of personal research interests of the provider? What has the referring provider said to the patient? What role does the family play in decision-making? A rapidly evolving issue is whether this cancer is inheritable and whether relatives are in the "zone of risk." Key elements of an informed consent document are disclosure of risks vs. benefits, alternatives, and the worst and most common effects of treatment. All wording and information must be tailored to the patient's competency. Can the patient understand the relevant information and appreciate the consequences of their decision? Can they answer routine questions, such as "What are the name and nature and stage of the cancer, the therapy, the benefits and risks?" Was the principal of voluntariness—no coercion or pressure—in play? Desperate patients will be very heroic. They need time and truth-telling, especially regarding prognosis.

In 1961, 90% of physicians as a routine practice did not disclose all the relevant information about a patient's cancer. It was more commonly parsed out in paternalistic packages. Today, thankfully, honesty is the general rule, as is patient autonomy. Physicians must never make secret pacts with the patient or family. Clinicians must be on guard not to make the mistake of inundation by exhaustively telling all at one sitting, unless patient and family comprehension cognitively and emotionally is clear.

Statistics are extremely helpful, but they must be balanced against the reality of individual responses. Statistics are derived from patients whose outcomes are already determined. They should be used to set the tone, the gravity, and the probability of limits on response and palliation. What patients hear and what the oncologist thinks they said or wrote down are not always synonymous. Physicians must be very specific about treatment details; this is a common pitfall. There must be emphasis on risks versus harms. Here is another great truth: doing nothing is an oxymoron; it has consequences. All "collateral damage" should be clearly articulated slowly and repeatedly.

Scholarly research into the value of hope was arguably begun at least a century ago. I fall on the side of argument that says there is an obligation to encourage hope. We must acknowledge the poorly understood synergy between mind and body. Increasing numbers of studies are pointing to this. Doctors should embrace that. Patients reliably will tell you that a provider's perceived attitude in this arena has immense impact on the probability of legal action being sought. Trust is presumed. As has been said previously in this book, the whole family should be encouraged, if the patient agrees, to be involved. They should be encouraged to take notes, but in a nonthreatening way, and the oncologist should help them review their notes to be sure all are on the same page. I am of the opinion that oncologists and their healthcare teams do best when they are masterful teachers. Overall, initial time-intensive meetings with the patient and family will save time and heartache. Most importantly, it is "the right thing to do," and it is viewed favorably legally.

Documentation is key. If it is worth saying, physicians should write it down and copy it into records. They would also be wise to considering holding on to phone logs, calendars, appointment logs, and literature given to the patient. They would be wise to keep a pad at home and in the car, as important communications can occur at those times with either the patient, the family, or members of the health-care team. Care should be taken to carefully train nurses and front-office staff on what they say, where they say it, to whom they say it, and how to document it all. Thorough, secure office files should be maintained long-term, including research protocols with informed consent.

The doctor is largely legally responsible for his or her employee's actions, within reason. This is often referred to as the concept of "parent agency," "borrowed servant," and "captain of the ship." This is actually simple in concept. The oncologist is not responsible for the acts of a competent consultant their patient is referred to as long as there is not overlapping competency. However, in oncology, the oncologist often assumes a further role, and thus acts as the "captain of the ship." It is common for excellent oncologists to know a great deal about another field of medicine, as cancer has no one-organ limitation and involves multiple diagnoses, stages, and treatments. This is not deification or arrogance. It is reality, and thus courts increasingly expect broader and deeper levels of awareness from oncologists than many other subspecialists.

Patients' employment rights under the American Disabilities Act (ADA) versus reality very frequently come up as issues. Patients and oncologists should be clear on the drafting of very explicit letters. Cancer survivors can be considered disabled under the ADA on a case-by-case basis. Patients may be covered whether cured, controlled, or in remission.

Patients typically come under the care of an oncologist for the long term and frequently for a lifetime or at least many years. Termination of this relationship is more often due to death than in other fields of medicine. No other field of medicine comes close to this level of frequency of intensity. This unique relationship frequently must address the issue of withdrawing or withholding active treatment, as previously noted. Providers routinely struggle with inappropriate distinctions between withholding and withdrawing care. The first step is for the patient and the family to be mutually clear as to what the patient's informed, realistic expectation is. Issues of futility are best addressed in advance, and that is actually frequently possible with attention to detail and planning.

The patient has the right to refuse therapy. Nutrition and hydration are essentially ethically and legally the same, as is starting and stopping them. Emotionally, this may not be seen as the case by some physicians, of course, and more so their patients and their patients' family members. Conversations in advance regarding the anxiety caused by new interventions and the possibilities of misadventures because of diagnostic exuberance can be enormously helpful. Common sense coupled with expert knowledge of the nature of the cancer and the status of the individual patient actually does provide many opportunities to prospectively do a cost/benefit analysis with the patient and family as to the prudence of a new test or some other intervention. All must be wary against doing too much out of desperation and not discernment.

Palliation and beneficence are as the patient sees them. Withdrawing support is not physician-assisted suicide or euthanasia. Oncologists, as well as patients and families, have an ethical duty not to prolong death. The best deterrent is healing and heaping helpings of knowledge and conversation long in advance of the reality of end-of-life care becoming an issue. A guiding ethical principle is whether the patient is experiencing pain (not just physical) and is the physicians' response proportional to the pain. The action of the provider is *not* to relieve symptoms by primarily expediting the patient's demise. The family and providers should count the patient's pills if they suspect something amiss is brewing.

Genetic testing for susceptibility for cancer genes is probably not the same as other diagnostic tests. There are potentially enormous psychological and economic risks in lieu of the hoped for "reprieve." Most cancers are not inheritable, but for those that are, informing the family of heritable risk is now a duty. This requires an expert team usually at the university level, and early referral is very wise. Once again, although there are notable examples, such testing is not only not the norm for most cancers, but it is also psychologically harmful and emotionally and financially irresponsible until there is data to support it on a case-by-case basis.

Do so-called dual loyalties of economic or clinical profiling and incentives for economic care exist? This is the practice where the economic costs of how oncologists provide care are used to profile them based on expense. This is then used to tailor reimbursement, which of course may ultimately affect care. This may also potentially lead to payers attempting to shift care of a patient to a less expensive setting. Patients must be aware of how their oncologist is being reimbursed. A Pandora's box of inappropriate defensive medicine is waiting to snare both the oncologist and his or her patient. My advice is simple, and I am sure it is already followed by most, if not all, oncologists; do not do it when, in using your best clinical judgment, the risk of testing (both physical and psychosocial) will cause more harm than the risk of missing an unlikely event.

It may not be easy to spot the confrontational patient or family likely to sue. As always, communication and documentation while assuring comprehension is key. One type of patient that can be challenging is the one who is interpersonally inappropriate, narcissistic, and complimentary: the "We know you are the best doctor" type of patients who feel a special sense of entitlement. Conversely, occasionally patients will "kick the cat," meaning that they will take out their fear or anger against not only innocent others but also those who are trying to help them. This can be seen most often when there is displaced anger and fear regarding diagnosis. Although patients can handle a nonpersonable *procedural* physician, an oncologist should be prepared to assist in psychosocial, spiritual, familial, and daily living activities and issues and should be prepared for patients and families to expect that.

Three final special situations come to mind. The first situation occurs when an oncologist is the family member of a loved one with cancer. This can cause problems. The best solution is to not in any way assume the role or duties of a physician, but to get a competent colleague to do so.

The second situation is the VIP patient. A sure way to have missteps in such a situation is to treat the patient with kid gloves or in a special or different way than any other patient deserving the best in care.

Finally, there will be patients the clinician personally dislikes. If the doctor cannot be objective, he or she must disengage, but only after first ensuring adequate referral. Doctors are only human, and this will happen. The same is true for patients. They have a responsibility to both themselves, their families, and the treating physician to either be clear on their displeasure with the treating oncologist for whatever reasons or, if they choose to be silent, to request a referral to another oncologist. It is a largely a myth that the expression of displeasure will adversely affect care.

The special problem of pain is multifactorial, embracing cultural differences, preconceived ideas, and knowledge deficits regarding how effectively pain can be treated by following the World Health Organization step approach. Uncommonly, some non-oncologists have a hesitancy to prescribe powerful narcotics and either will not prescribe them at all or, more likely, will refer patients to those who more commonly treat severe, narcotic-requiring pain. Oncologists typically are expert at pain management, as over 90% of all of patients can be made comfortable with expert care. Pain is rightly now considered the fifth vital sign and must be addressed, as its chronic presence can have severe impact on patients. One of the most popular self-help books in the late '90s was *How to Commit Suicide*. We must not underestimate the power of pain. Physicians must believe their patients. Addiction, drug selling, etc. is rare. Fortunately, the trend to delay the use of strong opiates is improving dramatically.

Complementary and Alternative medicine is tried by somewhere between 20–50% of all cancer patients. We really do not know as much as we should about this unregulated, $20-billion industry that can profoundly interact with a patients' health, treatment, and confidence. There are many resources available to learn about these issues, and I find it wise for oncologists and patients to do so. There are numerous reputable texts and web sites. Perhaps a leader is the site provided by the publishers of the Physician's Desk Reference. The National Cancer Institute web site is also excellent.

Although eventually a very small number of these unapproved potions are added to our armamentarium, it takes an average of six years and $600–700 million to complete carefully done research and then submit the treatment for FDA approval.

Clinicians are responsible for giving their patient a sense of control and hope. In my career, although not frequently, I have heard of patients feeling "unattached to an impersonal physician." Doctors are legally courting a disaster and spiritually damaging both themselves and their patients in such relationships. Patients want guidance and are frequently afraid to ask for in-depth knowledge, as they are paralyzed by their understandable fear, which is fuelled by ignorance and not an inability to learn.

In conclusion, the modern practice of oncology is a fertile field for the application and understanding of medical ethics and medical law.

Frequently, the stakes are very high as well. It is wise to remember that oncologists and patients are making a contract in which they promise to address the following: active listening, pain, weakness, daily activities, teaching, sleep, truth-telling, being available, bowels, family rules, how to handle answering machines, anxiety, nausea, vomiting, progress reports, and so much more that has been covered. Patients have the duty to tell the truth at all times, be clear, express their feelings, and comply with mutually agreed-to, reasonable interventions that were explained to them. Patients expect clinical excellence. They need time, patience, permission, listening, appropriate touch, security, honesty, humor, and respectful compassion. If all get the basics right, excellent care will follow and the courts will stay clear.

THE INTERNET

In prior sections, I have given you a number of web sites you can refer to using the World Wide Web. I urge you to try to do this in harmony with your physician and be critical about what you read. Nonetheless, everything you could want is out there, and the list presented here is fairly comprehensive regarding reputable sources for any information I have ever imagined a need for, but it is by no means complete. You will notice I have repeated some of the clinical trials sites for emphasis.

- CALGB Cancer and Leukemia Group B
  www.calgb.uchicago.edu
- ECOG Eastern Cooperative Oncology Group
  ecog.dfci.Harvard.edu
- NCCTG North Central Cancer Treatment Group
  ncctg.mayo.edu
- NSABP National Surgical Adjuvant Breast and Bowel Project
  www.nsabp.pitt.edu
- POG Pediatric Oncology Group
  www.pog.ufl.edu
- RTOG Radiation Therapy Oncology Group
  www.rtog.org
- Southwest Oncology Group
  www.swog.saci.org
- European Organisation for Research and Treatment of Cancer
  www.eortc.be

- National Cancer Institute of Canada Clinical Trial Group
  www.ctg.queensu.ca
- National Cancer Institute
  http://rex.nci.gov
- American Society of Clinical Oncology
  www.plwc.org
- American Society of Clinical Oncology
  www.asco.org
- American Cancer Society
  www.cancer.org
- CancerGuide: Steve Dunn's Cancer Information Page
  www.cancerguide.org/
- Cancer News on the Net
  www.cancernews.com/
- Cancernet
  http://cancernet.nci.nih.gov/
- CanSearch
  www.cansearch.org/
- Huntsman Cancer Info Service
  www.hci.utah.edu/
- Medicine Online
  www.meds.com/
- New York Online Access to Health
  www.noahhealth.org/
- Oncolink
  http://oncolink.upenn.edu/
- University of Texas MD Anderson Cancer Center
  http://utmdacc.uth.tmc.edu/

The National Cancer Institute has many materials to help you understand your medications and diagnosis. The US government sponsors this. The NCI coordinates the government's cancer research program and provides information in both English and Spanish for patients, the public, and the media. Information is available about advances in cancer treatment and research, ongoing clinical trials, specific types of trials (many on campus), specific types of cancer, and managing adverse effects of treatments. Cancernet, PDQ, and the Cancer Information Service are all provided by the NCI. They publish many monographs and booklets, among which are *Chemotherapy and You* and *Helping Yourself During Chemotherapy.*

The American Society of Clinical Oncology has a number of new resources available for practitioners to share with patients. As the leading professional society for professionals who treat people with cancer, ASCO is committed to providing patients and their families with information that is accurate, timely, and oncologist approved. Some of their materials are *The Cancer Handbook,* second edition; the *Cancer Advances* annual meeting newsletter; *ASCO Patient Guide: Understanding Tumor Markers For Breast and Colon Cancers*; *ASCO Technology assessment: Aromatase Inhibitors for Early Breast Cancer*; and "People Living with Cancer," which is the new patient-education website from ASCO. This offers easy-to-understand cancer information that is accurate, up-to-date, and oncologist approved. There are sections devoted to cancer types, clinical trials, symptom management, cancer news, family and friends, coping, discussions, and much more.

The American Cancer Society has many local programs to support their patients with cancer and their patients' families. They will connect you with the office nearest you. The American Cancer Society is a voluntary organization with national and local offices that may be able to provide patient services, including transportation, lodging, cancer information, support groups, and oncology camps. They have information and catalogs for cancer-related products, such as hats, turbans, hairpieces, wigs, prostheses, and breast forms. They lobby for cancer-prevention legislation and conduct education and awareness programs, such as Man to Man (prostate cancer), Reach to Recovery (breast cancer), and "Look Good Feel Better."

Steve Dunn's website is maintained by a cancer survivor and provides information specifically for patients. It tells patients how to find information, the pros and cons of researching their cancer, when and why to get a second opinion, and how to maintain a positive outlook. Alternative and unconventional therapies are discussed in a practical, balanced manner, and patients are cautioned to make careful decisions.

A nuclear medicine physician who works with cancer patients edits Cancer News on the Net. It can provide articles on many forms of cancer.

CancerNet is an international online service provided by the National Cancer Institute. This information is for patients, families, the public, health-care providers, and researchers. It covers cancer detection, prevention, treatment, and research. Users may research CancerLit, a bibliographic gold mine of a database that indexes cancer-related articles from the medical literature. It does not provide articles but helps users decide which will be the most useful. PDQ, the NCI's comprehensive cancer database, can be accessed from CancerNet.

Cansearch is a site sponsored by the National Coalition for Cancer Survivorship for both survivors and patients. It provides information about meetings and events, survivorship programs, and a systematic guide to cancer resources on the Internet.

Huntsman Cancer Institute at the University of Utah provides patients and providers with information about cancer detection, prevention, and treatment. Referral to local programs is also provided.

Medicine Online is sponsored by Ultitech and funded by Glaxo-Wellcome and Pharmacia. It provides information, education, the *Daily Oncology News Digest*, discussion groups, and meeting reports.

New York Online Access to Health is provided by the City University of New York and has information for both patients and providers on cancer and other diseases.

OncoLink is sponsored by the University of Pennsylvania and contains information for patients and providers about specific diseases, medical specialties related to cancer treatment, chemotherapy, psychosocial support, clinical trials, financial issues, international cancer meetings, and other topics.

The University of Texas MD Anderson Cancer Center, which is an enormous institution, provides information about cancer prevention and detection, clinical trials, and basic information about cancer and its treatment.

Another completely different and more personal approach is offered by radio and is called *The Group Room: A Worldwide Virtual Support Group*. It airs every Sunday from 4–6 p.m. eastern time and can be reached at 1-800-GRP-ROOM (1-800-477-7666). For a list of radio stations that carry *The Group Room*, or to listen to the Internet broadcast, please visit www.vitaloptions.org.

Information is available from many sources about specific types of cancer. Patients may wish to join cancer-specific support groups or find vendors, such as vendors for prostheses for bone cancer or breast cancer, or ostomy bags. The following is a good sampling of cancer-specific resources available by telephone or the web. Remember, these may not be as reliable or accurate as those sponsored by the NCI or major institutions.

- American Brain Tumor Association
  1-800-886-2282 http://www.abta.org
- Brain Tumor Society
  1-800-770-8287 http://www.tbts.org
- Cure for Lymphoma Foundation
  1-800-235-6848 http://www.cfl.org
- International Myeloma Foundation
  1-800-452-2873 http://www.myeloma.org
- Leukemia and Lymphoma Society
  1-800-955-4572 http://www.leukemia.org
- National All Br Ca Org
  1-888-806-2226 http://www.nabco.org
- National Hospice Organization
  1-703-243-5900 http://www.nhpco.org/body.cfm
- National Ovarian Cancer Coalition
  1-888-682-7246 http://www.ovarian.org
- Support for People with Oral and Head and Neck Cancer
  1-800-377-0928 http://www.spohnc.org/
- Y-ME National Breast Cancer Organization
  1-800-221-2141 http://www.y-me.org

Sources of National Cancer Institute Information

Cancer Information Service:
Toll-free: 1-800-4-CANCER (1-800-422-6237)
TTY (for deaf and hard of hearing callers): 1-800-332-8615

NCI Online:
Use http://cancer.gov to reach NCI's website.

LiveHelp:
LiveHelp link on the NCI's website.

PROGNOSIS

It is natural for anyone facing cancer to be concerned about what the future holds. Understanding the nature of cancer and what to expect can help patients and their loved ones plan treatment, anticipate lifestyle changes, and make quality-of-life and financial decisions. Cancer patients frequently ask their doctor or search on their own for statistics to answer the question "What is my prognosis?"

Prognosis is a prediction of the future course and outcome of a disease and an indication of the likelihood of recovery from that disease. However, *it is only a prediction.* When doctors discuss a patient's prognosis, they are attempting to project what is likely to occur for that individual patient. The doctor may speak of a favorable prognosis if the cancer is expected to respond well to treatment, or an unfavorable prognosis if the cancer is likely to be difficult to control.

A cancer patient's prognosis can be affected by many factors, particularly the *type* of cancer the patient has, the *stage* of the cancer (the extent to which the cancer has metastasized, or spread), or its *grade* (how aggressive the cancer is or how closely the cancer resembles normal tissue). Other factors that may also affect a person's prognosis include the patient's *age* and *general health,* or the *effectiveness* of treatment.

Statistics are also used by the doctor to help estimate prognosis. Survival statistics indicate how many people with a certain type and stage of cancer survive the disease. The five-year survival rates are the most common measure used. They measure the effect of the cancer over a five-year period of time. Survival rates include persons who survive five years after diagnosis, whether in remission, disease-free, or under treatment.

Shorter and longer durations may be used depending on the cancer and original stage. It is important to understand that statistics alone cannot be used to predict what will happen to a particular patient, because no two patients are exactly alike.

Patients and their loved ones face many uncertainties when dealing with cancer. For some, coping is easier if they know the statistics; for others, statistical information is confusing, fearful, and too impersonal to be of use. The doctor who is most familiar with the patient's situation is in the best position to discuss a patient's prognosis and to help interpret what the statistics may mean for that patient.

If patients or their loved ones feel they want to know prognostic information, they should talk with the doctor. At the same time, it is important for patients to understand that even the doctor cannot tell them exactly what to expect; in fact, a patient's prognosis may change over time if the cancer progresses, or if treatment is successful.

Seeking prognosis information and understanding statistics can help some patients reduce their fears as they learn more about what their prognosis means for them. It is a personal decision and the patient's choice about how much information to accept and how to deal with it.

WHAT IS A TUMOR REGISTRY?

A cancer registry (sometimes known as a tumor registry) collects and stores data on cancers diagnosed either in a specific hospital or medical facility (hospital-based registry) or in a defined geographic area (population-based registry). A population-based registry is generally composed of a number of hospital-based registries. Registries participating in the SEER Program are population-based.

Cancer incidence data presented since 1973 in the Central SEER Registry (CSR) come from nine SEER geographic areas that maintain population-based cancer registries in four metropolitan areas and five states across the United States. The registries cover Atlanta, Georgia (five counties); Detroit, Michigan (three counties); San Francisco/Oakland, California (five counties); Seattle/Puget Sound, Washington (13 counties); and all counties in Connecticut, Hawaii, Iowa, New Mexico, and Utah. Data are also presented for the two new registries added to the SEER Program in 1992.

Cancer mortality data on all deaths occurring in the United States are obtained from the National Center for Health Statistics (NCHS), which is a part of the Centers for Disease Control (CDC). The projections of the number of new cancer cases and cancer deaths in the United States are obtained from the American Cancer Society, and population data are obtained from the US Census Bureau.

These registries can now help us understand the behaviors of cancers and how populations will do as a mean (the middle) or the arithmetic average with relative statistical certainty. However, you are an individual, and you will fight, with your team, individually. Yes, at times you will fight against odds, but those odds are not edicts. The mean, or average, will give one a sense of how populations he or she resembles will do only if one is matched in all the relevant variables. Lance Armstrong had what should have been a curable malignancy, a somewhat uncommon and potentially lethal recurrence, and then he survived to accomplish incredible feats. So may you. Thus, although in a sense you are a number, the number is yours and unique.

Another excellent text to evaluate survival odds in every conceivable way and understand the tools used to do so is *Cancer Medicine,* fifth edition, edited by Holland and Frei. Chapter 4, "Cancer Epidemiology" focuses on this aspect. As you can now see, it would take quite a large amount of computing to consider all of your individual variables, but your general odds can be found and are known. Again, these are odds, not edicts.

SOME FINAL THOUGHTS

Just a few decades ago, cancer was the incubus, the pariah, and a death sentence. Through the scholarly cooperation of thousands of scientists of all manners, this is no longer the case, and enormous strides are being made. It is overwhelming how we have affected previously lethal leukemias, testicular cancer, lymphoma, breast cancer, lung cancer, and colorectal cancer, to name a few. The improvements in morbidity and palliative and supportive care are no less awesome thanks in large part to the pharmaceutical industry and the dedicated members of the entire oncology team.

It is my hope that this book has passed on a great deal of the information that you need as a cancer patient With it, you are much more prepared for the fight. You have the right and duty to expect full communication with your health-care team. I hope this work will increase the odds of excellent two-way communication. Get smart fast. Read the book. Look into clinical trials. Take charge of your life and engage fully. Seek out support from family and ancillary staff alike. Participate in your healing, which is far more than just of the body. You are so much more than mere pounds of flesh. Share fears and tears with your team.

Be wise about complementary and alternative medicine, and intelligently use the Internet and seek out the great sources that are there just for you, whether they are tumor-specific or survival-oriented such as the Livestrong Foundation. These are of immeasurable value, as are you to them.

Lobby for an always increasing NCI budget. Know and appreciate that the big pharmaceutical companies are made up of truly dedicated people, are the largest supporters of cancer charities. and are on your side. So is the FDA, which gets faster and better every year.

Be sure you receive in-depth knowledge of the follow-up in your care after treatment that is required. You know every test exacts a toll of anxiety, so be judicious; ask questions. Know your stage and how it was derived. Engage with all your vigor and understanding of the treatment possibilities, as well as what published data says are the probable prognoses. Understand the rules of the road for inpatient care and the ethical and legal issues as they relate to your care. Get the finest in supportive care and other pharmaceuticals for palliative care and avoidance of morbidity.

Strongly consider participation in cancer support groups, not only for what you can receive but also for what you will contribute.

Finally, understand that from the moment when tumor is the rumor all the way through the journey that commences once cancer is the answer, there is information out there that will suppress your anxiety, improve your care, and cherish and protect your autonomy.

THE HEROES

The Telling

Her voice was quavering and had the draped grayness of a funeral. "I thought these were supposed the good times." Her breath fogged the hospital room window as she stared hopelessly into a future this stranger had just given her reason to fear. Red-eyed, she turned to me, the stranger oncologist she had just met moments earlier, and she weightily sighed. "Why?" she asked.

June had just had explained to her in as many ways I could think of that she had an enemy deep in her marrow—an enemy she could not see, feel, or easily fight. Her tragedy was myelodysplastic syndrome. This was a kind of catch-all phrase for an angry and disrupted bone marrow where normalcy had collapsed into a slow but relentless chaos of dysfunction characterized by falling blood counts and the risks of bleeding, infection, and profound fatigue. Its endpoint for her stage was typically soon and would be either bone marrow failure or transformation into leukemia. For now, her situation was not quite marrow failure or scarring and not yet acute leukemia. Nonetheless, her bone marrow stem cells that made all cells in her blood had turned traitors. In her case, the main insult was anemia with a dragging fatigue that would require repeated transfusions for as long as she lived.

Even worse, her platelets, the little amazing cell fragments that rush to the rescue when a blood vessel wall is broached and form a primitive but effective patch, sending out the call for mortar to cement them together and plug the hole, were possibly impotent and permanently decimated in number. She had barely a tenth of the normal amount.

She gazed at her rock of a husband as one could tell she had done so many times over their forty-six-year union, looking for a solution he did not have. Earl sat motionless as his sorrow puddled in his eyes, refusing to fall. He stared at his timeworn cowboy boots, clearly shell shocked. His hulking square laborer's frame was cowed, and his ruddy complexion had been abandoned to chalky white. Earl's lips trembled as he spoke, as if not believing his own words, "She just came in with a little cold; I figured she was just tired from a cold, you know, the flu or something. Why"—he paused—"Doc, why did this happen to her?"

This is a large part of what I do, every day, every week, and I have been doing it for more than twenty-five years. I box with God. Occasionally he spots me a few rounds and keeps his fist open, just tagging me every now and then with the sting of reality. Not now. This was a brawl, and we were losing. This is what I do. I also see more heroes than are in a John Wayne movie. It is some measure of comfort that June, too, will amaze me with her courage and pluck. As almost all do, she will face her fears, transform her anxiety into fear through knowledge, and together we'll carve out her best battle plan. Now I am the quarterback with a limited playbook, and once again we started near the end of the game.

Too old for an attempt at bone marrow transplant and understandably unwilling to undergo the few chemotherapy regimens that have been tried with minimal success, June elected supportive care. The transfusions are working, but soon we will have to cope with her overloading with iron because of them. Her platelets are hanging in there, and she is not bleeding. For now, June will see another spring.

Hitting Home

"Wait a minute! That is not fair, it's not fair. That isn't how it goes." These and other heartfelt protestations of outrage we make when first diagnosed with cancer are impotent, holding no sway over the marauding malignant cell. Everyone knows—well, at least we cancer-killers confidently assume—that our fascination and fight against cancer immunizes us from being its next victim. Are we not special? Are not we physicians immune to cancer and specially empowered to wage war against malignancies? After all, we are doctors, not patients.

Any insight physicians have into the reality of their mortality is paid intellectual lip service at best, especially when they are in their prime. After all, it is only fitting that our membership in the healing guild seems to fittingly include a protective cloak, a shield from pestilence and disease. Cancer patients are them, not us.

He silently appeared in my doorway. His countenance was one of disbelief, his eyes bloodshot and pleading. It seemed remarkable that he had the ability to stand. I had seen this reaction before. I had felt it two decades earlier when I was diagnosed with melanoma.

The words from another consulting oncologist to him were still burning in his mind: "You have a lymphoma. I can't believe that such a little lesion on your skin is malignant, but all the experts have looked at the slides. That little skin lesion is a T-cell, large-cell, anaplastic lymphoma. We kill it or it kills you."

He was a surgical oncologist, a colleague, and a dear friend, and he knew this diagnosis was an enemy he could not attack with his knife. You did not whack this one out with the deft wielding of a blade. This was a malignancy that was notorious for being widespread but initially hidden, as well as difficult to fight. No, this cancer was the domain of the medical oncologist. There was staging to be done, consultations with experts to be made, and chemotherapy to possibly consider. Sometimes the mixture of only rudimentary knowledge of the cancer and the pending dependency of this rightfully proud and competent surgeon was breeding a deep fear—the fear of being out of control.

I am sure he never felt me gently guiding him to a chair next to me. I knew there was need for proximity, perhaps touch, as this was a frightened, devastated, surgeon just learning of his ominous diagnosis. It was the right thing to do. There would be no across-the-desk "professional distance" setting of a stage this time. This was my friend both personally and in the fight against cancer. He was a respected physician in his prime.

I had never had this particular experience before, and my thoughts automatically went to God, almost as an injured child unconsciously seeks Mom, a bastion of beneficence, grace, and comfort. I was also prayerfully pleading for guidance, knowing that my every nuance and inflection would have great weight and that these first moments could never be retrieved. I placed my hand on his knee and told him that the fight was on and that we could be in it together if he wished.

His jaw was tense, belying the quavering lip above as he quietly said, "I am not afraid to die. I knew I had to go sometime, and if God has decided it is time, then there is nothing I can do. I just thought it would be not so soon—my children; it's my children." He stopped for a moment to compose himself and then continued. "I am putting myself in your hands; I want you to be my doctor."

Something very fundamental and very sacred was occurring. This was as real as it gets. This was time to begin the education on what this diagnosis meant and what we had to do next. We had to find out whether the enemy had spread. We had to move swiftly, tireless and merciless in our counteroffensive, as cancer was no longer the rumor but, for now, the dreaded answer.

So much more was said, and I am sure it mattered. He wandered away to prepare the unthinkable moments he—and later I—would spend with his wife and family. I gently closed my door, fell into my chair, and, wet-eyed, prayed.

Snow Job

It snowed in my clinic today. How strange. The forecast for the oncology clinic was once again for increasing periods of foggy depression with precipitation sure to follow. These "bad weather" days in the oncology clinic can blanket one in disappointment and squelch the slightest iota of joy.

This was not so for Jake, a twentysomething US Air Force sergeant whose initial journey into the world of cancer brought good humors to the clinic. Despite his initial diagnosis of what was initially thought to be early-stage testicular cancer, life was in full bloom in Jake, and when first diagnosed, he excelled at engaging it.

However, today's clinic visit was a big one—*the* big one. His cancer was not early stage, and today we would decide if our last assault in the war against the worst testicular cancer anyone could remember had met with any permanent measure of success. The bad news meant it was time for raping his bone marrow, nuking his cancer with a bone marrow transplant, and running to the rescue with harvested bone marrow stem cells—the Adams and Eves of his blood. A full year had passed since the last of the intensive chemotherapy had coursed in Jake's veins. His chest wall had been partially removed, and his spine had weakened. My "robo-patient" sported space-age alloy mesh for his right chest wall, and two titanium rods strained to support his spine. He had started all this as a strapping six-footer. Although he stood tall in our eyes, we had mercilessly beaten him down to about 5'8", as if shrunken by a giant press of malignancy.

Today was the day, all right. After all the surgery and chemotherapy was done, Jake had said it was quits if the cancer came back again. There was no mistaking his battle-wearied seriousness as he said calmly to me before we reviewed the test results, "Doc, a man has to know what a battle is and what a war is. I am not going to confuse 'em. So we are at a year now, a year since the last chemotherapy. If it is back again, well, I just can't do no more. I won't do no more. I ain't afraid to die anymore; I have seen death." His eyes stayed fixed as if he were peering back and staring into the personal tour of hell he had taken in the past two years.

A little over two years before, Jake's saga that became legend was born. There was nothing typical about it. His traitorous testicular cancer cells had set up shop throughout the back of his abdomen, his pelvis, his brain, and his lungs. Markers of the cancer's activity in his blood were ascending like a ballistic missile. He probably had twenty pounds of the beast in him. The prognosis, even with the chemotherapy, aggressive surgery and radiation treatment, was poor, although not impossible to cure—but with a huge price and a reasonable chance treatment might not be survived.

Weaned in the rough-and-tumble barrios, Jake always had mountains to climb. He saw his initial diagnosis of the cancer as no greater peak than he had faced before. He embraced it with maturity beyond his years. In the beginning, he handled his chemotherapy with bravery and grace as he spent that initial hospital time socializing with other patients; he was a regular poster child for just how well intensive treatment could go. Then the dam broke and all manner of havoc let loose. The chemotherapy had exacted a toll of relentless nausea and vomiting so severe it ripped his esophagus. It had also caused both kidney failure and near-crippling lung disease. His diet, which he called "high-octane intravenous go juice," was administered via tubes and transfusions. The chemotherapy's assault on his bone marrow required many transfusions of red blood cells owing to profound anemia, as well as platelets to prevent him from spontaneously bleeding.

Masses still clung to his chest wall and spine after chemotherapy. Although markers in his blood of cancer activity were negative, it was likely that these masses, benign or not, would become locally invasive and result in a catastrophic outcome. All this left Jake simply too gaunt to even cast a shadow. Any more insults against this walloped warrior and he would be gone.

Yes, Jake loved to climb mountains. His dream was to conquer Half Dome in Yosemite before he "checked out." It became his quest, his daily obsession, and his reason to fight. We would talk of manly things: athletic escapades and the heroic exploits he would have when well. He loved our talks, hanging on each imagined adventure, wringing them for every precious drop of hope. When it first was clear that we might lose the battle, his initially engaging and courageous demeanor smote me. It was the right stuff of heady inspiration. In time, however, this demeanor gave way to one of simply surviving each moment, scratching out some modicum of feeble hope that one day he could really put one foot in front of the other and leave the hospital alive and well. The time came when Jake was pondering whether he should even try. He was tired and had had enough. He thought it was time to seal the contract and acknowledge defeat.

Rarely had I launched so fervently into supporting a patient with wavering will. All the stops were taken out. Every manner of cajoling, admonishing, preaching, challenging, cheerleading, and commiseration was thrown at him. In shameless desperation, I offered a contract for life: I would deliver him from his travail, and he *would* climb one last mountain.

I did the wrong thing. I promised he would live. I just knew a nasty exit was not yet in the cards. Jake did not. Yet somehow, agonizing in every moment, he plodded on.

His recovery from the removal of his chest and spine tumors was bloody trench warfare, gargantuan suffering to gain a shot at cure. Nevertheless, gain he did. I thought we would lose him, but there was the promise—our contract. He fumbled on until now it had been a year since the last of all the therapy—a crucial time at which, if he was cancer-free, it would portend well that he might remain so. We were in the clinic. This was the day.

I had seen him twelve weeks previously, and we hoped then that we would declare him cancer-free at the one-year mark. He was indeed cancer-free at that time, but he was a cane-assisted, barely walking testimonial to the melee and carnage of his journey. There may have been the faintest, almost imperceptible spark of life.

Today was different, very different. There was something impish, something teasingly spry this time. There was a lilt in his banter and swagger in his walk. An engaging hint of a wry smile flirted across his face. Crazy sprouts of curly black hair seemed to almost dance merrily on his once bald head. Something was up, and so was Jake. He was impatient for me to get on with the checkup routine, almost as if I were his dad making speeches rather than passing out the presents on Christmas morning.

That was when he produced his prize. Unbeknownst to me, he had gathered all manner of folk who had shared his saga over the past two years just outside the exam room. I think he even waved down passersby. Beaming and bouncing, he produced his treasure trove. It was a small, dirty, banged-up, seen-better-days cooler. With all the pomp and circumstance of a five-star hotel concierge, he bade me to open it. There, placed on a bed of mountain laurels and glistening, as were both our eyes, was a wet, weeping ball of ice—a snowball. Before I could connect the dots, he produced the prize—a photograph. Plain in God's sight, shirtless, with a deformed chest and rods in his back like bionic harpoons, was Jake, high atop Half Dome in Yosemite, his fists in the heavens, the snowball in his hand.

It snowed in my clinic today. I think I will go out and play.

The Lioness

"Be self-controlled and alert. Your enemy the devil prowls around like a roaring lion looking for someone to devour. Resist him; stand firm in the faith because you know that your brothers throughout the world are undergoing the same kind of sufferings. And the God of all grace who called you to his eternal glory in Christ after you have suffered a little while will himself restore you and make you strong, firm and steadfast" (1 Peter 5: 7–10). The biblical metaphor is enticing, is it not? There are those that believe that the prince of this world is given free rein to attack those he will with no more regard or respect to personhood than a terrorist. So it is with cancer: the great mimicker, the fooler, the tease, and worst yet, the sneaky and relentless assailant. For example, there is more than one poor soul who has heard herself say, "Well, my breast cancer was only stage one; my doctor said the odds of recurrence are so low," only to succumb to recurrence up to decades later. Cancer can and does beat its own odds.

This is the story of the lioness, a terribly courageous pastor's wife who developed advanced widespread breast cancer when all the odds said such a thing was a remote chance. But a pastor's wife—how dare it? How dare the offspring of her original little clump of malignant cells arrive with a vengeance after being dormant for nearly a decade? Diagnosed more than eight years before with stage 1 limited breast cancer, our lioness was a robust evangelizer of God's word, especially to newly diagnosed and advanced-stage cancer patients. She presumed she had been "saved" for such a calling. She and her husband thought themselves fortunate being blessed by the low stage, the tiny tumor, and the positive estrogen receptor status, whispering a promise of a good prognosis. Even more, she was negative for Her-2/neu, a tumor marker that, if present on her cancer cells, would foretell anger and a higher risk of spread and growth. Thus, all pointed to a less aggressive disease. Removal of only a small portion of the breast (lumpectomy), radiation, and perhaps five years of the well-tolerated pill tamoxifen and all would be well. And it was well for eight years.

However, cancer is no respecter of persons. Within four years, against all the odds, there was painful spread of the cancer to multiple bones, lymph nodes throughout her body, and even the lining of her lungs, with sympathetic weeping of her organs, causing fluid accumulation in her chest cavity. Still, her faith was unwavering.

Her husband, Bill, was the senior hospital chaplain. He was complex, intelligent, and devout. However, he was always questioning. Through entwining himself in the spiritual needs of others and wrangling with their complex issues, as well as overly involving himself in every test, he avoided his own issues with seeming nonchalance. Now he was powerless and, worst yet, not in control. I have seen this dilemma so often with the suffering servants and the professional helpers who in part quench their need to control and cope by resorting to such behavior. They give quite sincerely to others when they are themselves in profound need. He had withdrawn to a personal "thought hell" of the potential loss of the lioness. His dwelling on everything and attempting to "captain the ship" was his ever-present burden, prodding him incessantly. Thus, communication was not what it could be with these no-doubt lifetime lovers as fear had them in its grip. She feared he could no longer handle her death, and he feared somehow he would miss something that he could fix and make it all go away.

There was a popular period of employing bone marrow transplants for the treatment of widespread breast cancer; it occurred right when the lioness received the unthinkable news that she had widespread disease. The procedure was accomplished with intensive chemotherapy and rescue with bone marrow thought to be clean of tumor cells. There was (and remains) no known cure for widespread breast cancer. Thus, in those days, the pendulum was swinging favorably for insurance plans to reimburse attempts at transplant. Those were exciting times rich with the hope that transplant might finally be the elusive potential cure for widespread disease.

She related to me how the voices of the enthusiastic transplant team still banged about in her head: "Why, it will be toxic and, well, yes, a few transplant patients will die from the attempt, but most will make it through and recover to feel better with hopefully no tumor left." As with any potential new breakthrough therapy for a common cancer previously thought incurable, the rush was on to enroll as many patients as possible in clinical trials in hopes of getting results as soon as possible and finally announcing a potential cure. Thus, as was considered appropriate for that time, she underwent a bone marrow transplant. In her case it was a tandem transplant. Two transplants were crammed in as soon as those who gave it said the patient had recovered sufficiently and it was okay to proceed.

The lioness and her husband survived the enormous trauma. For four years after that, they danced away from a recurrence without too many peeks over their shoulders. As breast cancer is known to often do, the beast that had never left came back at all the prior sites where the disease had spread to before transplant recurred—no more and no less. Blessedly, it did so amazingly without the curse of pain or need for radiation to imminent fractures due to spread to multiple bones. Despite there being a great deal of tumor in the spinal column, there was miraculously no threatening compromise of the nerve roots or the spinal cord.

Tamoxifen failed to control the tumor. The next hormonal type of therapy, the aromatase inhibitors, resulted in only a transient response by our lioness. Amazingly, although all this tumor was readily visible by various types of scans and X-rays, the lioness felt fine and spent most of her time fighting to convert souls and comfort those with cancer and spiritual unrest. Months turned to years as the lioness nearly glowed in the dark from all the trips to the radiology department. Finally, the press of overall tumor burden—which was slowly progressing, aided and abetted by the growing anxiety of the patient and, in particular, her husband—pushed us toward chemotherapy.

The choices were multiple, with diverse toxicities, though none held promise of a cure or a long progression or relapse-free interval of time. Toxicity in such a previously heavily treated individual could be great, and the bone marrow might not be able to handle the assault on its ability to make blood, infection-fighting white blood cells, and bleed-fighting platelets. Yes, we have made enormous strides in terms of toxicity. Nonetheless, it would be disingenuous to not acknowledge that the oncologist's view of "modest" toxicity can understate what patients experience. Toxicity aside, the intent for a chance to return to a more functional life was irrepressible, and therefore chemotherapy was selected and the drama continued.

Over forty weeks, the lioness pressed on with her visits to her second family in the outpatient infusion center as we dripped Taxotere into her veins. She was treated every Thursday and was responding. Then bad things began to happen. She developed a life-threatening clot in her lungs, a pulmonary embolus, from which she recovered. Then followed a clot in the leg, and a filter was placed in the great vein to her heart to protect the lungs. She recovered again. The often unstoppable toxicity of Taxotere at first came like a wolf in the night. It was just as relentless and ignored what meager steps there are for prevention. Her body became flooded. She developed anasarca—total-body fluid retention.

So there we were. Now, the spouse, the hospital senior chaplain, was flying in ever-tightening concentric circles of anxiety. Understandably, he did not realize that in these emergent moments, his place was to not be hovering over every medical consultant's conversation and peering into the dark beyond of every ultrasound and scan and test. It was to accept help himself and support his wife

The lioness was ready to quit. There was no mistaking the look; it was not one of fear, but of abject resignation forged from immense and unrelenting suffering and buttressed by a true faith of a better place with her creator. However, each carefully planned study and test showed that the tumor was on the run; the prior clot in the lung was gone, and there was no new threatening clot, new tumor, or failure of her anticlotting medicine.

Her anasarca was a result of her not having enough of the major protein of the blood, albumin. It was capillary leak syndrome, wherein the albumin, the granddaddy protein of the blood, had microscopically leaked out everywhere because of damage to her vessel walls from the chemotherapy. Yes, this could be fatal, but with meticulous attention to detail, it need not be. Nonetheless, she was admitted to the medical intensive care unit for a third time in fewer months.

I felt I needed to convince her to reconsider that this battle might also be won if we did everything right. I was quite clear with her. If she wished to quit, all she needed to do was deny her professed faith, take a right her faith tells her she does not have, and go home and die. The choice was hers, and the time was up to make it. That was the just the right recipe. Our reluctant warrior agreed, so we bundled the lioness off to the ICU with her agonizing husband bravely trying to put his arms around that which he could not control.

It all worked. The kidneys did not fail; the albumin came up as the tides of body fluids waned, and her weight plummeted to a healthier level. Most importantly, for the first time in months, our lioness smiled. That meant she was living, not merely surviving. Her quality of life improved every day.

It came time for her to return home and take in some much-deserved R & R, as the tumor had been transiently beaten into submission. I am told she even crossed the living room floor to empty the dishwasher under her own power while only one day out of the medical intensive care unit.

I suspect we will readdress the tumor in good time, but for now our lioness is very much alive and well, and not in winter.

The Flood

John frantically clawed at the air in which death hung impatiently over him, tearing at the flesh of some invisible assailant that would give no comfort to the wounded, no hint of honor in defeat. Between the indecipherable gasps and soul-stirring death rattles, he repeatedly spit out a terminal mantra: "C'mon, let's go, let's go. C'mon. Doc, please. Doc, please no more. No more; let's go." His body writhed in some sort of macabre death dance as the leukemia cells did what they do, rapidly dividing and flooding every organ, his brain, and even his skin, pushing against every pain fiber of his disease-ravaged body. John was in excruciating pain. John was dying.

Ours had been a twelve-year affair. He was one of the medical miracles. A real one-in-a-million case and fodder for numerous parables I had told to many of my students. John had chronic myelogenous leukemia (CML), and he had broken all the records. Over thirty years, his body was witness to our wading in the dark, employing one marrow poison after another to effect some sort of truce with his cancer without causing him any toxicity. The almost guaranteed conversion of his disease to a typically incurable acute phase typically occurring in five years was like the sword of Damocles, whose blade we avoided for thirty years.

A few decades ago, a key part of the magic decoder ring of this disease was deciphered. We still do not know why, but in CML two of those miraculous little think tanks called chromosomes break and realign as a new hybrid. They call it the Philadelphia chromosome. In one of the many bizarre twists of science, this disease, more so than many, has fostered innumerable careers and breakthroughs into the fog of why cancer cells kill. This hybrid chromosome harbors a lethal set of instructions for the parentage of all the previously normal blood cells: Make this protein; make it mimic the normal protein. It will fool them. Make this protein, and all the new children of the marrow will live forever. That is the seduction that was played out at the molecular genetic level against John's marrow cells: Make too many cells, take over, and never mind the rules of propriety and cell growth. Take over! Turn into acute leukemia.

Without a transplant, there was no cure, and transplant without at least a close match could easily be lethal. There was no match for John. Thus, it was marrow mayhem. In time, everywhere was overrun as the disease blasted off into acute leukemia, angry and recalcitrant to our best efforts. John had seen all the treatments in vogue over the decades and had wrestled an easy truce. He endured the flulike symptoms of daily self-injections with interferon and enjoyed a hematological remission whereby his chronic leukemia appeared to disappear. The miracle oral pill Gleevec of the twenty-first century was not even on the drawing board yet. Furthermore, this was acute leukemia now, and it came in bansheelike furor.

There was never a more simple congenial man, a more trusting and loyal patient, than he. He got along to get along. He was one of the folks where A plus B really does equal C; he was very direct, simple and straightforward, and enormously kind. There was no algebra to figuring John out. Having retired after a pleasant and nurturing twenty years in the air force, he worked the night shift at a manual-labor job and lovingly tended to his family. I had come to believe the totally unscientific sentiment that his cancer was seemingly paying homage, a sort of tribute in his body. Could it have been held in abeyance by his simple honesty and gentle demeanor?

We felt the conversion to acute leukemia coming long before the first snippet of hard evidence. It was as palpable as a pulse and equally relentless. Initially without objective evidence, John began to have sweats, low-grade fevers, bone pain, and generalized fatigue and weakness The transformation to acute leukemia was one of the nastier I had seen, as if revenge were being exacted and the toll of a twenty-five-year pardon from the typical recurrence at five years were now payable in full.

John was now in agony with terminal disease. He was growing increasingly resistant to escalating doses of morphine. This happens with accelerating chronic narcotic-requiring pain. As the nurse prepared a massive dose of intravenous morphine, I stood in the hospital room doorway with young doctors in training, describing the nuances of intravenous pain control and that the issue here was pain relief and mercy. I formally and fully briefed them and the family on the aspects of euthanasia versus death by secondary effect—the necessary alleviation of pain leading to a pain-free death.

I prayed for his peace as I pressed down on the syringe, gauging his pain relief as my guide. A lifetime reduced to this single act is surreal to imagine but quite real when you are in it, as the physician must do the best in terms of good versus harm. I prayed as his family said their goodbyes and the morphine pulsed through his veins.

I said to the residents, "Never forget what you have seen." I already knew they would not. Good-bye, John, and thank you.

The Gift

It was as if her soul had cruelly been branded "Kick Here" at birth. It was not that she was dealt bad cards so much as she never had much of a prayer to be in the game of life. Alcoholic and abusive parents spawned this only child almost three decades ago and rendered havoc on her congenitally frail spirit and teetering health. Not surprisingly, she was cursed from the beginning as a severe diabetic. This had withered away her adolescence in angry diabetic comas and multiple illnesses as her family rambled helter-skelter across the country, lashed to the whims of a drunken, oft-unemployed father.

Now a mother herself, Maria was at most a trembling waif of a young woman. She had been murderously robbed of childhood innocence, weaned on despair, suckled on disappointment. Against the odds for severe diabetics, she had amazingly survived pregnancy with very healthy twins.

She had escaped her hell of a family only to find herself in a ramshackle marriage to a pestilence, not a man. A wife beater and child abuser, her enlisted military husband was a belligerent, brooding hulk for which fatherhood was a grave inconvenience and a blot on his life.

I have come to believe that it was not by chance that one of our sage senior physicians happened to pull ER duty the day she walked the miles to our hospital carrying her precious cargo shivering in her arms. Both of her babies had fevers, and to the discerning eye, it was clear that evil had pitched its tent in their home. Incessant apologies from a terrified, tearful mother, as well as classic fractures and scarred, blistered skin from burning cigarettes having been pressed into innocent skin, wailed as a wounded plaintiff cry for a savior, for justice. Clearly both she and her children had been abused. She collapsed out of catharsis and experienced at least a momentary reprieve from fear and overwhelming grief when the emergency-room team were marshaled to gather them all into our protective bosom. Simultaneously, the search was set for her stain of a husband.

In short order, it became painfully clear that the tragedy had no bounds. It was soon obvious that Maria was ill. Evaluation in the emergency room showed that she had rapidly worsening kidney failure from what was soon learned to be malignant masses in her abdomen that were choking off her kidneys and eating voraciously through her pelvis.

I was drawn to this wounded pup. The ache of seeing such unfairness from a world that offers no guarantee of freedom from suffering was a constant companion for many of us tending to her care. Our clinical bond and trust falteringly evolved. Leveraging the lifeboat of her children, I painstakingly strained to encourage in her a glimmer of hope, and perhaps flame, the fading flicker of her fight for her life, for her children.

We all have bucket lists of dreams unfulfilled and longed for. Her dream was common enough. She longed to simply play with her children, to frolic with fantasy, unburdened by dread. Now she was resigned to a painful death; it was all she expected. Only the irrepressible devotion to her babies and the possibility of their future being so uncertain carried her on. However, it quickly became clear that the cancer would agonizingly strain the last beats of life from her.

We raced through the diagnostic evaluation and made a hurried dash to save her kidneys and numb what had to be blinding pain. There was never the slightest whimper, the faintest flinch from her. Through wounded eyes, she watched, disaffected, rallying only when her babies were safe and near. It was for them that she allowed the tubes to be inserted into her kidneys; for them she tolerated the invasion of her belly to knit together her perforated, strangulated bowels; for them she bloodlessly whispered a vacant yes to chemotherapy. If only she could have had just a moment's peace.

A few years ago, I suffered through the disaster of a rental condominium in Orlando that only Erma Bombeck could rightly do justice. It was absolute architectural anarchy. If water should have passed through it, it did not, if designed to support weight, it would not, if it had been controlled the environment, it could not. It was simply a massive disappoint and grand inconvenience.

Therefore, one day the stuff of fairy tales landed in my mind. I fashioned a story and made the calls. Perhaps I was serving my need to somehow save her, perhaps not. By the time the smoke cleared, it was all arranged, clearly by the hand of a force far greater than mine: airfare, a rental car, lodging, and Disney World admission was waiting, free of charge for Maria and her babes.

Yet she was giving up and dying. I eagerly told her of the scheme to whisk her away to fantasyland. I was stupefied by her visceral response. Life beamed in her eyes, and for the first time of what was to become an adorable habit, Maria smiled. I could almost hear her soul snap into action, barking orders to finally fight the beast eating her body. Her husband safely spirited away, a battered and bruised young, very alive mommy made it home for a long weekend for the first time. Irrespective of my personal faith, I was ill prepared for what lay ahead for Maria and her children.

A few Mondays later, my nurse hovered in my doorway, seemingly buoyed by joy, wet-eyed, and spiritually transfigured. Stammering, she said, "It is Maria ... Maria, she ... ah ...she is so alive." I am sure I fumbled out something only to have my nurse say, "No, it's Maria; you don't understand what's happened." In an instant, she was gone and I was confused.

Then I saw the glow of life as never I have seen before. Guided by grace, this beautiful woman glided into my office and settled into the chair. I was steeped in the warmth issuing from this vision. It looked like the Maria God would have fashioned were he to meddle mercifully in her miseries. She spoke serenely. "I stopped taking the narcotics; they made me sleepy. And I have no more pain. I am eating everything in sight, and my sugars seem okay. Doctor? Doctor? Are you okay?" Aghast and afraid that I might burst the bubble, I beckoned her in to the exam room. It was normal, unbelievably normal.

A lump was growing in my throat, and my voice grew strangely hushed. I vaguely remember calling the chief of radiology for the urgent CAT scan, but I do remember his return call after it was done He was incredulous, questioning me. "I do not know what you pulled, but the scan I have here—well, it's normal. No tumor, and healing bone." Gone, too, was the bowel obstruction, the blocked kidneys—all of it, gone. The physical exams, CAT scan, blood tests—all were normal. Softly, before I could gather myself, she spoke as if the hand of God were gently stroking my disbelief. "I know," she said. And then she was silent. I was in the presence of grace.

I had no problem getting through on the phone to make all the arrangements final, and in moments, it was done. She would leave for Orlando that weekend. The sweat of my soul slid down my face as my nurse handed me a tissue and floated out with our miracle.

On a Monday, some weeks after the joy of a lifetime with her children in Orlando, Maria appeared in my office. She was gaunt, wasted, and desperately pleading. "Tell me my babies will be okay," she said. "Tell me what will happen to them. Tell me." We spoke until the ache lifted from her spirit and she reached some manner of closure with the cancer that had so quickly returned to ravage her body. Abruptly, she stopped, rose to face me, and gently put her arms around my neck without a word. I saw that she knew it was over and her children would be safe.

There was no sorrow that Friday in the hospital. Her babies lay besides her in her arms, sleeping, as God called his angel home.

A Leprechaun's Laser Light of Life

As I made rounds, lilting laughter punctuated a ragtag vocal ensemble's singing of "Danny Boy." It ebbed and flowed from the oncology ward lounge, warmly filling a sterile hallway, but not my heart. It was the twentieth St. Patrick's Day since small-cell lung cancer had riddled and devoured my tough, son-of–Hell's Kitchen, World War II–veteran Irish dad. Although he died during the dreary, wet, frozen rains of a New England fall, he was etched into my heart's memory owing to one very magical St. Patrick's Day.

As I have done on every St Patrick's Day since his death, I was reminiscing about a time when I, a newly minted, wet-behind-everything medical student and a second lieutenant in the US Air Force in the Health Professions Scholarship Program, visited my dad at work as General Electric's chief labor relations negotiator in Manhattan. The day ended at a midtown Irish bar with me accompanying him on the tavern's beer soaked upright as he crooned "Danny Boy." You could feel the century-old pub wood weep as a sonorous tenor voice I had never before known he had lifted hearts, minds, and glasses. Mutually uninhibited, but not inebriated, father and son were in tune.

So here I was, decades later, on another St Patrick's Day, rounding on the oncology ward, tired and tied to a bittersweet memory. Regaining focus for the duties of the day, I began to thumb through the chart rack. Suddenly, intruding through the funk was the unmistakable sound of a Buck Rogers ray gun. It was right behind my left ear, magically mixing with leprechaun-like chortling and giggles.

I spun on my heels and was bowled over by the impish grin and theatrical posturing of my toy-toting assailant. Hopping and toe-dancing as lightly as a shamrock blown by faerie breath, and half naked in hospital regalia with toy cosmic carbine in hand, retired USAF Chief Master Sergeant O'Reilly squealed, "Ah-eee! Gotcha, doc"!

O'Reilly had whistled and skipped to an easy truce with his sleepy follicular non-Hodgkin's lymphoma for sixteen years prior to this admission. His blarney charmed the beast called anxiety. His acceptance of the capriciousness of a life filled with the Damocles sword of a strong probability of an aggressive transformation of his disease was like a therapeutic balm of Gilead for not only himself but also the many patients he befriended and bolstered.

His checkups were always happy routines rife with fabulous tale-spinning, unabashed limerick-singing, and other sound medical practices. Clinic visits from the sage retired chief leprechaun of the USAF always ended with a pat on my head, a wink at the nurses, and his trademark squeezing off of a couple laser beams of magic from the now infamous toy gun at whomever he thought needed it most. It never hurt, it often helped, and, more than once, it seemed more powerful than my prescription pad. An emeritus professor of mirth and mentorship, O'Reilly was one of the wisest men I knew.

Shortly before this final admission, the limber leprechaun interrupted plans to visit family in Ireland because, as he said, "Me shillelagh's telling me something ain't right." A thorough history and physical revealed nothing. The complete blood count showed a slight drop in his usually robust hemoglobin, and his platelet count had fallen considerably. So did my heart when review of the peripheral blood smear suggested what an immediate bone marrow examination confirmed—myelopthisis. His lymphoma had transformed aggressively and was exploding in bansheelike furor. It was replacing his bone marrow. Further staging showed broad lymph node, boney, spleen, and meningeal dissemination. An incredibly bright man, he fully understood the limits of therapy and the grave prognosis. Typically unafraid and more concerned for his family, he was annoyed at the change in travel plans. He sprightly assured me, "I have a few things yet to do, so let's have a go at it."

We did. After a rocky course consisting of intensive systemic and intrathecal brain chemotherapy, massive transfusions, considerable assistance from colony-stimulating factors to support his white blood cell count and fight infection, and the use of erythropoietin to help him make blood, this knobby-kneed leprechaun of a man was zapping my dour spirits. Bald and beaming and headed toward a major clinical response, he was working his magic on this very special St Patrick's Day.

It was his family in the lounge warming the ward with lilts of laughter. Spying my doleful drudge as I began ward rounds, he had left the comfort of family and friends to fire a laser beam of life my way. Clearly unfazed by the enormous odds of a rapid and refractory-to-treatment recurrence of his cancer, he often grandly showcased his plastic phaser, quipping something to the effect of, "If it comes back, we'll zap me cancer with this thing; it's better than those poisons, eh?"

O'Reilly was one of the gifts clinical oncologists can garner in decades of clinical practice if they are open to receive them. He was one of those wonderful "doctor-patients" put in our path to minister magical wisdoms just when we oncologists need them most. Being touched by such patients' special zest, zeal, and wisdom is one of those easy medicines to swallow. Souls such as these are precious jewels in the growing treasure chest of a clinician's experience, and the luster of the clinical pearls they impart are often both illuminating and transformative. So it was with O'Reilly.

Unbeknownst to me, he had more things than fighting his cancer on his agenda. He had taken particular notice of one of my young clinic nurses. She was a seemingly emotionally cold and somewhat intense second lieutenant nurse that was "too young to act such a tough nut and too talented not to try and crack," according to O'Reilly. She had requested transfer to the inpatient oncology service. This coincidentally put her on the ward—and in O'Reilly's service and sights—when the aggressive transformation of O'Reilly's lymphoma occurred. Both I and the senior nursing staff were concerned for her, believing her far more fragile than her implacable demeanor might suggest, but our "tough nut" showed no signs of trouble and, sadly, few signs of warmth, even when O'Reilly's improbable clinical remission occurred.

Shortly after that St Patrick's Day, the probable occurred. O'Reilly was readmitted with signs and symptoms of a rapid recurrence. He was quick to grasp his situation, calmly and confidently summarizing my lengthy delivery of sad news to a family unwilling to believe the unacceptable, saying gently to all, "It's been a great run, so now, soon, I'll be with sod and saints." In his final days of a rapidly progressing malignancy that would not be denied, he had three simple requests: some intimate uninterrupted time with the missus, a steady supply of Guinness Stout, and "one last shot at some unfinished business." Curiously, and without any explanation offered, he decreed that the "tough nut" young nurse be assigned to his care, and furthermore she was to be the only medical staff he wanted in his room—no one else, no exceptions. Somewhat bewildered, but always admiring of his wisdom, the charge nurse and I warily agreed. On hearing his request, the young lieutenant almost condescendingly agreed, seemingly fashioning it as some sort of dramatic last wish. After all, she thoughtlessly quipped, it was "probably [her] turn anyway." She would be in his service, having no idea how true that would prove.

I was shaken upon news of his passing the next morning. However, deeply appreciative of O'Reilly's gifts, I was both concerned and curious as to the impact, if any, his passing had made on the young "tough nut" nurse. No worries. I no sooner strode onto the ward than she ran up to me glowing, seemingly transformed and weightless, her eyes brimming with tears of joy. She reached into her pocket and produced our leprechaun's little laser gun. Smiling, she told me that he had called her to his room, eschewing all others. She bubbled joyously about how they had chatted for hours about secret things—special things about love and the rich life. She was bursting with the pride and surprise of one who had been picked above all others as something special and lovable. Tugging at my white coat like the impatient, exuberant child she then was, she announced triumphantly that she was the last target he aimed a final salvo of saving love at. He then bequeathed his otherworldly potion in a pistol to her, saying, "I can go now. You'll know when to use it and when it's time to pass it on."

Death is not always so kind or so graceful in its gifts. When we healers and helpers are absorbed in our sorrows, perhaps lost in the fog of sadness over the limits of our skills or other concerns, we may also be most vulnerable to the laser beams of life from those who by all rights should be sorrowful and yet are not.

The Connection

I had heard of, and worse yet felt, "the wall" some medical residents place around their feelings like a moat that somehow will keep out the pain inevitably experienced in an internal medicine training program.

God, they had so much to wade through. "Dr. Plumber" (an assumed name, as she refused to use her first name lest it crack her wall) had much work yet to be done on the fortress around her heart. The windows to her soul were shuttered too tightly. Though superb in her clinical care, she was deficient in her caring.

Her call to me was crisp in presentation, thorough, and clipped at a staccato but calm and self-assured pace. Her voice was more like the Dow ticker than the beat of a heart telling me one of my heroes had fallen, both literally and figuratively.

Felipe was a brave and devoted Filipino husband, father, and patriarch who had served dutifully in the air force and his community after his retirement, before he was felled by one of nature's cruel immunologic tricks, the usually innocuous Epstein-Barr virus. It is best known because of its association with mononucleosis, but it could also insinuate its DNA deep in the belly of some cells and work out a darker fate, from nasopharyngeal carcinoma to lymphomas. Felipe had the former.

There was no braver or truer "Yes, doctor" uttered by a patient in my twenty plus years than when we told him how we would combine the powerful cis-platinum with 5-FU and radiation. In savage synergy, they would attack the cancer and exact a toll of leathery skin, diminish the ability to taste or even produce saliva, and, in his case, possibly depress his hearing to the point that even devices would only moderately help. The prize was a real shot at survival, but in a world requiring enormous adjustment and sacrifice. He focused on those odds on every day of therapy and for the three years since with zeal

It was three years later that the news of his prostate cancer landed. Once again, he stood up to the beast and beat it. It was local stage, and the potentially emasculating surgery was painfully accepted by this proud patriarch.

So now this clipped voice, referring to herself always as "Dr. Plumber," never by her first name, was telling me the tale of rapidly deteriorating strength in Felipe's lower extremities and other widespread neurologic findings in a manner not quite following the blueprint of our neurological wiring. There was, of course, more. The lesion on the MRI of his brain had revealed a probable area of foreign tumor in the brain, and its location was quite likely to have seeded cells throughout the whole wiring diagram and central computer—the brain and its covering. His tumor was bathing the lining of the brain and spinal column; it was meningeal carcinomatosis. Only a spinal tap could confirm what I knew had to be. This often treatable, sometimes curable, and frequently fatal condition could be a third cancer. It was—a non-Hodgkin's lymphoma.

The positive spinal tap is not the point of the story. First was "the telling." All of the family was there, including two who were nurses—a difficult position, to be sure. Often in such situations, personal grief must do battle with a sense of duty to engage as a health-care provider, spokesperson, and some form of second authority.

Happily, the spanking-new one-stripe airman who had been with my wounded warrior since admission boldly asked to be with me through the "telling talk," all the way. The family agreed. In we paraded, MDs in training in tow. I stopped in front of every family member, particularly noting the somewhat starched but not really distant demeanor of one of the older daughters as she called me colonel, not doctor.

I took special care with this family. After a warm, strong embrace of my patient's hand, I motioned for his acceptance to sidle up to and hunker down my six-foot-three, 220-lb frame next to this former marine weighing in at barely 145 pounds. There is a personal, intimate space for every patient; it changes with every doctor, as well as throughout the relationship. The time was now to sit hip-to–bony frame, eye-to-eye, grasp a wasted hand firmly, and search deep into the heart behind those steely eyes veiled with a mist of tears. I leaned close to his ear, as his hearing had been ravaged as predicted, and grunted "Oorah! Semper fi." " He grasped my hand tightly and responded in kind. My heart has never heard the call so ready for the fight.

We began. "Okay, Felipe, this is a big one. You sloshed through the fetid swamp of Vietnam and stood tall in blazing, burning oil fields. You faced a cancer that threatened to take your face and your life, and you accepted surgery that left you unable to be the man you saw yourself as; you were forced to adjust. This one is bigger." I paused to take his measure. He was unwavering, his grasp locked.

The true essence of the physician is much more than an ounce of teacher. Be it by metaphors, parables, and the like, you must meet patients at their ground, on their turf, or you are never in the game and could do great harm. It is may be hard to think about what you are about to say, but to say only what you are thinking and what you know they will hear—that is the rub. That is the art of the teacher-physician.

"Felipe, your car has oil, and you know why?" He nodded. "And it goes all through the critical engine parts. It must be pure, clean—no dirt, right?" Again a nod. I grabbed the nearest piece of paper and drew a brain and a stalk, sort of like a lopsided sideways broccoli or cauliflower. I then drew a long cord from the stalk ending in what looked like a horse's tail with hairs splayed out in a fan shape. I explained the anatomy of the central nervous system to him in the most basic of terms.

I gave dramatic pause to let the picture and metaphor begin to grow in the mind's eye of Felipe and family—all eleven that were there at his request. Gesturing to all with my free hand, I said, "Let's open the broccoli and learn that there are chambers that hold fluid and a canal that connects it all and it is all in one long sac. The meninges cover the brain and reflect downward to the stalk and cord and horse's tail, the cauda equina. There is fluid that bathes the brain and the cord and is pumped around in a circular manner, up and down and back, and absorbed by cells lining the rooms, or ventricles, in the brain. Just like oil has a certain set of necessary characteristics, so does this fluid; in this case, they are sugar, protein, and pressure. Do you see?"

As I waved my hand through the imaginary circulating cerebral spinal fluid in their mind's eye, I turned to Felipe. "We cannot have any foreign debris, or dirt, or foreign bad cells here, can we?" He was unmoved. "We cannot have those cells grow and multiply." He was still unmoved. I continued knowing he was processing the inevitable conclusion and racing ahead of me. "Now stay with me", I said. " We cannot have those cells grow in a closed, tight space like the one I explained, for if they do, they will damage whatever function wherever they land."

His eyes cleared, and he stared at his emaciated legs. "So that is why I can barely walk now, doctor, and maybe one or two places it is worse than others; maybe it can go anywhere in that canal system or my skull cannot take the pressure eventually, is that it?"

I simply said a quiet yes.

Unshaken, he said, "This is very bad, doctor. Can we treat it? Can we cure it? Do we know its name? Is it from my nasopharyngeal cancer or prostate?"

Slowly I explained to him the vagaries and mysteries of the amazing immune system, the role of normal white blood cells and the types, using the military as my metaphor and the rise of Nazism as my parable of the malignant, unarrested clonal growth of a lymphoma, a third cancer that was seizing his senses and threatening a painful death. We waded carefully through the many types and what difference it made to him. I explained he had a third cancer, possibly related in ways we had not yet fully discerned to that same Epstein-Barr virus. It was primary to his central nervous system, which he now understood, and it had seeded his meninges like stucco sprayed erratically by a whipping hose in a closed space.

He got it, and they got it. I explained that there was a realistic chance of recovery of some or, uncommonly, all of his leg function because it was a lymphoma and that the very potent high-dose steroids we were using were in part killers of these cells.

He would need a catheter connected at one end to a small port about the size of a quarter that led into the ventricles in his brain so that chemotherapy could bathe his brain. I explained the risk of the procedure and told him that we could do that all here but that he also needed radiation treatments for his entire central nervous system and high-dose chemotherapy with very close monitoring. I asked him if he got the science of it all after reviewing endlessly the metaphor and the treatments; they all did. I then turned to the young doctor and said, "That was the longer and easier part." Turning back to my patient, I said "Now let's talk, Felipe. Let us talk about the fear, as the anxiety—fear of the unknown—is gone. We killed it with knowledge, didn't we? Let us talk as men and children of God, of fear. Talk to me, Felipe." He lessened his grip and gestured to his wife, who was bereft but very present.

In angelic strains only heard between true lovers, she said, "It is your decision, my love, and I know what it will be. I will be here and there and with you always." She gained strength and momentum. "You are my man; no prostate surgery changed that. You must talk to God, and he will hear you. You are a marine, and you know how to fight and when to surrender. My love, we will be the ones left behind." At this, Felipe broke down for just a moment. Admonishingly, she said, "We will be fine. There was no promise for forever, but until forever ended, and it has not. You know what to do; talk to Jesus."

The room had become a sacristy, and the Spirit was holding the very floor under all one dozen of us as we heaved each breath with heavy hearts. Felipe, the marine, fixed his jaw and set his eyes on mine. "Colonel, can we have a few days?"

"No!" was my response.

Without missing a pulse, his grip firmed again. "It is that fast?" he asked in disbelief.

"Yes," I answered sternly. "You always may have until forever comes, but to fight it, you must start now." With strength and uncommon valor, he declared he would talk to his family alone and give me his answer in ten minutes. The stage was set for our final dance, and the entourage of shaken medics left the room, gently closing the door. I intentionally separated myself from the others, as they needed to stew in the juices of the sweat of life's struggle privately for a moment, and we were not done.

Sufficient time had elapsed, and this time I stood astride, facing the family. I needed not speak. It was his show now. He spoke first, as I thought he would: "Let's do it."

I quickly spun on my heels and intentionally almost pinned Dr. Plumber in the direct line of sight of all, including the patient. Knowing how deep this man's faith ran, I knew we were not done. "Now Felipe, the most important part. You are a Christian, is that right? Are you praying?" I gently asked, and a chorus of yeses echoed through the room. I continued. "Felipe, do you think God is going to heal you or help you handle this?"

He said, "Life is not easy. He will not cure me; he can do anything, but he does not work that way. We know the love of Jesus and understand."

I asked, "Was he with you in Vietnam and Kuwait?"

Instantly he said, "Oh yes," and a smile that could fill the Philippine Sea warmed the room.

I asked, "Do you remember in the Garden of Gethsemane, what Jesus first said while praying to his father when he was alone without the disciples?"

His beam of faith grew brighter, and he excitedly replied, "Oh yes, he asked to get out of it, and he sweated blood."

At once my heart was less heavy as I softly said, "Yes, Felipe, yes, and we, too, may cry." And he did cry as our eyes met.

Through the corner of my eye, I unmistakably saw a right arm ceremoniously lifting into a salute. It was that of Felipe's sister, the starched one I had noticed before, standing more proud and erect. "Chief Petty Officer Angoco requests the honor of a return salute, Colonel, sir!" I felt I was on the USS *Missouri* in WWII and there was only one right response to this wet-eyed soldier obviously soon to assume command of the family. I abruptly turned and returned the greatest salutation I daresay I have had in many a year.

Turning back, I continued. "Felipe, you are a hero. I doubt I could ever do this even with the most beautiful family you have." He waved me away, but I sternly stared him down. "No! Dammit, you are a hero, and you will listen to me. Dr. Plumber, what is he, hero or not? Could you do it, can you even conceive of it?"

She was motionless, standing with her head down; she whispered, "No."

I continued and pressed her. "And tell me, have you ever had an attending physician do this?" She gave the same response. "And tell me,"—I parsed my words for maximum dramatic affect while in tempo staring at each family member in turn—"will you ever forget Felipe Angoco, ever?"

She again gave the same response: "No."

I stood taller and took in a commanding breath. "There is more, Felipe and Dr. Plumber; there is much more here."

Again, I began, but this time, with the fluttering of my eagle-wing epaulets almost audible, I challenged her. " Will you see cancer again?"

A meek yes was uttered.

In instant retort, again I challenged. "Will you see meningeal carcinomatosis as a possible differential diagnosis again."

This time she said, "Yes, yes, Colonel."

After taking a dramatic pause, I reached out for her hand, put it in Felipe's, and said as gently as I could, "Then thank the man on behalf of the thousand Felipes who will cross both your path and the paths of those you will teach in the next thirty years. Look in his eyes and tell him you will never forget"

Time stood still, although—thank God—their hands did not.

Postscript: While writing my note for the record in the on-call room littered with charts, and with Dr. Plumber burying her face in melting tears nearby, the young, black, single-stripe airman who had asked to be there during the "big talk" approached. He had undoubtedly raced in dangerous, screaming streets in earlier years, as was so apparent in his vernacular and visage. He walked in without a sound and cleared his throat from the tears he had obviously shed. Standing proudly at attention, staring through me at the wall behind me lest he break down, he passed me a note and searched my eyes for more than just a moment. He spun on his heels and solemnly faded away. It was written on a prescription pad and read as follows:

> To Dr. Plumber
> &
> The Colonel
>
> I am just writing this to thank you for everything you have helped me with today. Even though it may seem little to you, it was a great world to me. I appreciate it so much—more than you can ever know. It pushes me to

> strive and reach my dream to be a doctor also. May God bless you richly.
>
> Airman Jeff Smith

PPS: I waded over the moat of Dr. Plumber's Jericho walls and handed her the note. Softly, almost cooing, I said, "Here is your second of thousands of Felipe Angocos yet to come."

PPS: Felipe responded to all the therapy, and though modestly neurologically disabled from it, he survived. Dr. Plumber follows him in her clinic. Sometimes we win big.

The Quality of Mercy

In *The Merchant of Venice* by William Shakespeare, Portia, a brilliant Shakespearean heroine, impersonates a lawyer and pleads that mercy be granted a debtor in default to an abused moneylender who is demanding a rather gruesome repayment. Portia pleads that the quality of mercy is greatest when given freely and that mercy must have some weight on the scales of justice.

Leaving Martin Luther King Day and headed into Presidents' Day, my thoughts returned to a decades-old episode in my life in which similar words and sentiments of Shakespeare, Dr. King, and President Lincoln resounded.

Tom was a new air force sergeant with a mass in his chest. Almost everyone was convinced of the diagnosis. However, as I had often preached, "Although tumor is the rumor, tissue is the issue." Thus, a surgical biopsy was scheduled.

Garrison Keillor, of *Prairie Home Companion* fame, would be proud of this young Minnesotan sergeant. How Tom got to be noble and gracious at such a young age, I do not know, but this kid was something special.

The surgery went well. The biopsy looked extremely bizarre under the microscope, but our best pathologist was enormously confident about Tom's rare diagnosis. Something about that pathologist gnawed at me. Nonetheless, as we had a direction, I sat with the gracious sergeant and explained the intense therapy that lay ahead, the consequences of certain sterility and the high risk of permanent organ damage and possible death.

The therapy almost killed the patient. Many organ systems were severely damaged, perhaps permanently. Yet this young man's spirit only strengthened. When he was strong enough to speak in his many trips to the intensive care unit, his first words were always questions about how the other "older patients with families" were doing!

After Tom's final treatment, I received a hysterical call from our best pathologist. Between sobs, he told me how confident he had been about Tom's diagnosis. Because of his confidence, he hadn't checked on the all the special studies I requested. My colleague was wrong. Tom's tumor was an unusual variant of a highly treatable type of cancer. Although the mass was apparently gone, the drugs he received had never been tried before, and Tom would not survive more therapy. The pathologist's wife had suddenly shown severe mental health problems. His family was falling apart. His desire to "save somebody" had clouded his judgment.

I had to talk to Tom. I told him everything.

Tom understood and solemnly said, "We have to fix this." Moist-eyed yet resolute, he searched my face and asked, "Is he going to be all right?" He grabbed his IV poles like the arms of a helping comrade. He lifted himself out of bed and said he had to see the hospital commander "to tell him to forgive the pathologist and to remember all the good he has done and will do." I thought Tom could not walk; perhaps grace carried him to the commander—I could no longer see clearly through my own tears.

After over a decade of research, the previously untried treatment given by mistake was shown to be highly effective. The hospital commander, who was merciful in helping the pathologist recover, became surgeon general of the US Air Force and personally saved lives and commanded rescue efforts on 9/11 when a hijacked plane crashed into the Pentagon near his office. Tom survived. He is home in Minnesota, working as a union steward with his three children adopted from Ethiopia.

Portia was right. Mercy is not forced; "it droppeth as the gentle rain from heaven ... it is twice blest ... it blesses him that gives and him that takes."

The Power of We

Being a dyed-in-the-wool American, I never really bought into the "royal we" thing. The way the Queen Mum says "We are pleased" or "We are most miffed" always struck me as eerie. The same holds for those who think simply possessing a highly placed job warrants royal treatment or being held beyond reproach or approach. Some leadership positions clearly command respect, as they directly affect millions of lives, but the notion of the blue-blooded "royal we" never held its hue for this red-blooded American guy.

Then, in 2001, I met We.

Generals are where rubber meets the air. Chief master sergeants are where the rubber meets the road. We was a chief's chief. I will never forget that picture-perfect gentle warrior, a beautiful physical specimen of a man, cradling a Bible worn down by his "We-ness" as he sat in a chemotherapy chair on September 11, 2001.

After what seemed like every test known to man, I decided that the excruciating pain, progressive muscular weakness, and bizarre neurologic findings draining this blue-blood were due to a macabre tango between his immune system and a previously thought cured lymphoma that still somehow held a manipulating embrace of him immunologically and neurologically.

We had no disease we could follow or see, but we had definite muscle destruction and wasting along with the neurological findings not following any typical course. Thus we thought of an immune based attack of our own. We thought of using monoclonal antibodies. The team I was on years earlier was one of many trying to bring the 1975 Nobel Prize–winning guided-missile marvels known as monoclonal antibodies into the clinic in new ways. They home in on singular targeted cancer cells and thus assist in their destruction. Now, of all days, here were We and I, trying to negotiate a peace by controlling tumor terrorism using a novel approach to fight cancer we could not directly see.

We explained that his USAF-enlisted dad had first used the royal we. We used it ever since when things got tough. When he was eight years old, he was blocked by his race from entering housing and was complaining about having to hole up with five others in the family Buick. His dad said, "Son, we have a great nation with some wrong. We all have to get along to make it better. So remember, there is all the room in the universe in 'we.'" We junior gave his life to God that first Buick night. I think the transaction has clearly gone both ways.

We received the most prestigious USAF medal for heroism in peacetime as a new airman. In the black of night, this equally dark young man stopped his car, having spied a burning home in a neighborhood recently inflamed with racist hate. We rescued two wheelchair-bound former Klan members inside.

I remember him in the chemotherapy room, his eyes filled with laughter's mist as he related the story, saying, "Not too much more stupid than running into a burning building. Well, yes, running back in is pretty stupid." He was decorated again twenty years later when he careened his car into an embankment to so that he could tackle and subdue a massive knife-wielding man pummeling his naked wife, whom We saw run into the street while others simply watched.

It was We who, between chemotherapy treatments, in a wheelchair, flew to Iraq after 9/11 to support "our boys" while saying to his general, "We cannot send them where we would not go."

Normally the military will discharge those clearly not fit for full duty on a moment's notice. The medical evaluation board's response was one I had never seen. It stated simply and briefly in one sentence, "We still have need for this warrior, and we will find a way."

We recovered strength, retired after his two boys finished college, and moved back home to his dad's town, where I am told We, now a part-time minister, is "doing just fine, thank you."

I was too self-involved when studying those many years ago in the UK to understand there are bona fide "royal We's." I had the privilege of exchanging salutes with and serving one.

Station, position, and experience alone do not confer a crown. A '57 Buick Special can be a regal nursery, and royalty can be taught. The "royal We" is within the power of choice for you and me.

EPILOGUE

My surgical oncology colleague in "Coming Home" is doing well emotionally and physically. He occasionally worries over new little spots that show up on his skin, but after local therapy, he remains alive and well in a thriving practice.

Our hero in "Snow Job" is living the good life in Silicon Valley, recently married; very much in love and, as some thirtysomethings often do, nursing just a wee bit of a paunch.

The "Lioness" progressively deteriorated after a stable six months at home. It was not from her disease. In fact, even while not on therapy some of the tumor in her skin was shrinking. Her capillary leak syndrome and her leaking will to live both understandably took her home, which is what she wanted. To date, her husband seems okay. He is probably not okay, other than knowing where she is but he is not.

"The Flood" of acute leukemia took its victim as morphine successfully washed away his pain. The family keeps in touch and is grateful for the cleverly stolen decades of time. He has served as fodder for many a lecture and admonition to my medical students that sometimes nice people do fare better for some time. He died just a few short years before the wonder drug Gleevec, used for Chronic Myelogenous Leukemia, was in phase 1 trials.

The babes of "The Gift" have grown; one is a nurse and mother, the other still in college. They can still feel their mother's dying arms cradling and wrapped around them, as strong and graceful as boughs of redwood.

We are dancing with the devil and not yet paying our due with June of "The Telling." Very high dose Epogen, which stimulates red blood cell production, has eked out a remarkable come-from-behind, against-all-odds victory. She has a normal blood cell level and is independent of transfusions. Even more amazingly, although it should not have happened according to "science," her platelets rose to just under fifty thousand—quite a safe range. Here is the tricky part. We then made her slightly iron deficient by removing blood, and we kept pushing the marrow with Epogen to make blood. We hope we were fooling her marrow into thinking she was bleeding as we were making her ever-so-slightly iron deficient. Our best hope was that if her marrow thought she was bleeding because she was modestly iron deficient, the marrow might respond by making platelets, since they are needed to "plug" bleeds. It worked, and she now sports a totally normal platelet count and no longer has to live with immense risk of spontaneous or easy bleeding. How long will it last? Look up and ask. She is enjoying what she calls "her miracle," as well she should.

The laser-gun laddie from years ago is still standing at the pearly gates, passing out cosmic pistols and whipping off an occasionally spectacular trick shot at those passing by. He thinks it's funny and they giggle, sure and *begorra*.

Our good-looking young man of grace from "Mercy" married a good-looking woman, and his children are above average in a peaceful Minnesotan Lutheran town. Despite what we said could not be, he added two of his own to the adopted three. I will have to ask Garrison Keillor if our hero still frequents Bertha's Kitty Boutique, him being a cat fancier, don't ya know, eh?

Having made a final connection in the story of the same name, Felipe's steel-gray eyes remain open and cast upon a family phalanx of Philippine warriors of love. He is in complete remission.

We, from "The Power of We," has gained a great deal of strength, as unnecessary as that would be for such a man were I not speaking strictly anatomically. He is a part-time minister with some leg fatigue and no evidence of disease. It appears clear to him that the Rituxan monoclonal antibodies worked, and the physical exam supports that. I just cannot shake the image of We, cane in hand, later visiting Afghanistan just to support the troops.

INDEX/ PARTIAL GLOSSARY

A

Abandonment (see text) 72
Achilles' Heel (*of cancer cells*) 28, 32, 123, 129, 244
A Conclusion Should Not Be The Place You Reach When You Grow Tired Of Thinking (see text) 307
Active Listening (see text) 99, 280, 300, 336
Addiction (see text) 197, 211, 215, 218, 219, 305, 335
Addictive Technocracy (*overdependence on tests*) 69, 297
Adjuvant (see text) 26, 62, 108, 109, 126, 127, 133, 140, 174, 337
Affirmations (see text) 263, 269, 272
Age-Adjusted Rate (*statistics* [see text]) 177
Air Pollution (see text) 38, 43, 49
Alcohol (see text) 37, 38, 42, 43, 48, 50, 184, 186, 188, 190, 191, 201, 202, 205, 209, 246, 255, 320
Alkylating Agents (*type of chemotherapy* [see text]) 28, 29, 34, 131, 133
Allogeneic Transplants (HLA-*matched non-twin donors for bone marrow transplant* [see text]) 154, 156
Allopathic (*conventional medicine*) 222, 224, 238
Alopecia (*balding*) 183
Alternative Diets (see text) 230
Alternative Medicines (*unconventional unproven therapy*) 103, 105, 106, 110, 221, 222, 224, 225, 228, 234, 238, 239, 335, 347
American Academy Of Hospice And Palliative Medicine (see text) 315
American Board Of Internal Medicine (see text) 20, 293
American Brain Tumor Association (see text) 341
American Cancer Society (see text) 42, 176, 183, 184, 208, 230, 232, 239, 338, 339, 345
The American College Of Surgeons (see text) 42
American Disabilities Act (see text) 332
American Institute Of Cancer Research (see text) 42
American Joint Committee On Cancer (see text) 125
American Society Of Clinical Oncology (see text) 28, 321, 338, 339
Amino Acids (*DNA building blocks* [see text]) 230, 241, 252
Anecdotes (see text) 42, 89, 97, 107, 223, 238

Anemia (see text) 25, 61, 135, 147, 194, 320, 349, 354
Angels (see text) 68, 122, 291, 292, 366
Angel's Wing (see text) 292
Anger (see text) 79, 80, 94, 264, 277–279, 282–284, 310, 311, 315, 334, 356
Angiogenesis (*new blood vessel formation*) 150, 151, 152
Angiogenesis Inhibitors (see text and above) 151, 152
Antiangiogenesis (see text) 36, 146, 157, 236, 249
Antibodies (*proteins made by the immune system to fight specific antigens*) 32, 32–34, 117, 118, 121, 143–145, 146, 147, 149, 150, 157, 158, 244, 247, 249, 379, 382
Anti-CD20/B Cell Monoclonal Antibodies (see text) 146
Anticytokines (see text) 244
Anti-EGFR (*see EGFR*) 146, 147, 149
Anti-Epidermal Growth Factor Receptors (*see EGFR*) 244
Antifolates (*type of chemotherapy*) 30
Antigenic (*see antigen*) 122, 144, 154
Antigen (*substance capable of eliciting an immune response*) 34, 35, 118, 121, 144–146, 147, 154, 247–249, 253
Antimetabolites (*type of chemotherapy*) 29, 133
Antitumor Antibiotics (*type of chemotherapy*) 31, 131, 134
Anxiety And Fear (see text) xviii, 11, 86, 280
Anxiety (see text) v, xiii, xiv, xvii, xviii, xx, xxi, 8, 11–13, 19, 37, 38, 47, 59, 66, 70, 71, 73, 77, 78, 80–83, 85, 86, 94, 96, 102, 105, 113, 183, 184, 187, 190, 194, 196, 202, 205, 208, 222, 228, 229, 239, 257, 260, 262, 271, 272, 279, 280, 283, 292, 300, 312, 320, 332, 336, 348, 350, 358, 359, 367, 374
Apoptosis (*programmed cell death*) 53, 139, 158
ASCO (*American Society of Clinical Oncology*) 28, 73, 321, 338, 339
ASCO Patient Guide: Understanding Tumor Markers For Breast And Colon Cancers (see text) 339
Aspirin (see text) 44, 186, 195, 207
Ativan (*sedating antianxiety medicine*) 214, 320
Atropine (*drug to dry secretions from mouth*) 319, 321
Attending Physicians (*physician primarily and ultimately responsible* [see text]) 258, 293, 330, 375
Attitude (see text) 2, 3, 86, 95, 208, 270, 275, 288, 300, 318, 331
Autologous Transplants (*self as donor for bone marrow transplant*) 155, 156
Autonomous (*see autonomy*) 7, 8, 111
Autonomy (*right to self-determination* [see text]) xvii, xxi, 7, 8, 41, 46, 79, 82, 85, 95, 98, 101, 104, 111, 167, 223, 323, 330, 348
Average Life-Years Saved (*statistic* [see text]) 180
Average Years Of Life Lost (*statistic* [see text]) 178
Ayurveda (*yoga*) 226, 227

B

Baby Steps (see text) 269, 272
BCG (see text) 150, 195
Being Engaged (see text) 83
Beneficence (*acting for the welfare of another*) 167, 238, 323, 325, 327, 328, 333, 352

Beta Carotene (see text) 44
Beta Interferon (*immune modulating substance*) 254, 255
Bevacizumab (*a monoclonal antibody*) 152
Bexxar (*a monoclonal antibody*) 147
Bioelectromagnetic-Based Therapies (see text) 232
Biologically Based Therapies (see text) 226
Biological Therapy (see text) 149, 150
Biologic Response Modifiers (see text) 36
Biopsy (see text) 22, 39, 40, 45, 46, 58–60, 77, 78, 108, 118, 119, 120, 124, 126, 128, 141, 142, 303, 377
Bleeding And Thrombocytopenia (*low platelets increasing risk of bleeding*) 185
Blind Trust (see text) 82
Bogeyman (see text) 92
Bone Marrow And Stem Cell Transplantation (see text) 152
Bone Marrow (see text) 25, 35, 36, 51, 56, 61, 115–117, 120, 124, 129, 133, 134, 138, 140, 149, 152, 153, 155, 156, 214, 242, 243, 251, 254, 303, 349, 350, 353, 354, 357, 358, 367
Bone Marrow Transplantation (see text) 36, 153
Bone Scan (see text) 119, 141, 171
Boost Volume (*boost of radiation dose to primary site*) 138
Borrowed Servant (*medical legal term*) 332
Bowel Obstruction (see text) 214, 319, 365
Brachytherapy (*implanted radiation therapy*) 137
Brain Tumor Society (see text) 341
BRCA1 (*prognostic tumor-associated markers* [see text]) 47
BRCA2 (*prognostic tumor-associated markers* [see text]) 47
Breast Cancer (see text) 22, 23, 24, 31–33, 39, 43, 44, 46, 59, 60, 62, 63, 109, 120, 121, 125, 126, 133, 142, 148, 159, 251, 339, 341, 347, 356–358
Burnout (*of Oncology staff*) xix, 63, 70, 74, 75
But What Do I Say? (*to those with cancer*) xix, 277, 279, 285

C

CALGB Cancer And Leukemia Group B (see text) 174, 337
CAM (Complementary and Alternative Medicine) (see text) 103, 103–106, 221, 222, 224–226, 227, 228, 230, 232–236, 238, 239, 335, 347
CAM Office At The NIH (see text) 239
Cancer Advances Newsletter 339
Cancer Guide: Steve Dunn's Cancer Information Page (see text) 338
The Cancer Handbook (see text) 339
Cancer Information Service (see text) 176, 339, 342
Cancer Is Precisely The Unraveling Of The Norm (see text) 246
Cancerlit (*cancer informational website*) 174, 340
Cancer Medicine, fifth edition, Edited By Holland And Frei (see text) 346
Cancernet (*cancer informational website*) 174, 239, 338–340
Cancer News On The Net (see text) 338, 340

Cancer Of Origin (*correct naming of tumors based on origin, not spread*) 58
Cancerous Cells In Situ (*noninvasive*) 59
Cancer Risk (see text) 37, 38, 43, 44, 50, 51, 179
Cancer Trials (*to treat and evaluate patients in a systematic, controlled manner*) 174
Cansearch (*cancer informational website*) 338, 340
Captain Of The Ship (*medical legal term* [see text]) 69, 332
Carcinogens (*substances known to cause cancer*) 49, 50
Carcinomas (*broad category of cancers*) 54, 57, 58, 59, 370
Cardiovascular Disease (see text) 23, 24, 41, 44
CAT (scan) (see text) 365
Causes Of Cancer (see text) 22, 37, 48
Celecoxib (*Celebrex anti-inflammatory drug*) 44
Cell Division (*to increase cell numbers*) 29, 30, 31, 52, 54, 55, 139, 147, 157
Cells Have A Life Cycle (see text) 130
Centers For Disease Control (see text) 345
Cervical Intraepithelial Neoplasm (*noninvasive*) 59
Chaplain (see text) 259, 315, 316, 357, 359
Chemotherapy (*types of* [see text]) xiii, xviii, 21, 22, 24–29, 31, 32, 36, 40, 54, 59, 62, 70, 105, 107, 111, 113, 116, 123, 129–136, 138, 140, 142, 143, 145–149, 152–154, 156, 157, 160, 162, 164, 166, 181, 183–188, 190–192, 194–197, 199–206, 208, 209, 211, 214, 228–230, 243, 247, 255, 291, 292, 314, 339, 340, 350, 351, 353, 354, 357–359, 364, 367, 373, 379, 380
Children (see text) xiii, 21, 24, 25, 51, 58, 101, 120, 130, 132, 154, 197, 247, 249, 271, 282, 313, 352, 361, 363–366, 374, 378, 382
Choice (see text) 7, 8, 37, 49, 58, 62, 86, 88, 89, 94, 106, 127, 188, 189, 194, 269, 272, 273, 278, 281, 323, 344, 358, 360, 380
Christ's Reported Interpersonal Skills (see text) 279
Chromosome (see text) 30, 35, 51, 52, 54, 130, 132, 158, 159, 241, 243, 252, 253, 361
Chronic Myelogenous Leukemia (see text) 35, 92, 250, 251, 303, 360, 381
Chronic Pain (see text) 194, 211, 212, 229
Cicely Saunders (*founder of hospice* [see text]) 314
Circulating Tumor Cells (see text) 255
Clarity (see text) xviii, 37, 60, 88, 100, 299, 304, 320
Clinical Staging (*spread of cancer based on clinical observations and scans/tests*) 116, 126
Clinical Trials In Oncology (see text) 167, 174
Clinical Trials (see text) xviii, 27, 28, 37, 66, 68, 93, 102, 103, 105, 113, 125, 127, 129, 130, 136, 137, 145, 149, 156, 157, 160–162, 167, 169, 171, 173, 174, 175, 216, 223, 227–229, 231, 234–238, 270, 303, 337–341, 347, 358
Clonagenic (*one cell dividing into identical clones*) 115
Code (*genetic* [see text]) xxi, 29–31, 35, 52, 53, 67, 132, 170, 242, 244, 245, 250, 252, 308

Code Of Life (*genetic instructions in every cell* [see text]) 244
Collateral Damage (*non-tumor cell damage from tumor therapy*) 331
Colon Cancer (see text) 43, 45, 126, 149
Common Manifestations Of Common Diseases (see text) 297
Communication (see text) xix, xx, 70–75, 86, 91, 100, 157, 181, 197, 208, 238, 263, 269, 279, 295–297, 299–301, 304, 305, 318, 319, 326, 334, 347, 357
Compazine (*antinausea* [see text]) 320
Complementary And Alternative Medicine (see text) 103, 105, 221, 224, 225, 228, 238, 239, 335, 347
Complete Human (see text) 258
Complete Physician (see text) 258
Complete Response (*statistical term—all evaluable disease is gone*) 63, 169
Complications (see text) 40, 41, 140, 152, 153, 156, 182, 183
Conclusions (see text) 12, 68, 88, 91, 125, 128, 265, 273, 280, 302, 307, 335, 372
Confidence Interval (*statistical term of certainty level*) 295
Confounding Variables (*factors affecting statistical outcome*) 170
Confusion (see text) 79, 118, 218, 319, 320
Consequence Of Dabbling In The "Black Arts" Of Complementary And Alternative Medicine (see text) 239
Conspire Against Your Emotions (see text) 272
Constipation (see text) 186, 186–188, 204, 215, 218, 319
Consultations (see text) 58, 87, 100, 257, 303, 312, 351
Controlled Study (see text) 170
Control (see text) vi, xiii, xvii, xx, 8, 19, 35, 37, 38, 53, 63, 69, 79, 81, 83, 88, 94, 95, 99, 100, 138, 140, 142, 149, 159, 170, 173, 176, 181–183, 186, 189, 197, 199, 202, 206, 213, 216, 218, 221, 222, 224, 237, 261, 265, 267, 268, 272, 283, 284, 311, 318, 321, 327, 328, 335, 343, 345, 351, 357, 358, 360, 362
Cowardice (see text) 92
COX-2 (*important enzyme* [see text]) 248
COX (*important enzyme* [see text]) 248
Creativity (see text) 3, 4, 70
Cross-Sectional Trial (*type of powerful clinical trial*) 168
Cultural Differences (see text) 45, 50, 101, 334
Cure For Lymphoma Foundation (see text) 341
Cure (see text) 2, 12, 25, 26, 35, 40, 43, 57, 62, 63, 91–93, 99, 104, 114, 116, 133, 135, 140, 143, 144, 172, 222, 223, 227, 230, 231, 233, 281, 317, 341, 353, 355, 357, 358, 361, 373, 375
Cutting-Edge Therapies (see text) 241
Cyclooxygenase (*see COX* [see text]) 244, 248

D

Daily Affirmations (see text) 269
Daze (see text) 79
Death By Double Effect (*resulting from ethically treating pain*) 218
Death By Secondary Intent (*resulting from ethically treating pain*) xviii, 327

Death Rattle (*end-of-life sound*) 321, 360
Decadron (*powerful steroid*) 214, 319–321
Delirium (*severely altered mental status*) 319, 320
Demagogues (see text) xix, 67, 298, 305
Dementia (*severely altered mental status, not competent*) 94, 319
Denial Syndrome (see text) 278
Dental Problems (see text) 188
Dependency (see text) 94, 95, 101, 116, 218, 351
Depression (see text) 61, 85, 94–97, 184, 187, 189, 190, 194, 196, 218, 230, 257, 262, 273, 284, 310, 312, 328, 352
The Diagnosis (*series of events likely to occur once the diagnosis of cancer is made* [see text]) xiii, xvii, xviii, 2, 3, 21, 37, 39, 46, 58, 59, 66, 77–79, 81, 85, 86, 89, 92, 93–97, 99, 102, 104, 108–110, 128, 189, 219, 257, 263, 267, 274, 291, 315, 377
Diagnostic Trials (*determine sensitivity and specificity of a test*) 168
Diarrhea (see text) 41, 60, 139, 149, 163, 182, 190, 191, 319
Dietary Supplements (see text) 225, 230, 231
Diet (see text) 38, 42, 43, 48–50, 50, 104, 185, 193, 221, 227, 228, 230, 231, 233, 235, 246, 267, 354
Differentiation Agents (*make cancer cells mature into normal cells*) 134
Discontinuing Care (see text) 326
DNA (*basic building block; code of all life*) 28, 28–31, 33, 35, 36, 49, 52–54, 130, 132, 133, 136, 138, 159, 160, 242–245, 250, 252, 253, 370
DNA Synthesis Phase (see text) 130
Documentation (see text) 69, 99, 288, 296, 326, 331, 334
Donor Lymphocyte Infusion (*type of therapy of administering immune cells*) 156
Dose Response (*change in response of cancer with dose change*) 138
Double Effect Of Medication (*see "death by double effect" above*) 328
Doubling Time (*of tumor cells*) 54
Dry Mouth (see text) 190, 209, 218, 319
Dual Loyalties Of Economic Or Clinical Profiling (*effect of money on care*) 333
Ductal Carcinoma In Situ (*noninvasive breast cancer*) 59
Durable Power Of Attorneys (*living wills, naming a decision-maker*) xviii, 326, 327
Dyspnea (*difficulty breathing*) 320

E

Eagles May Soar (*being first and fast is not always best*) 306
ECOG (*Eastern Cooperative Oncology Group*) 174, 337
Edema (*fluid accumulation*) 192, 193, 198
EGFR (*epidermal growth factor receptor*) 146, 147, 149, 246, 247
Electrochemotherapy (see text) 34
Emotions (see text) v, 2, 8, 12, 13, 42, 61, 67, 70, 73, 83, 94, 98, 257, 267, 271–273, 278, 279, 283, 300
Empathy (see text) xix, xxi, 71, 79, 262, 281, 308
End-Of-Life Care (see text) 317, 333
Engage Fully (see text) 111, 347
Engraftment (*of donated bone marrow*) 155
Environmental (see text) 43, 48, 49, 159

Epidermal Growth Factor Receptor (*seen on some cancer cells*) 147, 244, 246
Erbitux (*name of anti-EGFR drug*) 149
Erythropoietin (*natural blood-making hormone*) 135, 194, 368
Estimated Annual Percent Change (*statistical term* [see text]) 178
Estrogen (*female hormone*) 32, 39, 121, 158, 159, 199, 208, 356
Estrogen Receptor (*breast cancer cell receptor for estrogen*) 158, 356
Ethical Duty Not To Prolong Death (see text) 333
Ethical Principles (see text) 333
Ethics (see text) xviii, 167, 323, 328, 335
European Organisation For Research And Treatment Of Cancer (see text) 337
Euthanasia (see text) xviii, 218, 265, 323, 327, 333, 362
Event-Free Survival (*statistical term* [see text]) 169
Example Of Finding Just One Cancer Cell (*impact on diagnosis and treatment*) 113
Excisional (*type of biopsy to remove all tumor with clear margins*) 141
Exercise (see text) 41, 42, 43, 49, 81, 104, 186, 189, 190, 194, 197, 198, 200, 215, 227, 228, 237
Existential (*essential to core reasons for existence*) 97, 257
Extracorporeal Photopheresis (*treating sensitized blood outside body*) 166

F

Failure To Diagnose (*a medical legal issue* [see text]) xviii
Faith (see text) 4, 19, 79, 98, 287, 356, 357, 359, 360, 365, 374, 375
Family (see text) v, vi, xiii, xiv, xix, xx, xxi, 2, 11, 12, 35, 40, 42, 47, 48, 53, 63, 66–69, 71, 72, 77–79, 81, 82, 85, 86, 89, 90, 93, 95, 96, 98–101, 107, 110, 111, 145, 147–149, 181, 185, 189, 192, 198, 201, 211, 239, 259, 261, 263–265, 267, 268, 278, 280, 282, 283, 284, 287–289, 291, 292, 299, 304, 307, 309, 311–321, 325–328, 330–334, 336, 339, 347, 352, 359, 361–363, 367–369, 371, 372, 374, 375, 378, 380–382
Fasting (see text) 227, 231, 318
Fatigue (see text) 61, 135, 139, 147, 156, 181, 184, 189, 193–196, 208, 217, 294, 349, 362, 382
FDA (*Food and Drug Administration*) 24, 27, 103, 105, 122, 129, 130, 146, 148, 149, 151, 152, 157, 159, 166, 172, 174, 214, 223, 225, 230, 236, 238, 247, 250, 251, 294, 335, 348
FDA MedWatch (*cancer website*) 174
FDA'S Center For Food Safety And Applied Nutrition (see text) 225
Fear Not (see text) 270
Fear Of The Known (see text) 80, 86
Fear Of The Unknown (*anxiety* [see text]) 8, 11, 37, 86, 271, 280, 374
Fear (see text) xiii, xvii, xviii, 2, 5, 8, 11, 13, 16, 37, 66, 68, 71–73, 77, 79–81, 86, 89, 95–98, 100, 108, 167, 184, 212, 233, 234, 260–262, 270–272, 274, 279, 280, 283, 289, 292, 307, 310–312, 320, 334, 335, 349–351, 357, 359, 363, 374
Fecal Occult Blood (*test for nonvisible blood in stool*) 42
Federal Trade Commission (see text) 225

Ferrets Are Not Sucked Into Jet Engines (*methodical and steady can be best*) 306
Fiber-Optic Bronchoscopy (*flexible diagnostic tool to look into airways*) 39
Fiber-Optic Cables (see text) 166
The Fifth Vital Sign (*pain*) 211, 335
Finasteride (*hormonally related chemotherapy*) 44
Flulike Symptoms (see text) 191, 195, 361
Folic Acid (*essential vitamin*) 44
Food Supplements (see text) 223
Forgiveness (see text) 4, 274, 313
Fractionation (*divided doses of radiation*) 139
Front Office (see text) 287
The Future (*new advances at laboratory bench or just making it to bedside, future possibilities* [see text]) 13, 107, 125, 134, 136, 173, 197, 236, 241, 243, 246, 259, 274, 293, 300, 343
Future (*research and therapies* [see text]) xviii, 13, 71, 78, 95, 96, 107, 109, 120, 125, 126, 128, 134, 136, 168–170, 172, 173, 197, 235, 236, 241, 243, 246, 251, 259, 261, 263, 274, 293, 300, 343, 349, 364

G

Gamma Rays (*type of radiation*) 137
Gastrostomy Tube (*tube placed through skin into GI tract to feed or decompress obstruction*) 143, 319
G–CSF (*molecule genetically engineered to make white blood cells*) 135
Gene-Based Testing (see text) 255
Genes (see text) xiii, 33, 35, 37, 42, 47, 52, 54, 122, 132, 133, 159, 160, 161, 241, 242, 246, 252, 253, 256, 333
Gene Therapy For Cancer (see text) 159
Gene Therapy (see text) 159, 159–161
Genetically Engineered Drugs (see text) 134
Genetic Manipulation (see text) 36
Genetic (see text) 27, 36, 38, 39, 41, 47, 48, 51, 56, 63, 122, 123, 127, 128, 130, 135, 148, 154, 159–161, 242, 244, 246, 248, 250–252, 254, 256, 333, 361
Germ Cell Cancers (*type of cancer with specific embryologic background*) 157
Gerson Therapy (*type of unproven therapy*) 231
GIGO (*garbage in, garbage out*) 88
Gleevec (*treats chronic myelogenous leukemia and other tumors*) 92, 250, 361, 381
GM-CSF (*molecule genetically engineered to make white blood cells*) 135
Goals And Timing Of Treatment (see text) 62
Goals (see text) 12, 62, 93, 99, 138, 161, 172, 194, 229, 255, 269, 273, 311, 312, 323
God Gave You Ears (see text) 300
God (see text) v, xviii, 2, 8, 13, 15, 66, 67, 80, 81, 83, 89, 91, 100, 101, 215, 258, 260, 262, 265, 268, 270–273, 275, 278, 289, 291, 300, 305, 312, 313, 315, 327, 350–352, 355, 356, 365, 366, 370, 374–377, 380
Good Death (see text) 318, 327
Goods Versus The Harms (*ethical principle* [see text]) 323
Grace (see text) 279, 292, 308, 352, 353, 356, 365, 378, 382
Graft-Versus-Host Disease 153

Graft-Versus-Tumor (see text) 154
Gratitude (see text) 274, 275
The Group Room (*a cancer web site and chat room for support*) 341
Growth-Factor Inhibitors (*biological type of therapy*) 244
Growth Fraction (*percentage of cells actively multiplying in tumor*) 131
Guided Imagery (*mind technique to palliate symptoms*) 217, 228, 229, 232, 237, 310
Gynecologic Oncology (see text) 21

H

Haldol (*sedating drug, antipsychotic*) 320
Hasty Generalizations (see text) 302
Heart (see text) v, xiii, 3, 9, 22, 24, 38, 65, 73, 77, 97, 107, 139, 152, 156, 192, 193, 196, 218, 237, 257, 260, 262, 264, 269, 274, 275, 289, 292, 298, 310, 313, 314, 320, 329, 359, 366, 367, 370, 371, 374, 375
Heat Shock Proteins (*in cells, may be manipulated to cause cell death*) 253
Hematopoietic (*blood forming*) 135, 153
Her-2/neu (*tumor marker in some breast cancers, confers worse prognosis*) 39, 251, 356
Her-2 (see above) 39, 251, 356
Herbal Products (see text) 230, 231, 232
Herceptin (*drug to exploit Her-2/neu*) 33, 148, 149, 195, 251
Heroes (see text) xv, 8, 13, 66, 272, 349, 350, 370, 375, 381, 382
    A Leprechaun's Laser Light of Life 366
    The Connection 370
    The Flood 328, 360, 381
    The Gift 362, 381
    Hitting Home 350
    The Lioness 356–360
    Mercy 377, 378
    Snow Job 273, 352, 381
    The Telling 77, 349, 371, 382
    We 379, 380
High-Dose Chemotherapy (see text) 36, 153, 157, 373
Histological Grade (*degree of angriness or maturity of cells*) 128
HLA-Matched (*matching of donor and recipient for transplants in a major antigen way*) 155
Home Health Aides (see text) 316
Homeopathic (*unproven system of beliefs for therapy with small doses of substances alleged to be causing primary disease given as therapy*) 227
Homeopathy (see above) 226, 227
Homeostasis (*tendency of biological system to achieve balance and feedback coordination* [see text]) 246
Honor (see text) 271, 272, 310, 360, 375
Honor Your Thoughts (see text) 271
Hope (see text) xx, xxi, 25, 93, 96, 98, 106, 113, 117, 124, 144, 153, 172, 200, 222, 234, 236, 237, 248, 267, 298, 311, 331, 335, 347, 354, 357, 363, 382
Hormone Receptor Down-Regulators And Destroyers (see text) 244
Hormones (see text) 32, 44, 51, 52, 134, 158, 194, 208, 244, 250
Hospice Care (see above) 314
Hospice (*system of care focused on palliation in the terminally ill*) 13, 259, 309–311, 314, 315, 316, 317, 319, 327, 328, 341
Hospice Volunteers (see text) 316

How You Say It (*when telling the diagnosis or other important news*) 86
Human Epidermal Growth Factor Receptors (see text) 147
Human Genome Project (*coordinated project that mapped human DNA code*) 161
Human Leukocyte-Associated (HLA) Antigens (*important fingerprints of white blood cells*) 154, 155
Human Papilloma Virus (*associated with cervical cancer*) 44
Humor (see text) 4, 282, 336
Huntsman Cancer Info Service (*cancer website*) 338
Hydration (see text) 317, 318, 321, 332
Hyperthermia (*intentionally increasing temperature to kill cancer cells*) 161, 161–163
Hyperthermic Peritoneal Perfusion (*above done into abdomen*) 163
Hypervariable Portion Of An Antigen (*the unique identity area*) 249

I

Idiotype (*see hypervariable portion*) 249
IL-2 (*important white cells product, can be used to alter immune system to fight cancers*) 150, 159, 195
Imitate (see text) 16, 38, 269
Immune Surveillance (*elegant system to detect foreign substances and eliminate them*) 32, 48, 55
Immune System (*armamentarium of multiple cells and products to fight invasion by cancers and infections, foreign substances*) 16, 25, 32, 36, 50, 55, 114, 115, 134, 143–147, 149, 150, 154, 156, 157, 158, 166, 195, 233, 241, 242, 249, 253, 254, 256, 270, 373, 379
Incidence (*statistical term related to frequency of cancers in a population*) 24, 70, 176–178, 181, 219, 345
Incisional (*partial biopsy of tumor*) 141
Inclusion And Exclusion Criteria (*characteristics affecting eligibility for clinical trials*) 170, 175
Infertility And Sterility (see text) 196
Informed Consent (see text) 103, 167, 325, 330, 331
Informed (see text) xviii, xix, xx, xxi, 8, 19, 46, 80, 90, 92, 94, 99, 101–103, 167, 169, 182, 184, 196, 200, 219, 225, 295, 325, 330–332
Inhibitors (see text) 31, 36, 151, 152, 208, 244, 248, 251, 252, 339, 358
Inpatient Care (see text) 293, 317, 348
Inpatient Medicine (see text) 293, 294
Insomnia (see text) 94, 197, 229, 261
Interferon Alpha (*a naturally occurring as well as genetically engineered product of the immune system to try to fight cancers*) 150
Internal Medicine (see text) 20, 21, 72, 293, 370
International Myeloma Foundation (see text) 341
The Internet (*see list in text for use and effective reference sites for information and support online*) 2, 12, 78, 174, 225, 270, 337, 340, 341, 347
Internet (see text) 2, 12, 78, 174, 225, 270, 337, 340, 341, 347
Interphase (*a phase during cell division*) 54, 130
Intraluminal (*inside a tube or conduit or pathway*) 162

Introduction To Complementary And Alternative Medicine (see text) 103
Ionizing Radiation (*how radiation therapy works*) 51, 136, 137
I Really Do Not Want To Hear It (see text) 278

J

Jejunostomy Tube (*similar to gastrostomy tube but put percutaneously into small intestine*) 143
Jesus (see text) 293, 308, 374, 375
Judeo-Christian (see text) 327
Jumping To Conclusions (see text) 302
Justice (*ethical principle*) 167, 323, 363, 364, 377
Just One Cancer Cell (*what does that mean if found on testing*) 113, 115

K

Kindness (see text) 4, 86, 287
Knowledge (see text) v, xvii, xviii, xxi, 11–13, 27, 37–39, 47, 66, 67, 71–73, 80, 81, 86, 90, 94, 98, 104, 111, 125–127, 142, 148, 179, 208, 226, 239, 243, 250, 251, 256, 260, 263, 265, 272, 289, 292, 299, 300, 305–307, 318, 325, 333–335, 348, 350, 351, 374

L

Lactulose (*nonabsorbable sugar to treat constipation and high potassium*) 320
Laetrile (*dangerous compound once thought to have anticancer benefit*) 44, 232, 235
Laparoscopy (*using fiber-optics through skin to evaluate abdominal cavity*) 141
Laporotomy (*using open surgery through skin to evaluate abdominal cavity*) 141
Laser (*focused high-intensity light beam used for surgical interventions*) 27, 34, 35, 164, 165, 166, 247, 249, 366–369, 382
Laughter And Beauty (see text) 268, 269
Laughter (see text) 268, 269, 366, 368, 380
Lead-Time Bias (*Statistical term where early diagnosis makes it look like patient lived longer*) 46
Legal Aspects Of Oncology (see text) 329
Leukemia And Lymphoma Society (see text) 341
Leukemia And Lymphomas (see text) 57
Leukemia (*uncontrolled growth of primitive white blood cells*) 20, 21, 24, 30, 31, 35, 50–52, 54, 57, 58, 92, 116, 117, 120, 127, 134, 140, 146, 154, 156, 158, 174, 250, 251, 303, 337, 341, 349, 360–362, 381
Levels Of Evidence (*Internationally agreed-upon ranking of evidence needed to reach certainty or odds of a conclusion*) 173
Lies, Damn Lies, And Statistics (see text) 87
Life Cycle Of Cancer (see text) 53
Listening For Those Whispering In The Patient's Ear (see text) 89
Live The Moment (see text) 271
Living To Die And Not Dying To Live (see text) 273
The Living Will (*medical legal document stating desires of a patient when in an end-of-life scenario* [see text]) 326

Living Wills (*similar to durable power of attorney*) xviii, 311, 325
Longitudinal Trial (*clinical trial following enrolled patients over time*) 168
Look Good Feel Better (see text) 339
Loss Of Appetite (see text) 139, 156, 185
Loss Of Control (see text) xiii, xvii, 79, 94, 189
Love (see text) v, 2, 40, 67, 77, 82, 208, 257, 264, 270, 273, 274, 277, 284, 285, 291, 299, 313, 369, 374, 375, 381, 382
Low-Grade Neoplasia (*low-level malignancy with better prognosis*) 59
Lung Cancer (see text) v, 23, 24, 31, 43, 44, 49, 50, 79, 164, 178, 179, 246, 254, 277, 281, 347, 366
Lymphedema (*swelling owing to blocked or obstructed lymph channels and lymph nodes*) 198, 199
Lymphoma (see text) 20, 21, 33, 146, 147, 150, 154, 156, 159, 166, 341, 347, 351, 367, 368, 371, 373, 379

M

Macrobiotic Diet (*unproven dietary regimen to fight cancer*) 231, 235
Magic Decoder Rings (see text) xx, 67, 245, 293, 361
Malignant Transformation (*process by which normal cells evolve into cancer*) 48
Mammograms (see text) 39, 42, 47
Managed Care (see text) xviii, 108, 324
Man To Man (see text) 339
Marker (*some detectable substance or change indicative of underlying malignancy*) 39, 45, 56, 57, 59, 115, 117, 118, 121, 128, 130, 339, 353, 354, 356
Matrix Metalloproteinase Inhibitors (*inhibitors of substances cancer cells use to invade and spread locally*) 244, 251
Maurie Markman (*see foreword*) xiv, xv
Maximal Tolerated Dose (*of radiation, differs with each tissue*) 138
MD Consult (*medicine website*) 234
MD (see text) xiv, xv, 20, 67, 95, 176, 234, 236, 254, 305, 314, 338, 340
Media Matters (*impact of lay versus professional media*) 106
Mediastinoscopies (*fiber-optic scope inserted under breastbone for diagnostic purposes*) 141
Medical Director (see text) 315–317
Medical School (see text) 20, 65, 69, 72, 226, 258, 262, 265, 314
Medical Student (see text) 310, 366, 381
Medicare Hospice Benefit (see text) 315
Medicine Is Not A Contest (see text) 298
Medicine Online (*cancer website*) 338, 340
Medline (*medicine website and search service*) 234
Medscape (*medicine website and search service*) 234
Menopausal Symptoms (see text) 199, 200
Mesenchymal Stem Cells (*stem cells of a specific embryologic line*) 254
Metabolic Therapies (see text) 232
Metastasis (*cancer spread*) 26, 33, 49, 114, 124, 126
Metastatic (see above) 27, 31, 148, 149, 152, 163
Mind/Body Intervention (*systems to palliate symptoms* [see text]) 226, 228

Mini-Transplant (*lower-dose chemotherapy in bone marrow transplant*) 153, 156
Miracles (see text) 16, 98, 135, 281, 311, 314, 360, 361, 365, 382
Mixed Response (*a statistical term of some response, some progression*) 169
Molecular (see text) 28, 56, 122, 123, 127, 128, 138, 144, 157, 158, 243, 247, 248, 253, 255, 361
Monoclonal Antibodies (*antibodies with highly specific immunologically active targets* [see text]) 32–34, 117, 118, 121, 143–146, 145, 147–149, 157, 158, 244, 247, 248, 379, 382
Mortality (see text) 96, 176–178, 180, 280, 309, 330, 345, 351
MRI (*agnetic resonance imaging, used to scan the body diagnostically*) 42, 56, 119, 124, 126, 371
Mucositis (see text) 188, 200–202
Multidrug Resistance Gene (*confers resistance to some cancer cells to dispose of chemotherapy without being harmed*) 132, 133
Music Therapy (see text) 229
Mustard Gas (see text) 24, 25
Mutagens (*substances that can convert normal cancers to cancer cells*) 49, 50, 51
Mutations (see text) 47, 49, 51–53, 161
Myelosuppression (*suppression of the bone marrow in its function and amount*) 25

N

Nanoparticles (*exceedingly small particles being investigated for therapy* [see text]) 33, 34
Narcotics (see text) 187, 201, 202, 205, 218, 328, 335, 365
National Board Of Examiners (see text) 223
National Cancer Institute Cooperative Group (see text) 168
National Cancer Institute Of Canada Clinical Trial Group (see text) 175, 338
National Cancer Institute (see text) 24, 26, 42, 47, 90, 103, 114, 129, 168, 175, 176, 238, 335, 338, 340, 342
The National Center for Complementary and Alternative Medicine (see text) 221, 225
National Center For Health Statistics (see text) 176, 345
National Coalition For Cancer Survivorship (see text) 340
National Health-Care Budget (see text) xvii
National Hospice Organization (see text) 314, 341
National Institutes Of Health Office Of Alternative Medicine (see text) 224
National Institutes Of Health (see text) 24, 43, 93, 129, 221, 224, 228, 229, 231
National Ovarian Cancer Coalition (see text) 341
Naturopathy (*an alternative system of therapy based on nature—unproven*) 226
Nausea And Vomiting (see text) 41, 110, 148, 181, 182, 201, 202, 292, 321, 354
Nausea (see text) 12, 41, 110, 139, 148, 149, 156, 163, 181, 182, 195, 201, 202, 203, 207, 218, 228, 292, 319, 321, 336, 354

NCCTG North Central Cancer Treatment Group (see text) 174, 337
NCI CTC 2.0 (see text) 174
NCI'S Developmental Therapeutics Program (see text) 129
Nembutal (see text) 320
Neoadjuvant (see text) 26, 62, 133, 142
Neurological Symptoms (see text) 61, 204, 205
Neurosurgeons (see text) 22
Neutrons (*a form of advanced and new radiation therapy*) 137
Neutropenia (*low white blood cell count can occur from therapy*) 203
The Never-And-Forever Lie (see text) 12
New Diagnostic Tools (see text) 255
New York Online Access To Health (see text) 338, 340
Non-Cross-Resistant Chemotherapy (*treating with drugs that the cancer is not mutually resistant to*) 133
Nonverbal Communication (see text) 300, 304, 305
Normalcy (see text) 16, 52, 95, 280, 303, 349
Normal (see text) 12, 16, 17, 25, 29–31, 36, 39, 41, 44, 48, 52–56, 80, 114, 119, 122, 123, 128–131, 133, 134, 136–140, 145–148, 151, 152, 157, 159, 162–165, 185, 186, 190, 199, 206, 241, 243, 244, 246–249, 251, 252, 254, 256, 279, 282, 302, 303, 343, 350, 361, 365, 373, 382
Nothing Is Foolproof To A Talented Fool (see text) 307
NSABP (National Surgical Adjuvant Breast & Bowel Project) (see text) 174, 337
Nucleotides (*essential building block, unit of DNA*) 29, 30, 52, 54, 241, 252
Nucleus (*cellular organelles housing genetic material in the form of chromosomes*) 53, 54, 122, 130, 137, 145, 148
Nurses (see text) 68, 80, 108, 136, 170, 184, 203, 262, 263, 288, 291, 292, 309, 313, 314–316, 318, 331, 362, 365, 367–369, 371, 381
Nursing Staff (see text) 288, 368
Nutrition (see text) 42, 143, 185, 192, 194, 225, 230, 231, 243, 318, 326, 332

O

Obesity (see text) 37, 42, 49, 50, 246
Obstruction (see text) 60, 61, 142, 143, 202, 214, 319, 365
Octreotide (*substance used to treat severe diarrhea*) 319
Odds Ratio (*statistical term* [see text]) 179
Odds (see text) xvii, 12, 24, 37, 38, 40, 45, 48, 57, 59, 60, 63, 78, 87, 88, 102, 107–109, 110, 127, 128, 133, 168, 171, 175, 179, 207, 212, 247, 294, 295, 346, 347, 356, 357, 363, 368, 370, 382
Office Of Technology Assessment (see text) 239
Off-Label (*accepted practice of using proven chemotherapy drugs for other-than-original indications*) 105, 129, 130, 174
Oncolink (*cancer website*) 338, 340
The Oncologist (see text) xviii, 12, 26, 62, 63, 65, 66, 68, 69, 71, 77–79, 86, 93, 94, 100, 101, 113, 185, 238, 248, 265, 267, 292, 331–333, 358
Oncology Care Is Not A Commodity (see text) 292

Oncology Nurse Specialists (see below) 291
Oncology Nursing Society (*professional society of highly credentialed nurse experts in Oncology*) 291
Oncoviruses (*viruses known to cause cancer*) 50
The Opening Pitch (*the initial visit with the oncologist*) 85
Orthopedic Surgery (see text) 22
Other Biological Therapies (see text) 149
Otolaryngology (*ear, nose, and throat specialists*) 21
Outpatient (see text) 40, 165, 166, 254, 359
Overall Response (*statistical term measuring response rate to therapy*) 169
Overview Of Specialty (see text) 20
Own The Disease (see text) 81

P

Pain (see text) xiii, xviii, xix, 5, 8, 12, 39, 40, 61, 70, 71, 101, 106, 110, 136, 142, 163–165, 183, 186, 187, 189–191, 193–196, 198, 199, 202, 204, 206, 207, 211–215, 216–219, 222, 228, 229, 233, 239, 260–263, 268, 274, 280, 283, 289, 301, 303, 306, 307, 311, 312, 317–320, 323, 326–328, 333–336, 358, 360, 362, 364, 365, 370, 379, 381
Pap Smears (*analysis of cervical epithelial cells for cancer changes*) 42
Parallel Trials And Crossover Trials (*techniques of structuring clinical trial to get optimal validity of answers*) 168
Paralyzing Anxiety (see text) 292
Paralyzing (see text) 13, 80, 292
Parent Agency (*medical, legal, and ethical term*) 332
Partial Remission (*less than a complete response rate to therapy—a statistical term*) 63, 64
Partial Response (see above) 117, 169
Participant (see text) 67
Participate In Your Healing (see text) 347
Pathological Diagnosis (*diagnosis as a result of direct accessing of tissues*) 58
Pathologic Staging (*staging as a result of direct observation of tumor sites*) 126
Pathologist (see text) 39, 59, 120, 136, 324, 377, 378
Pathophysiology Of Cancer (*the biological how and why of the birth, growth, death, and overall functioning of cancer cells*) 52
Patient Communication (see text) 74, 91, 238
Patient Goals (see text) 93
The Patient Is The One With The Disease (see text) xix, 7, 8, 46, 83, 96, 99, 278, 280, 299
Patient's Bill Of Rights (*internationally accepted rules to establish patient rights*) 297
Pay It Forward (see text) 95
PDQ (*cancer search and web tool*) 174, 339, 340
Pediatric Oncology (see text) 21, 174, 337
People Living With Cancer (see text) 339
Percent Change (*statistical term* [see text]) 178
Percutaneous (*through the skin*) 143

Peripheral-Blood Stem Cells (*see above, capable of engrafting and restarting recipient bone marrow*) 153
Peripheral-Blood Stem Cell Transplantation (*marrow transplant using primitive stem cells harvested from circulating blood*) 153
Person Years Of Life Lost (*statistical term* [see text]) 178
Pessimists (see text) 38
PET Scans (*sophisticated functional scans used to track metabolic activity related to sites of tumor*) 119, 126, 141
Pharmaceutical (see text) 27, 104, 129, 172, 233, 250, 347
Phase 1 Trials (*standardized levels of trials used to develop new drugs—1 is toxicity assessment* [see text]) 130, 171, 172, 224, 381
Phase 2 (*assess possible benefit* [see text]) 171
Phase 3 (*compare to standard treatment* [see text]) 171, 172
Phase 4 (*after approval, marketing assessment and other possible uses* [see text]) 172
Phase Nonspecific (see text) 131
Philadelphia Chromosomes (*chromosomal rearrangement diagnostic of chronic myelogenous leukemia*) 35, 52, 158, 361
Photodynamic (see below) 165
Photodynamic Therapy (*irradiation of blood or tissues treated with an irradiation sensitizer*) 165
Photosensitivity Reactions (*sensitivity to sunlight owing to prior drugs or radiation*) 206, 207
Photosensitizer (*drug used to induce sensitivity of surface tissue or blood*) 165, 166
Physician-Assisted Suicide (see text) xviii, 218, 323, 327, 333
Physician–Patient Communication (see text) 238
Physicians' Desk Reference (*accepted authoritative text of all FDA-approved drugs*) 89, 239
Pious Platitude Syndrome (*a type of patient behavior* [see text]) 278
Placebo Effect (*real benefit seen despite therapy that is without activity being administered*) 223, 227, 238
Plant Alkaloids and Terpenoids (*types of chemotherapy*) 30
Platelets (*cellular elements important for blood clotting*) 25, 61, 135, 153, 155, 185–188, 303, 349, 350, 354, 358, 367, 382
Podophyllotoxin (*type of chemotherapy*) 33
POG Pediatric Oncology Group (see text) 174, 337
Polymerase Chain Reaction (*technique to detect genetic changes from a minute original amount of genetic material*) 250
Polypharmacy (*patients, often the elderly, taking a large number of drugs that are often unknown to each and every provider*) 294
Ports (*devices placed under or through the skin into large veins to facilitate delivery of drugs and drawing of blood samples*) 143
Positive And Negative Predictive Values (*where we measure ability of a test to predict truth or falsehood of a test's ability to predict outcome* [see text]) 178

Prayer (see text) 221, 226, 228, 233, 258, 260, 327, 362
Prevention Trials (see text) 168
Principles Of Surgical Oncology (see text) 140
The Problem Of Pain (see text) xviii, 211, 218
Pro-Drug (see text) 160
Productivity (see text) 3, 4
Progesterone (*female hormone, the receptor for which can be important in breast cancer prognosis and therapy*) 32, 39, 121, 199, 208
Prognosis (see text) 12, 61, 91, 96, 107, 117, 118, 124–128, 189, 233, 246, 255, 298, 319, 330, 343, 344, 353, 356, 367
Prognostic Score (*Mathematical statistic to calculate prognosis*) 127
Progressive Disease (see text) 169
Prometheus (see text) 305, 306
Prospectively (*to look forward before results are in to estimate*) 168, 333
Prostate Cancer (see text) 21, 23, 32, 42, 47, 48, 214, 237, 319, 339, 370
Proteasome (*important cellular garbage handlers that can be in excess in cancer cells, assisting in their immortality*) 159, 244, 251
Proteasome Technology (*to make antiproteasome therapy* [see above]) 244
Protons (*new and intense type of radiation therapy*) 137
Provider's Perceived Attitude (see text) 331
Psychological Issues (see text) 93
Psychosocial (see text) xviii, 41, 63, 75, 229, 309, 315, 334, 340
Pubmed (*medical literature search site*) 234
Purine Analogues (*types of chemotherapy meant to fool cancer cells*) 30
Purpose (see text) 3, 25, 65, 87, 225, 245, 257, 259, 261
Pyrimidine Analogues (*see "purine" above*) 29

Q

Quackwatch (*med site to watch and report on medical quackery*) 104, 226

R

Radiation Oncologist (see text) 22, 137
Radiation Recall (see text) 140, 206
Radiation (see text) xiii, xviii, 17, 22, 26, 32, 36, 41, 43, 45, 48–51, 56, 59, 104, 108, 113, 118, 121, 123, 130, 136–140, 145, 147, 153, 154, 156, 160, 162, 164, 166, 175, 181, 183, 184, 187, 188, 190, 191, 194, 196–203, 205, 206, 208, 209, 211, 244, 247, 321, 337, 353, 356, 358, 370, 373
Radiation Sensitizers (*drugs given in hopes their uptake by cancer cells primarily will increase odds of death of those cells upon radiation*) 36, 140
Radiation Therapy Oncology Group (see text) 175, 337
Radiation Therapy (see text) xiii, xviii, 136, 138, 139, 147, 153, 154, 156, 160, 162, 164, 175, 183, 188, 194, 206, 321, 337
Radioactive Isotopes (see text) 121, 137, 146
Radioimmunoconjugates (*monoclonal antibodies tagged with radiation for diagnostic or therapeutic purposes*) 244

Radioimmunotherapy (*see above; may use other biologic tags than monoclonal antibodies*) 146, 147
Raloxifine (*hormone treatment in primarily hormone-sensitive breast cancer*) 44
Randomization (*statistical technique to be sure treatment groups are well balanced in factors affecting odds of response*) 102, 170, 173
Rational Naming Of Cancers (*avoids confusion and assures uniformity*) 57
Reach To Recovery (*support group for breast cancer patients*) 339
React Angrily (see text) 80
Read (see text) xiv, xvii, xxi, 1, 2, 7, 29, 40, 41, 91, 92, 98, 106, 111, 173, 181, 183, 234, 238, 242, 252, 253, 268, 270, 281, 294, 301, 337, 347, 376
Reasoned Reflection (see text) 80
Receptor (*"keyhole" for specific molecules on cell surfaces*) 32, 121, 134, 147–149, 151, 152, 158, 159, 215, 244–248, 250, 251, 356
Recipe (see text) v, xvii, 1, 1–3, 5, 185, 272, 297, 299, 360
Recombinant Genetic Engineering (*altering or replicating genetic code*) 135
Red Blood Cells (*carry oxygen*) 135, 153, 155, 194, 245, 354, 382
Regional Perfusion (*infusion of therapy to local area that is isolated for treatment*) 163
Relabeling (*calling one behavior something other than what it really is*) 262, 265
Relative Risk (*statistical term of risk assessment, by percent*) 109, 179
Relative Survival Rate (*statistical way of measuring survival rates*) 177
Relaxation (see text) 197, 202, 221, 229, 232, 233, 237
Relaxation Therapy (see text) 232
Religious Affiliation (see text) 259
Religious Practices (see text) 260
Resistance (see text) 29, 131–133, 195
Respiratory Depression (see text) 218, 328
Resting (see text) 130
Retrospective (*to look back on events chronologically*) 168, 235
Right To Refuse Therapy (see text) 332
Rituxan (*monoclonal antibody used in lymphoma and some chronic leukemias*) 146, 147, 195, 248, 382
Rituximab (see above) 33, 146
The Role Of The Family (see text) 78, 98
Roundsmanship (*key insights to behaviors, policies, and rules while being an inpatient*) 293
RTOG (*Radiation Therapy Oncology Group—a cooperative research group*) 175, 337

S

Saint (see text) vi, 369
Sarcomas (*a class of tumor with similar embryonic background*) 57, 58
Scope Of Adult Oncology Practice (see text) 39
Scope Of Chemotherapy (see text) 24
Scope Of Lay Knowledge Of Malignancy (see text) 37
Scope Of The Problem (*of cancer*) 22
Scopolamine (*drug to assist in drying secretions*) 319, 321

Screening (*assays and studies used to find cancer before it is apparent*) xx, 23, 26, 38, 41, 42, 44–47, 129, 140, 178–180, 316
Screening Test Utility (*statistical measure of how useful a screening test for cancer is*) 179
Scribe (*someone appointed by the patient to take notes*) 82, 83
Second Mouse That Gets The Cheese (*metaphor for measured pace and not rushing for the sake of rushing*) 305
Second Opinions (see text) 12, 110, 340
Secret Handshake (*metaphor for specialized language and culture of oncologists*) xx, 67, 245, 293
Secrets (see text) xix, xx, 67, 104, 110, 233, 244, 245, 252, 293, 295, 330, 369
Sedation And Symptom Control (see text) 327
Sedation (see text) 204, 218, 327, 328
SEER (*national program to track cancer data and treatment results*) 175, 176, 177, 345
SEER Program (see above) 176, 177, 345
Selective Screening (*highly focused screening for cancer*) 45
Self-Talk (see text) xviii, 234, 237, 267, 272
Sensitivity (*a statistical term of how sensitive a test is to finding what it is aimed to look for when it is there—a measure of false negative results; the less, the more sensitive*) v, 32, 36, 45, 47, 118, 119, 135, 138, 144, 178, 179, 259
Sentinel (*a finding, usually a lymph node indicative of chance of cancer spread*) 126, 142
Set Goals (see text) 273
Sex And Significant Others (see text) 97
Sex (see text) 97, 158, 176, 177, 189, 200, 208, 241
Sexual Dysfunction (see text) 207, 208
Shocked (see text) 80, 215, 264, 350
Should I Enter A Clinical Trial (see text) 175
Sigmoidoscopy (*flexible fiber-optic tube used to visualize lower colon*) 42, 47
Significance (*a statistical term indicating results are not by chance and are reproducible*) 128, 178
Signs And Symptoms (see text) 60, 154, 181, 368
Single Blinding Or Double Blinding (*structure of clinical trial to ensure that bias before the trial is eliminated*) 170
Sinner (see text) vi, 308
Sisters Of Charity (*original group to systematically start hospice*) 314
Small-Molecule Rationally Designed Drugs (see text) 244
Small Molecules (see above) 33, 133, 247, 248
Smoking (see text) 22, 23, 38, 43, 48, 49, 51, 179
Some Final Thoughts (see text) 347
Southwest Oncology Group (see text) 175, 337
Specific And Related Fields (*to medical oncology*) 21
Specificity (*a statistical term indicating how well a result or test means what it says with few false positive results*) 45, 118, 178, 179
Spiritual Care (see text) 257
Spirituality (see text) xviii, 12, 97, 228, 233, 237, 257–259, 297, 298, 311

Stable Disease (*a statistical tool of tumor assessment indicating neither progress nor remission*) 64, 116, 169
Staff (see text) xix, 68, 71, 74, 75, 79, 138, 226, 260, 262–264, 287, 288, 289, 299, 311, 313, 317, 324, 331, 347, 368, 369
Stage (*degree of advancement of tumor using internationally accepted uniform criteria*) xviii, xxi, 16, 19, 22, 29, 30, 54, 59, 61, 62, 77, 78, 87, 117, 124–127, 128, 129, 133, 169, 170, 267, 277, 305, 314, 318, 330, 343, 344, 348, 349, 351–353, 356, 370, 374
Stage Grouping (see above and text) 126
Stage Of The Cancer (see above and text) 61, 330, 343
Staging Criteria (*rules internationally accepted applied to determine stage*) 62, 127
Staging (*the process of determining stage*) 12, 62, 87, 116, 117, 124–127, 128, 141–143, 255, 351, 367
Standard Error (*a statistical tool used to determine certainty of test results*) 178
Statistics (*Mathematical tools used to determine truthfulness of result* [see text]) 87, 87–89, 108, 109, 175, 176, 294, 295, 329, 331, 343–345
Stem Cell Research (see below and text) 243
Stem Cells (*primitive potent "Adam and Eve" cells in bone marrow, peripheral blood, and embryonic cord blood capable of maturing into normal cell constituents*) 58, 152, 152–155, 157, 160, 243, 254, 255, 349, 353
Stem Cell Transplantation (*infusion of most primitive and capable cells from a donor to rebuild a bone marrow depleted from chemotherapy*) 152, 153
Stents (*tubes used to connect or keep open vessels or other conduits*) 142
Steve Dunn's Website (*a cancer web tool and research site and blog*) 339
Stinking Thinking (see text) 96
Stool Softener (see text) 186, 187, 218
Stratification (*organizing risks and patients in clinical trials to have treatment groups balanced in all relevant criteria that could affect outcome*) 170
Stress (see text) xvii, 38, 49, 50, 53, 68, 70, 71, 75, 83, 96, 97, 101, 185, 187, 190, 194, 196, 205, 208, 222, 227–229, 237, 246, 260, 263, 270, 274
Subcutaneous (*under the skin*) 143, 191, 194, 201, 215, 319
Substituted Judgment (*Medical legal term wherein when a patient is incompetent, an assigned other is asked to decide for the patient as if he or she were the patient, rather than being asked what he or she would do*) 98
Summaries Of CAM Therapies (see text) 239
Summaries Of Various CAM Modalities (see text) 239
Support Groups (see text) 40, 232, 237, 264, 273, 274, 339, 341, 348
Support (see text) v, xix, 25, 26, 40, 52, 63, 68, 82, 85, 88, 106, 107, 117, 123, 129, 133, 135, 136, 161, 173, 216, 232, 235, 237, 264, 265, 273,

274, 277, 283, 298, 310, 315, 325, 333, 339–341, 347, 348, 353, 359, 364, 368, 380, 382
Suppressor Genes (*genes that suppress expression of other genes and their activity* [see text]) 52, 53
Surgical Oncologists (see text) 136, 140, 142, 143, 351
Surgical Oncology (see text) 22, 140, 381
Survival Rate (*statistical measure of survival at typically five years*) 52, 63, 177, 343
Suspect The Diagnosis (*events that transpire when suspecting a cancer diagnosis*) 77, 78
Symptomatic Relief (see text) 102
Symptom Control And Side Effects (see text) 181
Syngeneic Transplants (*transplants with donor being identical twin*) 154, 155

T

Take The Time And Avoid Timelines 108
Tamoxifen (*a breast cancer receptor blocking drug and type of hormonal therapy effective in hormone-positive breast cancers*) 44, 59, 208, 356, 358
Tandem Transplant (*two transplants of lower intensity given sequentially*) 153, 156, 157, 358
Targeted Cancer Therapies (*specifically aimed cancer therapies* [see text]) 157, 158
Targeted Therapies (see above and text) 27, 35, 122, 123, 145, 157, 158
Taxanes (*types of chemotherapy drugs*) 31
Teach (see text) 12, 101, 110, 118, 285, 291, 296, 313, 315, 316, 376
Team Approach (see text) 40, 263, 328
Thalidomide (*chemotherapy drug effective in myeloma; prevents formation of new blood vessels*) 150, 157, 249
Therapeutic Monoclonal Antibodies (*see "monoclonal antibodies"* [see text]) 143, 145, 146
Thoracic Surgery (see text) 22
Three-Dimensional Planning (for below) 139
Three-Dimensional Radiotherapy (*planning to give radiation considering all three dimensions in space of tumor and normal tissue*) 244
Thymus Therapy (*unproven therapy* [see text]) 232
Timelines (see text) 108
Tissue Diagnosis (*never diagnose malignancy without tissue confirmation unless impossible to obtain*) 39, 59
Topoisomerase Inhibitors (*type of chemotherapy*) 31
Toxic Stress (*an emotional drain on patients* [see text]) 270, 274
Traditional Chinese Medicine (see text) 226, 228
Training Requirements (*for professionals in oncology and related fields*) 20
Tranquilizers (see text) 265
Treatments (see text) xiii, xiv, xviii, xix, xx, xxi, 3, 8, 12, 17, 19, 21–28, 30, 31, 33, 34, 36, 38–41, 45, 46, 56, 58, 61, 62, 64, 68, 69, 71, 77–80, 87–89, 91–93, 95, 100–103, 105, 107–109, 111, 113, 114, 117, 119, 122–125, 127–129, 133, 134, 136, 138–140, 143, 146–149, 151, 152, 154–156, 157, 159–161, 163–172,

174, 175, 181–185, 188, 194–197, 200, 206, 207, 211–214, 216, 218, 221–223, 227–232, 234, 235, 237–239, 243, 248, 249, 251, 254, 255, 262, 263, 268, 279, 295, 297, 306, 312, 315, 317, 325, 330–332, 335, 337, 339–341, 343, 344, 348, 353, 354, 357, 361, 368, 373, 378–380

Truth (see text) xx, 7, 82, 109, 110, 183, 236, 279, 284, 302, 310, 311, 324, 329–331, 336

Tumor Cell Growth (*some general principles of how tumor cells grow*) 55, 131, 146

Tumor Growth Characteristics (see above and see text) 55

Tumor Registry (*A systematic repository of vital information on all cancer patients treated at a particular institution* [see text]) 345

Tumor-Specific Antigens (*specific proteins on a cancer cell surface that identify it immunologically* [see text]) 247

Tumor Vaccines (*anticancer cell vaccines meant to trigger an immune response against the cancer cell, various types* [see text]) 244

Types Of CAM (*see "CAM" and "complementary and alternative medicine"* [see text]) 104, 226, 227

Tyrosine Kinase (*an important workhorse enzyme for normal and cancer cells, can be overactive in cancer cells*) 35, 52

U

Ultrasound (*Use of special-frequency sound waves to see into the body according to density characteristics and thus image tumors or organs*) 36, 42, 119, 126, 162, 359

Unconventional Chemotherapies (see text) 232

Understanding Cutting-Edge Therapies (see text) 241

Union Against Cancer (*website and cancer organization*) 37, 126

Universal Screening (*screening entire populations, useful only when frequency of screened for cancer in population is very high*) 45

University Of Texas MD Anderson Cancer Center (*premier enormous cancer center in Houston*) 338, 340

Urology (see text) 21

US Census Bureau (see text) 345

V

Vaccines (see text) 35, 44, 130, 150, 242, 244, 249, 254

Valium (*sedative and antianxiety drug*) 213, 320

Vascular Endothelial Growth Factor (*factor that promotes formation of new blood vessels, may be increased in cancer cells*) 150, 151, 249

Vectors (*vaccine or other small molecules used to carry antitumor entity directly next to or near cancer cells*) 159, 160, 161

VEGF (see "vascular endothelial growth factor") 151

Venous Access Port (*ports placed subcutaneously and run into large veins to assist in drawing blood and infusing chemotherapy*) 291

Vessels (see text) 16, 36, 55, 115, 140, 150–152, 157, 160, 164, 166, 192,

198, 236, 243, 246, 247, 249, 250, 349, 359
Viruses (see text) 32, 44, 48, 50, 52, 134, 159–161, 203, 242, 370, 373
Vitamin C (see text) 44, 235
Vitamins (see text) 30, 44, 191, 205, 230, 232, 235
Vocabulary Of Survival (see text) 63
Vomiting (see text) xiii, 12, 41, 110, 148, 156, 163, 181, 182, 201–203, 218, 292, 318, 319, 321, 336, 354

W

We Know Self As Self (see text) 242
What About Oncologists (see text) 67
What Did They Hear (see text) 304
What Did You Spend (see text) 303
What Is A Tumor Registry (see "tumor registry" above) 345
When An Oncologist Is The Family Member Of A Loved One With Cancer (see text) 334
White Blood Cells (*important diversified infection-fighting cells*) 25, 61, 134, 135, 149, 153–156, 187, 195, 203, 204, 358, 368, 373
Whole-Body Hyperthermia (*heating the tumor and entire body to kill cancer cells*) 162, 163
Why Me (see text) xiii, 48, 80, 98, 267
Why Oncology (see text) 65, 66
Withdrawing Support (*see above—end-of-life decisions*) 333
Worry (see text) 5, 98, 103, 189, 264, 268, 270, 275, 288, 289, 369, 381

X

Xerostomia (*dry mouth from chemotherapy and possibly radiation*) 188, 209

Y

Y-Me National Breast Cancer Organization (*why me, etc ...*) 341

CPSIA information can be obtained at www.ICGtesting.com
Printed in the USA
LVOW08*0513080114

368519LV00001B/63/P